ISBN 978-0-331-07640-0
PIBN 11011281

THE

# FAMILY PHYSICIAN;

OR,

## *Domestic Medical Friend:*

CONTAINING

## PLAIN AND PRACTICAL INSTRUCTIONS

FOR THE

## PREVENTION AND CURE OF DISEASES,

*According to the newest Improvements and Discoveries;*

WITH

A SERIES OF CHAPTERS ON COLLATERAL SUBJECTS;

COMPRISING EVERY THING RELATIVE TO

*The Theory and Principles of the Medical Art,*

NECESSARY TO BE KNOWN BY

THE PRIVATE PRACTITIONER.

---

THE WHOLE ADAPTED TO
THE USE OF THOSE HEADS OF FAMILIES
WHO HAVE NOT HAD A CLASSICAL OR MEDICAL EDUCATION.

---

BY

ALEXANDER THOMSON, M. D.

AUTHOR OF A TREATISE ON NERVOUS DISORDERS; OF DIALOGUES IN A LIBRARY
AND OTHER PRODUCTIONS.

---

New-York:

PRINTED BY JAMES ORAM, AT HIS PRINTING-OFFICE,

NO. 102, WATER-STREET,

THIS first American Edition of *Thomson*'s FAMILY PHYSICIAN, 'tis hoped will meet the approbation of the Public, and of those Gentlemen in particular, who have favored the publisher by subscribing to the work, and to whom he tenders his most grateful acknowledgments for the same. In addition to what the Author has said in his Preface, it may not be amiss to publish the following Certificates from Medical Gentlemen of the first respectability of our own Country, to testify their Opinion of its merits.

## CERTIFICATES.

SIR,

*I HAVE perused Dr. Thomson's* "FAMILY PHYSICIAN," *and from the variety of valuable Matter it contains, as well as the agreeable Manner in which it is given, I believe it better calculated for the purpose it is intended, than any other Book of the kind we now have —I think it a work worthy the Public Attention and wish you much success in its Publication.*

*I am, Sir, Your's, &c.*

*JOHN R. B. RODGERS, M. D.*

Mr. JAMES ORAM.

New-York, March 29, 1802.

---

*THE FAMILY PHYSICIAN; or,* DOMESTIC MEDICAL FRIEND, *by Dr. Thomson, in comprehensiveness of plan, as well as in learning and general execution, is superior to former medical publications designed for popular use. The Preliminary matter is well adapted to communicate those elementary and essential principles which are requisite to prepare the reader to understand the precepts and cautions concerning the treatment of diseases, in the subsequent parts of the volume. The Author has much merit for the conciseness and perspicuity with which he describes diseases, and distinguishes such as are most apt to be mistaken for one another. He is duly attentive to modern discoveries and improvements, especially when they are practical, established upon competent evidence, and approved by experience. In a word, this work may be confidently recommended as one of the most judicious, accurate, and instructive of all the productions intended to divest Medicine of its technical and mysterious garb, and to render it familiar to the understanding of the unprofessional reader.*

*EDWARD MILLER, M. D.*

Mr. JAMES ORAM.

New-York, April 2, 1802.

THIS first American Edition of Thomson's Family Physician, it is hoped, will meet the approbation of the Public, and of those Gentlemen in particular who have favored the publisher by subscribing to the work, and to whom he tenders his most grateful acknowledgments for the same. In addition to what the Author has said in his Preface, it may not be amiss to publish the following Certificates from Medical Gentlemen of the first respectability of our own Country, to testify their Opinion of its merits.

## CERTIFICATES.

*I HAVE perused Dr. Thomson's "Family Physician," and* [illegible]

JOHN R. B. RODGERS, M. D.

Mr. James Oram.

New-York, March [illegible], 180[illegible].

---

*THE FAMILY PHYSICIAN of Dr. Thomson* [illegible]

[illegible] M. D.

Mr. James Oram.

New-York, April 2, 180[illegible].

# PREFACE.

THE work here offered to the public is ſo intimately connected with human happineſs, that little need be ſaid in favour of its general utility. To preſerve the health of the body, and to cure its diſeaſes, have ever been regarded as objects of great importance to mankind; and a knowledge of the means for promoting theſe ſalutary purpoſes can never be too widely diffuſed. The art, however, of preſerving health is, in general, ſo little cultivated, as well as imperfectly underſtood, that more diſeaſes proceed from a violation of its precepts than from all other cauſes whatever; and, with regard to the cure of them, an early obſervance of their approach, and a prompt application of medicine, are circumſtances which, if unfortunately neglected, no ſubſequent ſkill or exertion may ever afterwards be able to retrieve.

Another circumſtance alſo contributes greatly to favour the progreſs of diſeaſes. People often, from various motives, are diſinclined to call for the aſſiſtance of a phyſician, until the diſorder has ſo far advanced, that neither the diſtreſs of the patient, nor the apprehenſions of his friends, can admit of any longer procraſtination. Whether the diſeaſe be chronic or acute, this delay proves equally pernicious. If chronic, the diſeaſe may become ſo fixed in the habit as to reſiſt the utmoſt efforts of medicine; and if acute, the rapidity of its progreſs may not only bid defiance to all reſtraint, but utterly preclude every reaſonable hope of recovery.

Nothing, therefore, can ſo effectually obviate theſe inconveniences as a work of the preſent kind, which not only teaches to diſcover a diſeaſe at an early period, but to apply the proper means, as well for preventing its increaſe as, if poſſible, for its total extinction.

The author's principal care has been to deſcribe the various diſeaſes with accuracy, and to recommend ſuch a method of cure as is conformable to the lateſt eſtabliſhed improvements in medical practice. In executing this plan, he has every-where endeavoured to be ſparing in the uſe of technical expreſſions; but the total excluſion of them being incompatible with preciſion of ſentiment, an explanation of all ſuch terms is given in a Gloſſary.

It was originally intended to give a liſt of the moſt uſeful ſimples and medicinal preparations for a medicine cheſt; but this idea was at laſt relinquiſhed, upon the conſideration that the uſual aſſortment of thoſe cheſts would render the object unneceſſary.

As many readers may be totally unacquainted with the nature of ſome claſſes of medicines, ſuch as abſorbents, alkaline ſalts, &c. an explanatory account of theſe different ſubſtances is given in the Appendix; and it is confidently hoped that the various articles contained in that part of the volume will be found not only to afford much uſeful information, but greatly to facilitate the accompliſhment of the purpoſe which is the chief object of the work.

To point out any particular part as more intereſting than another, where the whole is equally practical, might be deemed an arbitrary diſtinction; but, among the preliminary chapters, the reader will perhaps be peculiarly gratified with the hiſtorical view of the theories which have ſucceſſively prevailed in medicine: the phyſical account of the air or atmoſphere; and the copious medicinal detail of all the principal articles of diet.

Upon the whole, if extenſive reſearch, important obſervation, and practical utility can ſtamp an inconteſtable value on a medical production, there is reaſon to think that the preſent treatiſe has, more than any other work of the kind, either foreign or domeſtic, ſuch juſt pretenſions to the approbation and favour of the public as cannot but enſure its ſucceſs.

*A. T.*

*London,*
*June* 12, 1801.

# CONTENTS.

## BOOK I.

### INTRODUCTORY CHAPTER.



## BOOK II.

### OF CHILDREN.

### THEIR MANAGEMENT AND DISEASES.

## BOOK III.

FEBRILE DISEASES.



## BOOK IV.

ON INFLAMMATIONS.

PAGE

## SURGERY.

## APPENDIX.

---

## APPENDIX.

THE

# FAMILY PHYSICIAN.

## INTRODUCTORY CHAPTER,

*Containing ſome General Obſervations on the Structure of the* HUMAN BODY.

BEFORE we enter upon the prevention or cure of diſeaſes, it may not be improper to take a curſory view of the human body, reſpecting the functions immediately connected with life. So wonderful is the ſtructure of our frame, as diſplayed by anatomy, that atheiſtical perſons, obdurate to every other evidence of the exiſtence of a God, who created the univerſe, have, on witneſſing a diſſection, been inſtantly convinced of their miſtake, and have acknowledged with equal aſtoniſhment and ſhame, that nothing leſs than a Being of infinite wiſdom and power could have contrived and executed ſuch a wonderful piece of mechaniſm as that of the human body.

The primary agent in the circulation of the blood is the heart, a large muſcle ſituated in the left ſide of the breaſt (thorax,or cheſt) and endowed with great irritability. In the firſt rudiments of animal life, even before the brain is formed, the *punctum saliens,* as it is called, points out the embryo heart in miniature, and marks its primæval irritability as a ſure preſage of its future importance in ſupporting the vital motions. As this ſingular organ exhibits irritability the firſt, ſo it never relinquiſhes it till the laſt; whence it has been called the *primum mobile,* and *ultimum moriens,* that is, "the firſt part that moves, and the laſt that dies," of the animal machine. It is obſervable, that the motion of the heart not only survives that of the organs of voluntary motion, but continues a conſiderable time even after it is ſeparated from the body of many animals. Hence, in drowning, or ſuffocation, though the pulſe be imperceptible, and apparently extinguiſhed, yet the heart ſtill preſerves this latent power or ſuſceptibility of motion, and wants only to be gently excited by ſuitable means to renew its action.

This organ is ſurrounded by the pericardium, or heart-purſe, an exceeding ſtrong membrane, which covers the heart, even to its baſis. Its uſes are to keep the heart from having any friction with the lungs, and to contain a fluid to lubricate or moiſten its ſurface.

From the right ventricle or cavity of the heart, the irritability of which is excited into action by the circulating fluid, the blood is propelled through the lungs, which are situated on the right and left side of the heart, from which they differ on appearing to be void of irritability. They are divided into two lobes, and these into more divisions, three on the right side, and two on the left. The trachae, or wind-pipe, descends into the lungs, and forms innumerable cells, which have a communication with each other, and give the whole the appearance of a honey-comb or sponge.

The blood, after passing through the lungs, arrives again at the heart, and from the left ventricle is expelled into the *aorta*, or great artery; which dividing into two branches, one upwards, and the other downwards, distributes the blood through the whole body; from the extremities of which it returns, by various veins, through the ascending and descending cava,* and is transmitted again to the heart.

The heart is the grand organ which actuates the vital functions; and to this purpose it is admirably fitted by its own irritability; but it is necessarily supported in its action by the powerful influence of the nerves, which are the ultimate instruments both of motion and sensation, and have their origin in the brain.

The diaphragm or midriff is a large broad muscle, which divides the thorax from the abdomen† or belly. In its natural state, it is concave or vaulted towards the abdomen, and convex towards the thorax.‡ Haller calls it "the most noble bowel next to the heart;" and, like the latter, it is in constant action. At the time of inspiration it approaches towards a plane. Besides being a muscle of inspiration, it assists in vomiting, and the expulsion of the fæces.§ From the exertion of this muscle likewise proceed sighing, yawning, coughing, and laughing. It is effected by spasms, as in the hiccup, &c. It is both a muscle of voluntary and involuntary action. We may observe in this muscle strong characters of admirable contrivance. It separates posteriorly into two slips, between which the descending aorta passes. A little above this, and towards the left side, in the most fleshy part of the midriff, there is a direct opening for the passage of the *œsophagus* or gullet. There is also on the right side a large triangular hole for the passage of the ascending *cava*.

* Cava is the large vein which conveys the refluent blood to the heart.

† Abdomen, from *abdo* to hide, as its contents lie hidden.

‡ Derived from the Greek, signifying the breast.

§ This word with chemists is used to express the ingredients and settling after distillation and infusion; here it means excrement.

The gullet is composed both of longitudinal and circular fibres, but chiefly circular, much more so than the intestines; because this has no foreign power to assist it, and because it is necessary that the food should make a shorter stay in the throat than in the bowels. The inner surface is a smooth membrane, well supplied with mucilage, to sheath the organ, and render the passage of the aliment or food easy.

The stomach lies across the upper part of the abdomen, and is covered by the liver; when distended it presses on the spleen. It nearly resembles in figure the pouch of a bag-pipe, its upper side being concave, and the lower convex. Its left end is the most capacious. On the left side is the entrance from the gullet; on the right is the opening, called *pylorus*, by which the chyle passes into the intestines. Here is a circular valve, or sphincter-muscle, which prevents a regurgitation of the aliment. The stomach has circular and longitudinal fibres, and its inner membrane is covered with a strong viscid mucus.

The liver, the largest gland in the body, is situated immediately under the vaulted cavity of the midriff, chiefly on the right side, and somewhat on the left over the stomach. Exteriorly, or anteriorly, it is convex, inwardly it is concave; very thick in its superior part, and thin in its inferior. The upper side adheres to the midriff; and it is fixed to this, and the *sternum*, or breast-bone, by a broad ligament. It is also tied to the navel by a ligamentous band, which is the umbilical vein of the unborn infant, degenerated into a ligament. Both these bands serve to suspend it, while lying on the back, from bearing too much on the subjacent *cava*; otherwise it might press on this important returning vessel, stop the circulation, and put a period to life. Dogs and cats, and other animals who are designed for leaping, have their liver divided into many distinct lobules, to prevent too great a concussion of the organ. The liver is the viscus or bowel which performs the secretion of the bile.

The gall-bladder is situated under the great lobe of the liver, a little to the right. In a standing posture it lies forwards and downwards. Its bottom is raised by a fulness, and depressed by the emptying of the stomach. The use of the gall-bladder is to serve as a receptacle for the bile.

The intestines are destined to receive the food from the stomach, and after exposing the useful part of it to the *lacteals*, a sett of extremely small vessels, to convey the remainder out of the body. The intestinal canal is usually five times the length of the individual: it is curiously convoluted in the abdomen, and is extremely irritable. Anatomists have divided this canal, although one continued pipe, into fix portions, three of which are termed the *fmall* inteftines,* and the three laft, the *great.* In the fmall inteftines there are numerous plaits to detain the food, and allow a larger furface for its abforption. Thefe are larger, and far more numerous near the ftomach, where the food is thinner, than they are towards the other extremity. At the entrance of the *ilium* into the *colon*, there are two very large valves, which prevent the regrefs of the fæces into the ilium. The *cæcum* and *colon*, two of the inteftines towards the lower extremity, befides having ftronger mufcular coats than the fmall inteftines, are furnifhed with three ligamentous bands, running lengthwife on their outfide, dividing their furfaces into three portions nearly equal. Though appearing externally like ligaments, they are compofed, in their inner ftructure, of true mufcular fibres. The ligament-like bands, which in the cæcum and colon are collected into three portions, are fpread equally over the furface of the *rectum*, or lower extremity of the inteftines. This is a wife precaution of Nature, that no part of it may be weaker than another, left it fhould give way in the efforts for expelling the *fæces.* The plaits are confiderably fewer in the great inteftines. They have all an inner membrane, covered with an infinite number of arteries or glands, which difcharge a lubricating fluid. They are furnifhed with mufcular fibres, both circular and longitudinal.

The fpleen, or milt, is fituated immediately under the edge of the midriff, above the left kidney, and between the ftomach and ribs. In figure, it refembles a depreffed oval, near twice as long as broad, and almoft twice as broad as thick. Chefelden informs us, that it has been taken from dogs without any obfervable inconvenience to them. Its ufe is ftill problematical.

The pancreas, or fweet-bread, is fituated tranfverfly under the ftomach. Its fhape refembles a dog's tongue. Along the whole length of it there is a duct, which terminates in the upper part of the inteftines near the ftomach. The pancreatic juice refembles the faliva, but is lefs vifcid or flimy, and contains a larger proportion of the falts of the blood. It is probably intended for the folution of our aliment.

The kidneys are two oval bodies, fituated in the loins, contiguous to the two laft fhort ribs; the right under the liver, and the

* The three fmaller are, the *duodenum*, from its length being about that of the breadth of twelve fingers), *jejunum*, and *ilium*, from the Greek, fignifying to turn about, becaufe it makes many convolutions.

The three larger are, the *cæcum*, or blind gut (so called from its being perforated at one end only); the *colon*, fignifying hollow, a word from the Greek; and the *rectum*, or ftraight gut.

left under the ſpleen. The ſtructure of the kidneys is curiouſly fitted for ſecreting the urine, which is carried from each of them by canals termed the ureters, into the bladder, the reſorvoir of that fluid, ſituated in the lower part of the belly. They enter the bladder near its neck, running for the ſpace of an inch obliquely between its coats, and forming, as it were, to themſelves, two valves; ſo that, upon the contraction of the bladder, the urine is directed along the urethra, which is its proper paſſage out of the body.

Over the upper part of the abdomen is ſpread the *omentum*, or caul, conſiſting of two broad, thin, and tranſparent membranes, joined together by cellular texture, in the cells of which a quantity of fat is depoſited. The uſes of it are to interpoſe between the *peritonæum*,* or lining, the inteſtines, and the ſtomach, to keep all theſe parts moiſt, warm, ſlippery, and to prevent their adheſion.

Laſt of all comes the peritonæum, a ſtrong membrane, which confines, as in an incloſure, the inteſtines and contents of the abdomen.

Such, in a general view, are the contents of the cavities of the breaſt and belly, which perform, reſpectively, the vital motions, and thoſe natural functions that are ſubſervient to the ſupport of our frame. But there remains to be mentioned another eſſential cavity, with its dependent ſyſtem, to the primary influence of which all the other parts of the body are indebted for their action and energy. The cavity to which I allude is the ſkull, the receptacle of the brain. The brain is divided into two portions; namely, the *cerebrum*, and *cerebellum*;† the former ſituated in the upper part of the ſkull, and the latter under it, in the hind part. The brain is a ſoft pulpy ſubſtance, ſurrounded by two membranes; one called *dura*, and the other *pia*, *matter*. It has alſo a third, called *arachnoid*, from its fineneſs, as being ſimilar to a ſpider's web. It contains ſome *ſinuſes*, which are nothing more than large veins or receptacles for blood, and four cavities called *ventricles*; moiſtened, in a healthful ſtate, with a fine vapour, which increaſing gives riſe to diſeaſes. Like other parts of the body, it has a variety of arterial branches from the heart, which are diffuſed through its ſubſtance, and on the membranes. The brain is the great elaboratory, where the animal ſpirits, or nervous influences which actuate our frame, are ſuppoſed to receive their exiſtence. The nature of this fluid, if really a fluid, has not yet been ſufficiently inveſtigated. It is certain, however, that from this ſource the nerves derive their

* Signifying near to, stretching round, or about, as *peri*osteum, *peri*carpium, near to the bone, heart, &c.

† *Cerebellum*, the little brain as it were: both are often called thus, when the brain is spoken of in small animals.

origin. These are white, firm, solid cords, which arise from the brain and spinal marrow, which is only an elongation of the brain, and are spread over every part of the body endowed with sensibility, by innumerable filaments. Ten pair of nerves issue from the brain itself, and thirty from the spinal marrow. Those that go to the organs of sense are considerably larger than the rest, and are in part divested of their outer covering.

Whether an immaterial and invisible Being can positively be said to exist in any place, it might appear presumptuous to determine; but it is a prevailing opinion in physiology, that the brain is the seat of the soul; and the *pineal* gland, in the *penetralia* of the brain, has been assigned as the sacred mansion of this immortal inhabitant. Human vision can discover no signs to confirm this opinion; but the man would be blind, and utterly void of understanding, who could not trace through the whole of the animal system the most evident marks of Divine Intelligence and Wisdom; of intelligence which excites admiration, and of wisdom beyond conception.

The wonderful contrivance exhibited in the human frame is, if possible, still more manifest from the curious formation of the eye and ear; of which only a very imperfect idea could be conveyed by verbal description. I shall therefore not attempt to delineate those admirable organs: nor need I mention the construction of the limbs; of the arms and legs; of the hands and feet; so nicely united with joints, and so happily supplied with muscles and tendons, with ligaments and nerves, that they are adapted to all the various purposes of convenience and utility in motion.

I shall conclude this imperfect sketch of the human body with a brief account of digestion, that important process in the animal economy, by means of which the continual and unavoidable waste of the constitution is regularly supplied.

The aliment being received into the mouth, the first operation it undergoes is to be masticated by the action of the teeth and several muscles. This mastication is of greater moment than is generally imagined; and the good effects of it are further promoted by mixing with the food a quantity of saliva, discharged from the glands of the mouth, and which is greatly conducive to digestion. When the food is carried down the gullet into the stomach, it there meets with an additional supply of juices, called the gastric juices, of a nature yet more efficacious than the former, besides a small portion of bile. During its continuance in the stomach, it experiences the effects of heat and muscular action, from the coats of that organ, and the motion and warmth of the surrounding parts. It thence passes out gradually by the right orifice of the stomach, and there meets with an additional quantity of bile from the gall-bladder and liver; besides the pancreatic juice, or that of the ſweet-bread, of a nature ſimilar to the ſaliva, but rather more thick, and the fluids ſeparated by the inteſtines. It now receives the action of the bowels, or the periſtaltic motion, by which they churn, as it were, the whole maſs, minutely mixing together the food, and the different juices, collected in the paſſage from the mouth. A fluid is now produced called chyle, which is ſeparated from the groſſer materials, and taken up by a ſet of extremely ſmall abſorbent veſſels called lacteals. Theſe have their origin in the inner coat of the inteſtines, and, paſſing thence, diſcharge themſelves into a duct named the receptacle of the chyle, whence this fluid proceeds along the *thoracic* duct*, which terminates in the left ſubclavian† vein. In the paſſage from the inteſtines to the receptacle, there is a number of glands, which ſeparate a watery liquid, for the purpoſe of giving the chyle a thinner conſiſtence. To prevent the chyle from falling back in its progreſs through the lacteals, the conſtruction of theſe veſſels is admirably contrived. They are furniſhed with a number of valves, which open only forwards, and are ſhut by any fluid preſſing backwards. From the ſubclavian vein, the chyle is poured into the blood, and thence immediately thrown into the right auricle and ventricle‡ of the heart; from which, now mixed with the blood, it paſſes into the lungs. It undergoes in that organ a conſiderable change from the act of reſpiration. From the lungs it proceeds through the pulmonary vein to the left auricle of the heart, and then into the left ventricle; whence, at laſt, endowed with all the qualities of blood, it paſſes into the aorta, and is diffuſed univerſally through the frame; the wants of which it is fitted to ſupply by the addition of nouriſhing particles. —Is it poſſible to contemplate this admirable mechaniſm without breaking forth in the exclamation of the Pſalmiſt, that "we are wonderfully made?" I may juſtly add, that, conſidering the great variety of ways in which the human body may be affected, both from without and within, with the neceſſity for the perpetual motion of the vital powers, and the millions of veſſels, inviſible to the naked eye, through which the fluids ought to paſs, it is a matter of real aſtoniſhment that we ſhould ſubſiſt a ſingle day. And doubtleſs it would be impoſſible, were not the machine conſtantly ſuſtained by the ſame Almighty and Beneficent Being who formed it.

* From thorax the breaſt.

† A term applied to any thing under the arm-pit or ſhoulder.

‡ Two muſcular bags, one on each ſide, are termed its auricles, from the Latin ſignifying ears.

## CHAP. II.

### *Of the Science of Medicine, and of the prevailing Theories among its Professors.*

FROM the account given of the human body in the preceding chapter, it will not appear surprising that it should be liable to many disorders; such a number of circumstances being requisite to the harmonious operation of the whole. The process of digestion alone, by which the aliments are converted into blood, is of a nature so complicated, that a defect in any of the organs or fluids requisite for that purpose is sufficient to lay the foundation of a variety of diseases.

In the early ages of the world, when the diet was simple, and the climates inhabited by the human race were of a mild and genial temperature, the seeds of disorders were seldom sown either by irregularity or accident, and never were fostered by the baneful influence of effeminate and luxurious gratification. It is probable, therefore, that, while the pastoral life continued, men generally experienced an uninterrupted state of health; but when, ceasing to sojourn in rural scenes, they assembled together in towns, and formed more extensive societies, they began to degenerate from their former habits, and fell into the corruptions usually incident to a promiscuous mass of inhabitants. Vice then succeeded to innocence, intemperance expelled sobriety, and health was daily sacrificed to the prevalence of sensual depravation.

Natural causes likewise concurred to engender and foment deviations from the standard of health. The bulk of the people, who had abandoned the pursuits of agriculture and the rearing of cattle, were under the necessity of having recourse to manual occupations for subsistence; and many of these being of a sedentary kind, the constitutions of men, which before were liable to be relaxed by the warmth of the climate, would contract a still greater disposition to disorders arising from that cause. To such constitutions, formerly inured to the wholesome air of the country, the polluted atmosphere of populous towns, neither ventilated by the gales nor refreshed by the showers of other latitudes, would prove extremely prejudicial; while, in addition to this powerful influence, the indelicacy common to a rude state of society in manufacturing towns, the want of soap for the purpose of washing, and the want likewise of the periodical rests of a sabbath, to induce a change of apparel; all these causes, operating in conjunction, could not fail to give rise both to internal and external diseases.

From this epoch, therefore, of the human race may be dated the origin of diseases; which, by weakening individuals, and entailing on their offspring an hereditary disposition to infirmities, would extend the boundaries of morbid affection, and disseminate among the people distempers of various kinds.

It may well be supposed, that a people who had been accustomed to see men die only of unfortunate accidents, or the effects of old age, would be surprized at the novelty of diseases which terminated in the extinction of life. Entirely ignorant of physical causes, they would probably ascribe such extraordinary incidents to some supernatural power; and superstition giving birth to a thousand phantoms of the imagination, charms and enchantments became the means by which they endeavoured to cure, as well as prevent, every malady. In process of time, however, experience and the result of observation, the sole rational guides in the cure of diseases, began to have an influence on the public mind. A general similarity in the cases of different patients afforded presumption that they were affected by the same specific causes; and wherever accident discovered, or was imagined to discover, any virtue in herbs, which perhaps were first tasted in the manner of aliment, the precious remedy was held in veneration, and recommended to every person whose complaints had any resemblance to those in which it was supposed to have produced beneficial effects.

Such was the manner in which the use of medicine was first introduced; but many ages were required to bring to perfection a science which can be completed only by faithful observation and experience. The importance, however, of health, to the happiness of mankind, soon rendered the knowledge of curing diseases an object both of fame and emolument; and there arose, in different quarters of the globe, a number of practitioners, who devoted their attention solely to the cultivation of this abstruse and important subject. Among those who afterwards appeared in the capacity of professed physicians, the most illustrious was Hippocrates, a Greek, who is supposed to have flourished about four hundred years before the birth of Christ. This extraordinary man may be regarded as the first that ever attempted to erect the science of medicine upon a solid foundation. In the treatment of diseases, his chief object was to observe the progress of nature with a scrupulous attention, and, according to the indications thence arising, to accommodate the method of cure. The numerous writings which he composed on medicine are extant at this day, and remain a monument of his penetration and judgment, as well as of unparalleled induſtry, and ſevere application, to promote the advancement of medical knowledge.

But to tread in the footſteps of Hippocrates required a mind like his own. It was eaſier, as well as more expeditious, to preſcribe fantaſtic and arbitrary laws to Nature, than to receive them from herſelf, and co-operate with them, as the great Hippocrates had done. In ſubſequent ages, therefore, it became a frequent cuſtom among phyſicians to be governed in their practice by ſome viſionary hypotheſis or ſyſtem, invented by their own imaginations, and ſo much unconnected with fact, as to be even utterly repugnant to the plaineſt dictates of obſervation and experience. Among thoſe who adopted this extravagant plan, we find Eraſiſtratus condemning in the ſtrongeſt terms the uſe of bleeding and purgatives, as remedies equally infamous and dangerous.

Aſclepiades, who purſued a ſimilar predilection for hypotheſis, ſuppoſing that health depends on the juſt proportion between the pores of the body and certain corpuſcles which they are deſtined to tranſmit, and that it is impaired whenever theſe corpuſcles are obſtructed in their paſſage, preſcribes exerciſe on horſeback in the moſt violent fevers. He advances it as a maxim, that one fever is to be cured by raiſing another; and that the ſtrength of the patient is to be exhauſted by watching and the endurance of thirſt. The practice of Aſclepiades was ſtrictly and ſeverely conformable to his principles; for he would not allow his patients to cool their mouths with a drop of water during the two firſt days of the fever, but he indulged thoſe who were phrenitic in the uſe of wine, even to intoxication.

Galen, who flouriſhed five hundred years after Hippocrates, followed the plan of that celebrated ancient in the treatment of diſeaſes, but differed eſſentially from him, by indulging in the moſt extravagant notions and idle diſputations reſpecting medical theories. He introduced a falſe and baneful theory, concerning the primary qualities of hot and cold, dry and moiſt, which probably led him into dangerous errors in the compoſition of medicines. The reputation of Galen, however, continued for many ages to ſupport the ſyſtem which he invented, and his authority was almoſt as great in medicine as that of Ariſtotle in the ſchools of philoſophy.

After the downfall of the Roman Empire, and when the inundation of Goths and Vandals had almoſt completely exterminated literature of every kind in Europe, medicine, though a practical art, ſhared the ſame fate with more abſtract ſciences. Learning, in general, baniſhed from the ſeat of arms, took refuge among the eaſtern nations, where the arts of peace ſtill continued to be cultivated. To the Arabian phyſicians, as they have been called, we are indebted both for the preſervation of medical ſcience, as it ſubſiſted among the Greeks and Romans, and likewiſe for the deſcription of ſome new diſeaſes, particularly the ſmall-pox. Though, for the moſt part, only copiers of the Greeks, they made, nevertheleſs, ſome improvements. They were the firſt who introduced chemical remedies, though of theſe they uſed but few. They added a great deal to Botany, and the Materia Medica, by the introduction of new drugs, chiefly of the aromatic kind, from the Eaſt, many of which are of conſiderable uſe; but Anatomy was not in the leaſt improved by them.

With regard to their practice, in ſome few particulars they deviated from the Greeks. Their purging medicines were much milder than thoſe formerly in uſe; and even when they did preſcribe the purgatives of the more antient phyſicians, they gave them in a much leſs doſe than was uſual in the Greek and Roman practice. The ſame may be ſaid of their manner of bleeding, which was never to that exceſſive degree practiſed by the Greeks. They deviated from Hippocrates, however, in one very trivial circumſtance, which produced a violent controverſy. The queſtion was, whether blood, in a pleuriſy, ought to be drawn from the arm of the affected ſide, or the oppoſite? Hippocrates had directed it to be drawn from the arm of the affected ſide; but the Arabians, following ſome other antient phyſicians, ordered it to be drawn from the oppoſite one. Such was the ignorance of a later age, that the univerſity of Salamanca, in Spain, made a decree, that no perſon ſhould dare to let blood but in the contrary arm; and they endeavoured to procure an edict from Charles V. to ſecond it; alledging that the other method was of no leſs pernicious conſequence to medicine than Luther's hereſy had been to religion.

When, after many ages of darkneſs, which had deſtroyed almoſt the whole of antient literature, learning was reſtored in the fifteenth century, it was the ſyſtem of Galen alone that the phyſicians of thoſe times became acquainted with, and during the century following the ſtudy of phyſicians was almoſt entirely employed in explaining and confirming that ſyſtem. Early in the ſixteenth century, Paracelſus had laid the foundation of a chemical ſyſtem, which was in direct oppoſition to that of Galen; and, by the efficacy of the medicines employed by himſelf and his followers, his ſyſtem came to be received by many: but the orthodox phyſicians continued to be chiefly Galeniſts, and kept poſſeſſion of the ſchools till the middle of the ſeventeenth century.

Various revolutions in the theory of phyſic have ſince taken place, and each of them, while it ſubſiſted, has been held in the highest esteem. One sect endeavoured to account for the phænomena of diseases upon the principles of mechanism; another maintained the general law of nature, respecting diseases, to be that of actual fermentation; a third, in explanation of morbid phænomena, asserted the universality of spasm; the great Boerhaave ascribed diseases to rigidity or laxity of the fibres, and acrimony or *lentor* of the fluids; and the reigning doctrine, at present, is, on one hand, a *debility* of the fibres; and, on the other, a *susceptibility* of *excitement*.

It is to be regretted, that, in a science of so great importance to the world as that of physic, men should, in the ardour of forming systems, adopt, as the basis of their superstructure, opinions which have no foundation in the animal economy, and some of them even manifestly repugnant to fact and observation. A strong imagination may give, to almost any system, an air of great plausibility, which will render it current for a time; till some inquisitive genius, either dissatisfied with its foundation, or pregnant with a system of his own, shall powerfully exert his efforts, and produce a fresh revolution. It is indeed often extremely difficult to pronounce a positive opinion on the truth or fallacy of a system in physic. The only test by which to judge of it, is by an appeal to its UTILITY IN PRACTICE; yet the experiment is so liable to indecision, from various circumstances, that the result, unless confirmed by a number of trials, and indubitable testimony, must still be regarded as problematical. In an internal disease, the *causa proxima*, as it is called, is an invisible object, and can be judged of with certainty only by its effects. At the same time, it is probable that there are general laws of nature, which operate uniformly in the course of diseases, though on account of various circumstances, they cannot be clearly ascertained.

Of all the transactions recorded in the history of physic, the most important is the discovery of the circulation of the blood, which will transmit the name of Harvey to the latest posterity. This single discovery has tended more to the improvement of medicine than all the hypothetical visionary systems that ever were invented.

Notwithstanding the fallacy of the various theoretical systems which have successively prevailed in medicine, the use of ratiocination, or just reasoning, in physic, is absolutely indispensable; and without it, the science would be nothing more than a mass of empiricism, or, at best, a system of vague, dubious, and unsupported conjecture. But, in order that the mode of reasoning employed may be of real utility, it must necessarily have its foundation in established and incontrovertible facts. It is such facts, and such reasoning, that constitute the essence of physiology, or the knowledge of the laws by which the animal economy is conducted. This knowledge, indeed, is only to be acquired by the ſtudy of the profeſſion of phyſic, and muſt have for its baſis a competent acquaintance with anatomy. But, without the advantage of ſuch erudition, it is poſſible for a perſon of good underſtanding both to learn and practiſe the general rules of phyſic in the greater part of common diſeaſes. Such a perſon may be ſufficiently well qualified to obſerve the ſymptoms deſcribed in proper books of phyſic, and thence to acquire a probable opinion of the exiſtence and ſtate of a particular diſeaſe; though he may not be able to diſcriminate the operation of medicine from that of the malady, nor to trace the concatenation between cauſe and effect.

It is upon this principle that the preſent work is founded; and there is ground to expect that it will prove of no ſmall advantage to the public. It will afford the means of determining, at an early period, the nature of a diſeaſe, and of applying the proper remedies accordingly, without loſs of time. It appriſes the reader of the caſes in which there may be a neceſſity for calling in medical aſſiſtance; and even then it will have the effect of enabling him to form an opinion with what judgment and attention ſuch aſſiſtance has been exerciſed. It will likewiſe be attended with the further advantage of directing a proper regimen, or courſe of diet, from the beginning of a diſeaſe—a due obſervance of which alone is often ſufficient to extirpate the complaint; and, laſtly, by pointing out the different remote cauſes of every diſeaſe, it will tend to guard againſt the operation of the ſpecific cauſe that may appear to have given riſe to it. In addition to all theſe advantages, it will have that of economy; by which in many, perhaps in moſt caſes, not only to preclude the expenditure of medical fees, but to leſſen greatly the charges of the neceſſary medicines. In a word, in every point of view, it may be regarded as a work of uncommon utility.

## CHAP. III.

### *Of the Air or Atmoſphere.*

PREVIOUSLY to entering on the principal ſubject of this work, it will be proper to take a general view of a variety of eſſential cauſes, which affect the human conſtitution, and, according to their nature and operation, conduce to health or diſeaſe. The firſt I ſhall mention is Air, that elaſtic, inviſible fluid which every where ſurrounds our globe, and affords the means of reſpiration, ſo neceſſary to the ſupport of life. When we conſider the different qualities of this element, namely, its heat, cold, dryneſs, and moiſture, with the extremes to which the two former are frequently carried, and the ſudden changes they often experience, it will not appear ſurpriſing that the air ſhould be the moſt powerful agent in nature on the bodies of animals.

The moſt obvious effect of warm air is to relax the ſolid parts of the body, and occaſion a quicker circulation of the fluids. By this means, when too hot, it diſſipates the watery parts of the blood, and gives the bile ſuch a ſharpneſs as not only produces great diſorders in the bowels, but alſo fevers of a dangerous kind. It is alſo particularly injurious to perſons of weak nerves, whom it affects with a variety of complaints. Cold air, by conſtringing the ſolids, and condenſing the fluids, diminiſhes perſpiration, and gives riſe to many diſorders immediately connected with that cauſe; ſuch as rheumatiſms, catarrhs, and coughs, with affections of the throat and parts pertaining to reſpiration. Upon the whole, however, a cold ſtate of the air, if not exceſſive, and long continued, is favourable to bodily vigour, eſpecially in thoſe who are accuſtomed to take briſk exerciſe; but to the infirm and inactive it is not equally ſalutary. Of all the different conditions of the air, that of moiſture is univerſally the moſt productive of diſeaſes, not only by deſtroying the elaſticity of the ſolids, but by obſtructing perſpiration, and rendering the body ſtill more relaxed by the humidity which inſinuates itſelf into the pores from without. Hence this ſtate of the air is apt to produce intermitting fevers, dropſies, and all the tribe of diſorders that depend on a phlegmatic or debilitated conſtitution. But the moſt dangerous and fatal effects on the human body ariſe from a moiſt ſtate of the air accompanied with heat; which, operating jointly, increaſe in a proportionable degree the laxity of the ſolids, and diſpoſe to putrefactive diſeaſes. On the other hand, the conjunction of dry and cool air is attended with ſalubrious effects; though a dry and very cold air, by thickening the blood, produces inflammatory diſorders. Dry and hot air has the ſame inconveniences aſcribed to heat alone; but a dry air, not too warm, is of all the moſt agreeable and healthful. Great and ſudden changes, from a warm to a cold air, ſcarcely ever fail of producing a variety of complaints, which chiefly break forth in the bowels.

Winds, which are only ſtrong currents of the air, have likewiſe ſenſible effects on the human conſtitution. A long continued north wind is comparatively the moſt wholeſome; as it purifies the atmoſphere of noxious vapours, renders the air ſerene and dry, and thus imparts to the body unuſual vigour and activity; though to perſons of delicate habits it proves both ſevere and injurious. An easterly wind is sometimes scarcely inferior in coldness to that of the north; but with this difference, that while the latter is in general salubrious, the former is directly the contrary. It is cold without bracing; and instead of enlivening, seems to communicate to the spirits a sensible depression. To the asthmatic, and such as are disposed to intermitting fevers, it is particularly hurtful. The south wind, as blowing from the warmer regions, and frequently accompanied with a latent humidity, relaxes the body, and disposes to phlegmatic affections of the head and breast. The westerly wind is distinguished by no peculiar characteristic; but, passing in its course over the vast Atlantic Ocean, it often brings with it a load of vapours, which afterwards descend in rain, especially on the western coasts of this country.

Besides the effects arising from the natural qualities of the air, there are others produced by contingent causes, which exert a more powerful influence on the body than the former, and generally of a hurtful kind. The atmospheric air is incessantly corrupted by the respiration of men and animals, and by the dissolution and putrefaction of innumerable substances. This is chiefly the case in great cities, where it is loaded with sulphur, smoke, and a variety of other exhalations highly prejudicial to health. Nothing is more pernicious than the air of a place where a numerous body of people are collected together within doors; especially if to the breath of the crowd there be added the vapours of a multitude of candles, and the consumption of the vital air by fires in proportion. Hence it happens, that persons of a delicate constitution are liable to become sick or faint in a place of this kind. These ought to avoid, as much as possible, the air of great towns; which is also peenliarly hurtful to the asthmatic and consumptive, as it is likewise to hysteric women, and men of weak nerves. Where such people cannot always live without the verge of great towns, they ought, at least, to go abroad as often as they can into the open air, and, if possible, pass the night in the wholesomer situation of the suburbs.

Air that has long stagnated becomes extremely unwholesome to breathe, and often immediately fatal. Such is that of mines, wells, cellars, &c. People ought, therefore, to be very cautious in entering places of this description which have been long shut up. The air of some hospitals, jails, ships, &c. partakes of the same unwholesome and pernicious nature; and they ought never to be destitute of ventilators—those useful contrivances, for expelling foul, and introducing fresh air into its place. The same may be said of all places where numbers of people are crowded together. Nature, as well as art, has furnished the means of correcting air which has become unfit for respiration. Among the most powerful of these is the growth and vegetation of plants. For it is now found that air, rendered mortal by the breathing of animals that had expired in it, may be again so completely restored by the vegetation of plants, that, after an interval of some days, an animal may live in it with equal ease, and for the same length of time, as in a similar quantity of common air. But this observation holds not universally at all times. It is found that most plants have the property of correcting bad air within a few hours, when they are exposed to the light of the sun; but that, on the contrary, during the night, or in the shade, they corrupt the common air of the atmosphere. Hence, it is a dangerous practice to have shrubs in an apartment that is slept in.

Both in public and private buildings there are errors committed, which affect, in an extraordinary degree, the salubrity of the air. Churches are seldom open above once a week; they are never ventilated by fires, and rarely by opening the windows: while, to render the air of them yet more unwholesome, little or no attention is paid to keeping them clean. The consequence of which is, that they are damp, musty, and apt to prove hurtful to people of weak constitutions; and it is a common remark, that a person cannot pass through a large church or cathedral, even in summer, without a strong sense of coolness.

The great attention paid to making houses close and warm, though apparently well adapted to the comfort of the inhabitants, is by no means favourable to health, unless care be taken every day to admit fresh air by the windows. Sometimes it may be proper to make use of what is called pumping the room, or moving the door backward and forward for some minutes together. The practice of making the beds early in the day
may suit convenience or delicacy, is doubtless improper. It would be much better to turn them down, and expose them to the influence of the air admitted by the windows.

For many persons to sleep in one room, as in the ward of an hospital, is hurtful to health; and it is scarcely a less injurious custom, though often practised by those who have splendid houses, for one or two to sleep in a small apartment, especially if it be very close. If a fire be kept in it, the danger is increased; and many have by that means been stifled in the night when asleep.

Houses situated in low marshy countries, or near lakes of stagnating water, are likewise unwholesome; as they partake of the putrid vapours exhaled in such places. To remedy this evil, those who inhabit them, if they study their health, ought to use a more generous diet than is requisite in more dry and elevated situations.

It is almost every where too common to have church-yards in the middle of populous towns. This is not only reprehensible in point of taste, but, considering how near to the surface of the earth the dead bodies in many places are deposited, there must necessarily arise putrid vapours, which, however imperceptible, cannot fail to contaminate the air. The practice of burying in churches is still more liable to censure; and not many years ago, the pernicious effects of this custom were so severely felt in France as to occasion a positive edict against it.

In short, there is nothing in nature so pestilential and destructive as putrid air. Every possible means should be diligently used to prevent it; and where it has once taken place, the most active exertion is necessary to check or extinguish it. If the external air be pure and wholesome, the apartments of a house may generally be kept clear of noxious vapours, by having the windows open for some hours in the day; but in places crowded with inhabitants, and those dirty or diseased, or both, recourse should be had to more powerful means of purification; such as fumigating them with spirit of vitriol and nitre, or sprinkling them with acids, particularly vinegar. But of all preservatives from foul air, and consequently from putrid diseases, the most important is cleanliness, in the utmost extent, in persons, in clothes, in houses, and even in the public streets: for it is almost inconceivable what pestilential effects may follow a great neglect, or disregard of this salutary principle, which is not less important in a physical than in a moral point of view.

To form a just opinion of the qualities and effects of air, it will be proper to take a short view of some principles with which the subject is connected.

For the better understanding this part of the subject, it may be proper to inform the reader of the external powers which chiefly act upon the human body, and by which it is influenced in respect both of health and disease—and to this purpose I shall have recourse to the observations made by the learned Dr. Garnett, in his ingenious lecture on the preservation of health.

The powers then which produce the living functions in our frame are chiefly heat, food, and air. Without inquiring into the property of living bodies which renders them susceptible of external influence, we shall content ourselves with giving it the name of *excitability*. When the excitability is in such a state as to be very susceptible of the action of external powers, it is said to be *abundant*, or *accumulated*; but when it is found not very capable of receiving their action, it is considered as *deficient*, or *exhausted*.

The laws by which external powers act on living bodies are found to be the following:

First, when the action of the exciting powers ceases for some time, the excitability accumulates, or becomes more capable of receiving their action, and is more powerfully affected by them. Dr. Garnett illustrates this law by the following example, taken from the effect of light.

If a person be kept in darkness for some time, and be then brought into a room in which there is only an ordinary degree of light, it will be almost too oppressive for him, and appear excessively bright; and if he has been kept for a considerable time in a very dark place, the sensation will be very painful. In this case, while the retina, or optic nerve was deprived of light, its excitability accumulated, or became more easily affected by light; for, if a person goes out of one room into another which has an equal degree of light, he will feel no effect. You may convince yourselves of this law by a very simple experiment. Shut your eyes, and cover them for a minute or two with your hand, and endeavour not to think of the light, or of what you are doing; then open them, and the day-light will for a short time appear brighter. If you look attentively at a window for about two minutes, and then cast your eyes upon a sheet of white paper, the shape of the window-frames will be perfectly visible upon the paper; those parts which express the wood-work appearing brighter than the other parts. The parts of the optic nerve on which the image of the frame falls are covered by the wood-work from the action of the light; the excitability of these portions of the nerve will therefore accumulate, and the parts of the paper which fall upon them, must of course appear brighter. If a person be brought out of a dark room where he has been confined, into a field covered with snow, when the sun shines, it has been known to affect him so much as to deprive him of sight altogether.

Let us next consider what happens with respect to heat. If heat be for some time abstracted, the excitability accumulates; or, in other words, if the body be for some time exposed to cold, it is more liable to be affected by heat, afterwards applied. Of this also you may be convinced by an easy experiment. Put one of your hands into cold water, and then put both into water which is considerably warm: the hand which has been in cold water will feel much warmer than the other. If you handle some snow with one hand, while you keep the other in your bosom, that it may be of the same heat as the body, and then bring both within the same distance of the fire, the heat will affect the cold hand infinitely more than the warm one. This is a circumstance of the utmost importance, and ought always to be carefully attended to. When a person has been exposed to a severe degree of cold for some time, he ought to be cautious how he comes near a fire: for his excitability will be so much accumulated, that the heat will act violently, often producing a great degree of inflammation, and even sometimes mortification. We may by the way observe, that this is a very common cause of chilblains, and other inflammations. When the hands, or any other parts of the body, have been exposed to violent cold, they ought first to be put into cold water, or even rubbed with the snow, and exposed to warmth in the gentlest manner possible.

Exactly the same takes place with respect to food. If a person has for some time been deprived of food, or has taken it in small quantity, whether it be meat or drink; or if he has taken it of a less stimulating quality, he will find, that when he returns to his ordinary mode of living, it will have more effect upon him than before he had lived abstemiously.

Persons who have been shut up in a coal-work, from the falling-in of the pit, and have had nothing to eat for two or three days, have been as much intoxicated by a basou of broth as a person in common circumstances with two or three bottles of wine; and we all know that spirituous or vinous liquors affect the head more in the morning than after dinner.*

All these facts, and many others which might be brought, establish beyond a doubt the truth of the law which has been mentioned, namely, that when the powerful action of the exciting powers ceases for some time, the excitability accumulates, or becomes more capable of receiving their actions.

The second law is, that when the exciting powers have acted with violence, or for a considerable time, the excitability becomes exhausted, or less fit to be acted on. This may be proved by a similar induction. Let us take the effects of light upon the eye.

* This circumstance was particularly evident among the sailors who were in the boat with Captain Bligh after the mutiny. The captain was sent by government to convey some plants of the bread-fruit-tree from Otaheite to the West-Indies. Soon after he left Otaheite, the crew mutinied, and put the captain and most of the officers, with some of the men, on board the ship's boat, with a very short allowance of provisions, and particularly of liquors: for they had only six quarts of rum, and six bottles of wine, for nineteen persons, who were driven by storms about the South-sea, exposed to wet and cold all the time for nearly a month. Each man was allowed only a tea-spoonful of rum a day; but this tea-spoonful refreshed the men, benumbed as they were with cold, and faint with hunger, more than twenty times the quantity would have done those who were warm and well fed; and had it not been for the spirit having much power to act upon men in their condition, they never could have outlived the hardships they experienced.

When it has acted violently for some time upon the optic nerve, it diminishes the excitability of that nerve, and renders it incapable of being affected by a quantity of light that would at other times affect it. When you have been walking out in the snow, if you come into your room, you will scarcely be able to see any thing for some minutes. Look steadfastly at a candle for a minute or two, and you will with difficulty discern the letters of a book, which you were before reading distinctly; and if you happen to cast your eyes upon the sun, you will not see any thing distinctly for some time afterwards.

Let us next consider the matter of heat. Suppose water to be heated lukewarm, if you put one hand into it, it will feel warm. If you put the other hand into water, heated for instance to 120° or 130°, and keep it there some time, we will say, two minutes; if then you take it out, and put it into the lukewarm water, that water will feel cold, though still it will seem warm to the other hand; for the hand which had been in the heated water has had its excitability exhausted by the application of heat. Before you go into a warm bath, the temperature of the air may seem warm and agreeable to you; but after you have remained for some time in a bath that is rather hot, when you come out you feel the air uncommonly cool and chilling.

These facts, with innumerable others, which will readily suggest themselves, prove the truth of the second proposition, namely, that when the exciting powers have acted violently, or for a considerable time, the excitability is exhausted, or less fit to be acted on.

Upon the whole, there are, according to Dr. Garnett, three states in which living bodies exist: 1. A state of accumulated excitability. 2. A state of exhausted excitability. 3. When the excitability is in such a state as to produce the strongest and most healthy actions, when acted upon by the external powers. These leading principles are of great importance, in many cases, towards ascertaining more determinate rules of conduct relative to the prevention and cure of diseases.

Of the exciting powers which act upon the human frame, one of the principal is air—the source of heat and activity, without which our blood would soon become a black and stagnant mass, and the springs of life would stop. It is now known that only a part of atmospheric air is necessary for respiration. The atmosphere, near the surface of the earth, consists of two kinds of air; one, which is highly proper for respiration, and combustion, and in which an animal immersed will live much longer than in the same quantity of common air; and the other which is perfectly improper for supporting respiration, or combustion, for an instant.

The former of these airs has obtained the name of vital air, from its property of supporting life, and constitutes about one-fourth of the atmosphere. The other, from its property of destroying life, is called azote, and forms of course the remaining three-fourths of the atmosphere.

These two airs may be separated from each other by various methods. If a candle be inclosed in a given quantity of atmospheric air, it will burn only for a certain time, and then be extinguished; and from the rising of the water in the vessel in which it is inclosed, it is evident that a quantity of air has been absorbed. What has been absorbed is the vital air, and what remains the azote, which is incapable of supporting flame. If an animal be immersed in a given quantity of common air, it will live only a certain time, at the end of which the air will be found diminished, about one-fourth being extracted from it; and the remainder will neither support flame nor life.

Some metals, and particularly manganese, when exposed to the atmosphere, attract the vital air from it, without touching the azote; and it may be procured from these metals by the application of heat, in very great purity.

If we take three parts of azote, and one of vital air, we shall form a compound which is similar to the atmosphere, and which is the mixture best suited to support the health of the body. If there were a much greater proportion of vital air, it would act too powerfully upon the system, and bring on inflammatory diseases. It would likewise by its stimulus exhaust the excitability, and bring us sooner to death; and in the same manner that a candle burns brighter in vital air, and would therefore be sooner exhausted, so would the flame of life be sooner burnt out. On the contrary, if the atmosphere contained a much less proportion of vital air, it would not stimulate the body sufficiently: the excitability would morbidly accumulate, and diseases of debility would occur.

Combustion, putrefaction, and the breathing of animals, are processes which are continually diminishing the quantity of vital air contained in the atmosphere: and if the wise Author of Nature had not provided for its continual reproduction, the atmosphere would, in all probability, have long since become too impure to support life; but this is guarded against in a most beautiful manner.

Water is not a simple element, as has been supposed, but is composed of vital air, and a particular kind of air which is called *inflammable*; the same that is used to fill balloons. It has been found by experiment, that one hundred pounds of water are composed of eighty-five pounds of vital air, and fifteen of inflammable air.*

* Strictly speaking, water is composed of the bases of these airs, the greatest part of the caloric being given out on their union.

Water may be decompounded by a variety of means, and its component parts ſeparated from each other.

Vegetables effect this decompoſition. They abſorb water, and decompoſe it in their glands; and, taking the inflammable air for their nouriſhment, breathe out the vital air in a ſtate of very great purity.

The vital air is received by animals into their lungs, and communicates a red colour to their blood. When animals die for want of vital air, their blood is always found black.

From what has been ſaid, it is evident, that in large and populous towns, where combuſtion and reſpiration are continually performed on a large ſcale, the air muſt be much leſs pure than in the country, where there are few of theſe cauſes to contaminate the atmoſphere, and where vegetables are continually tending to render it more pure; and if it was not for the winds which agitate this element, and conſtantly occaſion its change of place, the air of large towns would probably ſoon become unfit for reſpiration. Winds bring us the pure air of the country, and take away that from which the vital air has been in a great meaſure extracted; but ſtill, from the immenſe quantity of fuel which is daily burnt, and the number of people breathing in large towns, the air very ſoon becomes impure.

Children particularly require a pure air. This fact is placed in the cleareſt light by the following inſtance. In the lying-in-hoſpital at Dublin, 2944 infants, out of 7650, died in the year 1782, within the firſt fortnight after their birth, which is nearly every third child. They almoſt all died in convulſions; many of them foamed at the mouth, their thumbs were drawn into the palms of their hands, their jaws were locked, the face was ſwelled and looked blue, as if they were choked. This laſt circumſtance led the phyſicians to conclude that the rooms in the hoſpital were too cloſe, and hence, that the infants had not a ſufficient quantity of good air to breathe; they therefore ſet about ventilating them better; which was done very completely. The conſequence is, that not one child dies now where three uſed to die.

Having conſidered the purity of the air, let us next take a view of the changes in the temperature which it undergoes, and the effects which theſe have upon the conſtitution.

We find the air ſometimes conſiderable below the freezing point; nay, even ſo much as 20 or 30 degrees: it is then intenſely cold; and, on the other hand, the thermometer ſometimes indicates a great degree of heat; we then find ourſelves much relaxed, and our conſtitutions exhauſted.

To underſtand how this happens, let us conſider for a moment the nature of heat and cold. Heat is one of thoſe ſtimuli which act upon the excitability, and ſupport life: for, if it was totally withdrawn, we ſhould not be able to exiſt even a few minutes; and cold is only a diminution of heat. When heat is preſent, in a proper degree, or the atmoſphere is about that degree of heat which we call temperate, it juſt gives ſuch a ſtimulus, and keeps the excitability exhauſted to ſuch a degree, as to preſerve the body in health: but if it continue for a conſiderable time to be much warmer than this temperature, the conſequence muſt be, from the laws already laid down, an exhauſtion of the excitability, and a conſequent relaxation and debility. For when the excitability has been exhauſted by the violent application of heat, long continued, the common ſtimulant powers which ſupport life cannot produce a ſufficient effect upon it, to give to the body that tone which is compatible with health. On the contrary, when the heat of the air falls below what we call temperate, or when cold is applied to the body, from the accuſtomed ſtimulus of heat being diminiſhed, the excitability muſt accumulate, or become more liable to be affected by the action of the external powers.

This, however, very ſeldom produces bad effects, unleſs the exciting powers be improperly or quickly applied: for we can bear a conſiderable diminution of heat without any bad conſequences; and, in all caſes, much more miſchief ariſes from the too great action of heat, than from the diminution of it.

People are afraid of going out into the cold air; but if they conduct themſelves properly afterwards, they will never be in the leaſt danger from it. Indeed the action of cold, unleſs it be exceſſive, never produces any bad effects upon people in health.

This remark may, to many, appear to be erroneous, but is nevertheleſs well founded. For if a perſon go out into air which is very cold, and remain in it for a very long time, he will never perceive any ſymptoms of what is called a cold ſo long as he remains there.

A common cold is attended with a running of the noſe, hoarſeneſs, and cough, with a conſiderable degree of feveriſh heat, and dryneſs of the ſkin. Now it is univerſally agreed, that this diſorder is an inflammation, or is of an inflammatory nature: it is an inflammation of the ſmooth moiſt ſkin which lines the noſtrils, and goes down the windpipe into the lungs: but as cold is only a diminution of heat, or a diminution of a ſtimulus acting upon the body, it is impoſſible that ſuch a diminution can cauſe a greater action or excitement; we might as well expect to fill a veſſel by taking water out of it. But let us ſee how a cold, as it is commonly called, is produced. When a perſon in cold weather goes out into the air, every time he draws in his breath, the cold air paſſes through his noſtrils and windpipe into the lungs, and, in thus diminiſhing the heat of the parts, allows their excitability to accumulate, and renders them more liable to be affected by the ſucceeding heat. So long as that perſon continues in the cold air, he feels no bad effects; but if he comes into a warm room, he firſt perceives a glow within his noſtrils and breaſt, as well as all over the ſurface of his body. Soon afterwards, a diſagreeable dryneſs and huſkineſs will be felt in the noſtrils and breaſt. By and by a ſhort, dry, tickling cough comes on. He feels a ſhivering, which makes him draw nearer to the fire, but all to no purpoſe; the more he tries to heat himſelf, the more chill he becomes. All the miſchief is here cauſed by the violent action of the heat on the accumulated excitability. For want of a knowledge of this law, theſe diſagreeable, and often dangerous complaints are brought on, when they might be avoided with the greateſt eaſe.

When a perſon comes out of a cold atmoſphere, he ſhould not at firſt go into a room that has a fire in it, or, if he cannot avoid that, he ſhould keep for a conſiderable time at as great a diſtance from the fire as poſſible, that the accumulated excitability may be gradually exhauſted, by the moderate and gentle action of heat; and then he may bear the heat of the fire without any danger; but, above all, he ought to refrain from taking warm or ſtrong liquors while he is cold. If a perſon have his hands or feet expoſed to a very ſevere cold, the excitability of thoſe parts will be ſo much accumulated, that if they ſhould be brought ſuddenly near the fire, a violent inflammation, and even a mortification, will take place; which has often happened; or, at any rate, that inflammation called chilblains vill be produced, from the violent action of the heat upon the accumulated excitability of thoſe parts: but if a perſon ſo circumſtanced was to put his hands or feet into cold water, very little warmer than the atmoſphere to which he had been expoſed, or rub them with ſnow, which is not often colder than 32 or 33 degrees, the morbid excitability will be gradually exhauſted, and no bad conſequences will enſue.

When a part of the body only has been expoſed to the action of cold, and the reſt kept heated; if, for inſtance, a perſon in a warm room ſits ſo that a current of air coming through a broken pane ſhould fall upon any part of the body, that part will be ſoon afflicted with an inflammation, which is uſually called a rheumatic inflammation.

From what has been ſaid, it will be eaſy to account for this circumſtance. The excitability of the part is accumulated by the diminution of its heat: but at the ſame time the reſt of the body and blood is warm; and this warm blood acting upon a part where the excitability is accumulated, will cauſe an inflammation; to which the more you apply heat, the worse you make it.—From these considerations we may lay it down as a fact, and experience supports us in so doing, that you may in general go out of warm into cold air without much danger; but that you can never return suddenly from the cold into the warm air with perfect impunity. Hence we may lay down the following rule, which, if strictly observed would prevent the frequent colds we meet with in winter. *When the whole body, or any part of it, is chilled, bring it to its natural feeling and warmth by degrees.*

## CHAP. IV.

### *Of Exercise.*

IN vain will the air expand the lungs, and the heart propel the blood to the extremities of the body, if their efforts are not seconded by exercise, for the preservation of life and health. That man was intended for action, is from nothing more evident, than from a consideration of the necessity of exercise or labour, to guard him against weakness and disease. Such is the nature of the human constitution, that, without the assistance of these powerful agents, the solid parts must be deprived of their due elasticity, and the fluids become too thick for circulating through the various orders of vessels of which the body is composed. Hence digestion must be rendered imperfect; nourishment be proportionably defective; the different necessary secretions must proceed with a languid pace; and perspiration, that important function in our frame, be so much obstructed, that the most dangerous and fatal consequences must unavoidably ensue.

The salutary effects of exercise may be anticipated from what has been already said. It strengthens the solid parts, and promotes the circulation of the fluids beyond any thing else within the compass of nature. Weakness of the nerves, and obstructions of the glands, never fail to accompany a life that is passed in inactivity. What dreadful effects proceed from these two causes, it would be tedious to enumerate. There are very few diseases incident to mankind which inactivity may not produce; and where it has once fixed its residence it is extremely difficult to expel. It is not only of itself a plentiful source of diseases, but when become habitual, is generally attended with watchfulness, which likewise has a pernicious effect on the health.

For preserving health there is no kind of exercise more proper than walking, as it gives the most general action to the muscles of the body; but for valetudinarians, and those who have weak bowels, riding on horseback is preferable. It is almost incredible how much the constitution may be strengthened by this exercise, when continued for a considerable time; not so much in the fashionable way of a morning ride, but of making long journies, in which there is the farther advantage of a perpetual change of air. Numbers of people who were reduced to a state of great weakness have by this means acquired a degree of vigour and health which all the medical prescriptions in the world could not otherwise have procured. But it is of importance, in travelling for health, that one should not employ his mind in deep reflections, but enjoy the company of an agreeable companion, and gratify his sight with the prospect of the various objects around him. In this exercise, as well as in every other, we ought always to begin gently, and to finish gradually, never abruptly.

Exercise is hurtful immediately after meals, particularly to those of nervous and irritable constitutions, who are thence liable to the heart-burn, eructations, and even vomiting. Indeed the instinct of the inferior animals confirms the propriety of this rule: for they are all inclined to indulge themselves in rest after food. At all events, fatiguing exercise, after a full meal, should be delayed till digestion is performed, which generally requires three or four hours after eating.

Exercise may be divided into two kinds; namely, the active and the passive. Of the former kind is walking, running, leaping, riding, swimming, fencing, &c. Of the latter are, riding in a carriage, sailing, friction, &c.

The more active kinds of exercise are best adapted to youth, to those of a middle age, and particularly to the corpulent, and those whose evacuations are not in due proportion to the quantity of food and drink. The passive kinds of exercise, on the contrary, are better suited to infants, to persons far advanced in years, to the delicate and weak, and especially the asthmatic and consumptive.

To read during a walk is a custom improper in itself, and detrimental to the eyes, besides the danger it occasions of falling. This practice not only deprives a person of the principal advantage of a walk, but people thereby accustom themselves to an unsafe and ungraceful manner of carrying the body. It is productive of hurtful consequences to the eyes, because the focus is continually shifted, and the retina thus extremely fatigued.

Dancing, under proper limitations, is a wholesome exercise, especially in winter; but the more violent dances are frequently attended with pernicious effects. The exertion of so many muscles, and the quick inspiration of a warm atmosphere in a crowded assembly, excite such a rapid circulation of the blood, as is equal to that in the hot stage of a fever. When to this we add the improper use of liquors, which, if of a heating nature, increase the motion of the blood, or, if cooling, restrain it abruptly, we can no longer be surprized that spitting of blood and consumption of the lungs are often the consequence of such excesses.

Riding in carriages is an exercise conducive to health, as the gentle jolts which it affords promote the circulation of the blood; but to derive all the good effects from riding in a carriage, the body of it ought not to be too nicely suspended in the straps and springs, nor should the motion be too slow. One of the windows at least ought to be kept open, that the perspiration and breath of several persons inclosed may not too much vitiate the air.*

Of the passive kinds of exercise, sailing is the most efficacious. Those who are unaccustomed to it generally experience giddiness of the head, nausea, and vomiting: on which account it is beneficial to an impure stomach. To consumptive patients it is highly advantageous, if they have recourse to it before their disorder is too far advanced to be curable. At all times, however, if there be a spitting of blood, the motion of the vessel must necessarily prove injurious. On the other hand, the relaxed, the nervous, and particularly the hypochondriac, will find from this kind of exercise extraordinary benefit.

Reading aloud is a species of exercise much recommended by the antient physicians; and to this may be joined that of speaking. They are both of great advantage to those who have not sufficient leisure or opportunities for other kinds of exercise. To speak very loud, however, or exercise the voice immediately after a meal, is hurtful to the lungs, as well as to the organs of digestion. Singing, as by the vibratory motion of the air it shakes the lungs and the bowels of the abdomen, or belly, promotes, in a remarkable degree, the circulation of the blood. Hence those sedentary artificers or mechanics, who, from habit, almost constantly sing at their work, unintentionally contribute much to the preservation of their health.

All wind-instruments are more or less hurtful to the lungs; which they weaken by introducing much air, and keeping that organ too long in a state of distention. On this account, persons of weak lungs, who play much on the flute, hautboy, or French-horn, are frequently afflicted with spitting of blood, cough, shortness of breath, and pulmonary consumption. Blowing those instruments likewise checks the circulation of the blood through the

* In bad weather invalids, or other persons, may derive great benefit from the use of *the Chair of Health*, lately invented by Mr. Lowndes.

lungs, accumulates it towards the head, and diſpoſes ſuch muſicians to apoplexy.

One of the moſt gentle and uſeful kinds of exerciſe is friction of the body, either by the naked hand, a piece of flannel, or, what is ſtill better, a fleſh-bruſh. This was in great eſteem among the antients, and is ſo at preſent in the Eaſt-Indies. The whole body may be ſubjected to this mild operation, but chiefly the belly, the ſpine, or back-bone, and the arms and legs. Friction clears the ſkin, reſolves ſtagnating humours, promotes perſpiration, ſtrengthens the fibres, and increaſes the warmth and energy of the whole body. In rheumatiſm, gout, palſy, and green-ſickneſs, it is an excellent remedy. To the ſedentary, the hypochondriac, and perſons troubled with indigeſtion, who have not leiſure to take ſufficient exerciſe, the daily friction of the belly in particular cannot be too much recommended, as a ſubſtitute for other means, in order to diſſolve the thick humours which may be forming in the bowels by ſtagnation, and to ſtrengthen the veſſels. But, in rubbing the belly, the operation ought to be performed in a circular direction, as being moſt favourable to the courſe of the inteſtines, and their natural action. It ſhould be performed in the morning, on an empty ſtomach, or rather in bed, before getting up, and continued at leaſt for ſome minutes at a time.

Standing, though uſeful as a change after long ſitting, is apt to occaſion accumulations of blood, or the thinner parts of it, in the lower extremities. Swelled legs are, therefore, common among people of ſome occupations. It is a poſture little calculated to relieve the ſedentary; and the body is, at the ſame time, more fatigued by ſtanding than ſitting. The common way of ſitting, with the head reclined, is extremely pernicious; for the circulation of the fluids in the belly is thus checked, the inteſtines are compreſſed, and the veſſels of the breaſt contracted. The head alſo ſuffers by bending it too much forward, the blood being thus carried to it more copiouſly than is conſiſtent with health. The preſſure of the belly may, in a great meaſure, be prevented by high tables and deſks, and by raiſed ſtools and chairs, upon which a perſon rather ſtands than ſits.

# CHAP. V.

## *Of Diet.*

IT has already been ſeen, in the chapter on the Human Body, in how admirable a manner the all-wiſe and beneficent Creator has ordained that the body ſhould be furniſhed with the aliment neceſſary for the ſupport of life. What kind of food we ſhall uſe, whether of the animal or vegetable kingdom, in what quantity, and how prepared, he has graciouſly left at our own diſpoſal; and happy were it for us that we ſubmitted in all theſe reſpects to the laws of temperance and prudence.

On the quantity and quality of the food, and conſequently the nouriſhment of the body, both health and life are dependant. In regulating the quantity, no determinate rules can be preſcribed; as it is a point which involves the conſideration of a number of circumſtances; ſuch as the age, ſex, ſtrength, ſize, and habit of different individuals. But in this, as in all other things, the golden rule of mediocrity is what ought to be obſerved; and though, in general, nature teaches every creature when it has enough, it is more ſafe to keep within the bounds of ſatiety than to tranſgreſs them. For what we are accuſtomed to take daily in ounces and pounds, cannot be a matter of indifference, in reſpect either of quantity or quality.

When we take food in too great quantity, or of too nouriſhing a quality, it will either produce inflammatory diſeaſes, ſuch as pleuriſy; or, by exhauſting the excitability, it will bring on ſtomach complaints, gout, and all the ſymptoms of premature old age. This follows ſo evidently, from the laws which have been inveſtigated, that it is ſcarcely neceſſary to ſay more on the ſubject.

The quality of food, abſtracting from what is natural, depends either on accident or on artifice. Thus proviſions may be rendered unwholeſome, either by bad ſeaſons, which prevent the ripening of grain, or afterwards by involuntary damage; but, unfortunately, of late years, the practice has become too common in this country, of hoarding them up till they ſpoil, for the purpoſe of enhancing the price; and the bad being afterwards mixed with the good, the whole, in its beſt condition, is only an adulterated maſs; if not always diſagreeable to the taſte, at leaſt pernicious to the health of the conſumers. If ever the power of legiſlation ought to be exerciſed with ſeverity, it is againſt the authors of ſuch deſtructive rapine and fraud, who contribute largely to the diseases, the misery, and even the mortality of mankind. The corruption of animal food is, perhaps, yet more destructive than that of vegetables. All animal substances have a constant tendency to putrefaction, which, beyond a certain degree, is extremely injurious to health. In this class of unwholesome food must be included diseased cattle, and such as die of themselves, the flesh of which ought never to be eaten; but, in many parts of the country, this caution is not sufficiently regarded. Even the eating of those which die by accident cannot be wholesome, as the blood being mixed with the flesh must increase the tendency to putrefaction.

It may safely be assumed as a fact, that no animal can be wholesome which does not take sufficient exercise, and is even excluded from the fresh air. This is precisely the case with all our stalled cattle; which, under the two circumstances just now mentioned, are crammed with gross food. By this means, indeed, they increase in bulk; but, in proportion as they become fat, their flesh is unwholesome; and the very smell of it, when brought to the table, is offensive to those who know the qualities of good meat.

Over-heating an animal, by driving it too fast, throws it, in effect, into a temporary fever, often even to a degree of madness; and if it be killed in this situation, the blood is so intimately mixed with the flesh, that it is impossible to separate them: whence the juices, which were corrupted by the previous ferment they sustained, are incapable of affording wholesome nourishment.

It is well known that the practice of filling the cellular membranes with air, or what is called *blowing* meat, is become very common among butchers. This abominable custom not only renders the meat unfit for keeping, but communicates to it a taint, no less loathsome in idea than unnatural, and may often be aggravated, for any thing we know to the contrary, by the worst of human effluvia.

A similar method is practised by butchers, of filling the cellular membranes of animals with blood. At the same time that this makes the meat seem fatter, it adds something to its weight; but has double the effect of rendering it unwholesome and unfit for keeping. If it be true that veal is most frequently spoilt in this way, it may partly be occasioned by carrying calves from a great distance to market; whence their tender flesh is liable to be bruised, and many of their vessels burst.

Exclusive of the quantity and quality of food, great attention is due to the kind of it, in particular constitutions and circumstances. Whatever may have been the common practice in the earlier ages of the world, when mankind lived in warm climates, and the earth spontaneously produced a variety of fruits in abundance, it is beyond a doubt that animal food, as well as vegetables, was intended by Providence for the ſubſiſtence of our ſpecies; and a mixture of the two, where neither of them diſagrees with the conſtitution, is certainly the moſt proper. Animal food in general is more nouriſhing than vegetables; and when it is not ſalted, nor hardened by ſmoking, is likewiſe more eaſy of digeſtion. On this account, it generally agrees beſt with delicate and weak conſtitutions. But a mixture of many kinds of meat at a meal is undoubtedly injurious to the health; both as variety of diſhes may tempt to exceſs, and as a number of meats, very different in their texture, cannot be equally well digeſted in the ſame ſpace of time; the conſequence of which will be, that a part of the chyle will become rancid and unwholeſome before the other is brought into a condition for paſſing into the lacteals; during which retention it will likewiſe become rancid in its turn. To eat of one diſh only ſeems moſt conformable to nature, and is doubtleſs the means of procuring the moſt healthy fluids.

The mode of dreſſing meat has likewiſe an effect upon its utility and wholeſomeneſs. Fleſh that is boiled is deprived of its nouriſhing juice, as the gelatinous ſubſtance of the meat is extracted into the broth. The latter indeed contains the moſt nouriſhing part of it; but it is taken in a form that tends to relax the ſtomach, and thereby retard the proceſs of digeſtion. In the mode of dreſſing meat by roaſting, its juices are leſs waſted, and as a cruſt is ſoon formed on its ſurface, the ſtimulant particles are prevented from evaporating. Hence, roaſted meat ſeems likely to yield more nouriſhment than the ſame quantity of boiled meat. It would ſeem, however, that ſtewing is ſtill better calculated to preſerve the more ſubſtantial parts of animal food; for, being performed in a cloſe veſſel, the juices are neither extracted by water, nor made to evaporate by the heat.

As ſimplicity in food is the moſt agreeable to nature, there is reaſon to believe that the luxurious arts of cookery render many things unwholeſome which in themſelves are not ſo. All poignant ſauces, and high ſeaſoning, are incentives to intemperance, at the ſame time that they excite the digeſtive powers to an action too rapid and tumultuous. People in health require no excitement to the reliſh of good and wholeſome meat; and to thoſe in the oppoſite ſtate the luxuries of the table are poiſon.

Though appetite for food be the moſt certain indication that nature requires a ſupply, yet the calls of appetite, eſpecially when irregular, ought never to be indulged beyond a moderate extent. There are, in fact, three kinds of appetite, which differ from one another with reſpect to the cauſes from whence they ſeverally proceed. Theſe are, Firſt, the natural appetite, which is equally ſtimulated and ſatisfied with the moſt ſimple food as with the moſt palatable. Secondly, the artificial appetite, or that which is excited by liquors, ſtomachic elixirs, pickles, &c. and which only laſts during the operation of thoſe ſtimulants. Thirdly, the habitual appetite, or that which ariſes from the cuſtom of taking victuals at certain hours, and often without any real appetite. The true and healthy appetite alone can aſcertain the quantity of aliment proper for the individual; but the other two appetites are liable to miſlead in this indication, particularly the habitual appetite. The ſtomach being too much diſtended by frequent exertions, will not reſt ſatisfied with the former quantity of food, but its avidity will increaſe with indulgence, and temperance alone can reſtore its natural elaſticity. The more ſuddenly this expanſion takes place, the greater is the violence with which the ſtomach is affected, and the more ſenſible likewiſe the relaxation thereby induced. Slow eating is the beſt preſervative againſt ſuch an effect; as the ſtomach in this caſe ſuffers a very gradual diſtention, and the food has ſufficient time to be duly prepared by maſtication, or chewing in the mouth. He who obſerves this ſimple rule will feel himſelf ſatisfied only after he has received a due proportion of aliment; while he who ſwallows his food too quickly, and before it is perfectly chewed, will be apt to imagine he has eaten enough, when the unmaſticated proviſions occaſion a ſenſe of preſſure on the ſides of the ſtomach.

A healthy appetite is alſo determined by the ſeaſon, to the influence of which the ſtomach is expoſed, in common with the other organs. Hence in ſummer, as heat, in general, relaxes the body, and diſſipates the fluids, the ſtomach cannot digeſt the ſame quantity of food as in winter. Some, however, have the greateſt appetite in the extreme heat of ſummer. The bile of ſuch individuals is naturally of a watery conſiſtence, and two ſparingly ſecreted; a defect which is beſt remedied by heat. Thoſe who take more exerciſe in winter than in ſummer can alſo digeſt more food. But as individuals leading a ſedentary life uſually ſuffer in winter from a bad ſtate of digeſtion, owing to a want of exerciſe, they ought in that ſeaſon to be more ſparing of aliment.

Too little aliment weakens the body, and haſtens the conſumption of the living principle. After long faſting, the breath is fœtid; and the blood being thence rendered liable to putrefaction, the body becomes diſpoſed to putrid fevers. When a perſon has ſuffered ſo much from extreme hunger, that his fluids are already in a putreſcent ſtate, much food ought not to be given him at once; for the ſtomach being contracted and feeble cannot digeſt it. He muſt be ſupported with liquid nouriſhment, in ſmall quantities, and be treated in the manner of a patient in a putrid or nervous fever.

Hence, no animal food of any kind, but vegetables of a mild acid nature, can alone be given with propriety.

With respect to the choice of aliment, those who abound with blood should be sparing in the use of what is highly nourishing, such as fat meat, strong ale, rich wines, and the like. Their diet ought to consist chiefly of the vegetable kind, and their drink to be water, cyder, perry, or small beer. People whose solids are weak and relaxed, should avoid every thing that is hard of digestion. A nourishing diet, and sufficient exercise in the open air, are what in point of health will most avail them. To use freely a nourishing diet, is improper for those who have a tendency to be fat. They ought likewise to be sparing in the use of malt liquors, and to take a good deal of exercise. Those, on the contrary, who are lean should follow an opposite course. Persons who are troubled with eructations or belchings from the stomach, inclined to putrefaction, ought to live chiefly on acid vegetables; while, on the other hand, people whose food is apt to become sour on the stomach should make the greater part of their diet consist of animal food. Persons afflicted with nervous complaints, or with the gout, ought to avoid all flatulent food, and whatever is hard of digestion; besides that their diet should be spare, and of an opening nature. The age, constitution, and manner of life, are circumstances which merit attention in the choice of proper diet; and sedentary people should live more sparingly than those who are accustomed to much labour. People who are troubled with any complaint ought to avoid such aliments as have a tendency to increase it. Thus, such as are scorbutic ought not to indulge themselves much in salt provisions; while one who is troubled with the gravel should be cautious in using too much acid, or food of an astringent kind.

Though due attention should be paid to the general classes of food, according to the particular tendency of different constitutions, the diet ought not to be too uniform, at least for any considerable time. A person, by long accustoming himself to dine only on boiled chicken, one of the most tender kinds of food, will habituate his stomach to such a standard of action as to become incapable of digesting any thing stronger. Indeed this is an error not very liable to be often fallen into voluntarily: for people are generally inclined to a change of food; and the variety which nature has provided renders it sufficiently practicable.

The diet ought not only to be such as is best adapted to the constitution, but likewise to be taken at regular periods, for long fasting is hurtful in every stage of life. In young persons, it vitiates the fluids, as well as prevents the growth of the body. Nor is it much less injurious to those more advanced in life; as the humours, even in the most healthy state, have a constant tendency to acrimony; the prevention of which requires frequent ſupplies of freſh nouriſhment. Beſides, long faſting is apt to produce wind in the ſtomach and bowels, and ſometimes even giddineſs, and faintneſs; though the ſtrong and healthy ſuffer leſs from long faſting than the weak and delicate.

All great and ſudden changes in diet are univerſally dangerous; particularly the tranſition from a rich and full diet to one that is low and ſparing. When, therefore, a change becomes expedient, it ought always to be made by degrees.

The practice is not uncommon to eat a light breakfaſt, and a heavy ſupper: but the latter of theſe is hurtful; and where it is not practiſed, there will generally be found a diſpoſition to make a more hearty breakfaſt.

It is a diſputed point, whether a ſhort ſleep after dinner be not uſeful for promoting digeſtion; and in ſeveral countries the praetice certainly is indulged with impunity, if not with evident advantage; beſides that it ſeems to be conſiſtent with the inſtinct of nature. It is, however, only among a certain claſs that the practice can be uſed with propriety; and whoever adopts it ought to confine the indulgence to a ſbort ſleep of a few minutes. For, if it be continned longer, there ariſes more loſs, from the increaſe of inſenſible perſpiration, than can be compenſated by all the advantage ſuppoſed to accrue to digeſtion.

Thoſe who uſe ſuch a cuſtom, which may be allowable to the aged and delicate, ought to place themſelves in a reclining, not a horizontal poſture; becauſe in the latter ſituation the ſtomach preſſes upon a part of the inteſtines, and the blood is conſequently impelled to the head.

In the general claſs of aliment an eſſential part is drink, the uſe of which is indiſpenſible to the digeſtion of food; and there is almoſt as great a diverſity among the kinds of beverage, as there is among thoſe of ſolid food. Water, however, is the baſis of moſt liquors; and on this account its quality is of great importance in diet. Paſſing originally for the moſt part through ſubterraneous channels, it is often impregnated with metals or minerals of a nature injurious to the conſtitution; and ſuch impregnation may be known by the ſenſible qualities of the water. The beſt water is that which is pure, light, and without any particular colour, taſte, or ſmell. Where water cannot be obtained pure from ſprings, wells, rivers, or lakes, care ſhould be taken to deprive it of its pernicious qualities by boiling, and filtering, but moſt effectually by diſtillation. Any putrid ſubſtances in the water may be corrected by the addition of an acid. Thus, half an ounce of alum in powder will make twelve gallons of corrupted water pure and tranſparent in two hours, without imparting a ſenſible degree of aſtringency. Charcoal powder has alſo been found of great efficacy in checking the putrid tendency of water. To the ſame purpoſe vinegar and other ſtrong acids are well adapted.

Whether water be uſed plain, or in the form of fermented liquors, a proper attention ſhould always be had to its quality, as well as to that of thoſe liquors, now ſo generally the common drink over a great part of the world. Fermented liquors, to prove advantageous to the health, ought not to be too ſtrong; otherwiſe they hurt digeſtion, and weaken inſtead of ſtrengthening the body: for when in that ſtate, and drunk in large quantity, they inflame the blood, and diſpoſe to a variety of diſeaſes. A certain degree of ſtrength, however, is neceſſary to adapt them to moſt conſtitutions in cold climates. For, if too weak, they produce wind in the bowels, and occaſion flatulencies; or if become ſtale they turn ſour on the ſtomach, and have a pernicious effect on digeſtion, as well as prove otherwiſe hurtful. If fermented liquors, made for ſale, were faithfully prepared, as there is too much reaſon to believe they are not, and were kept to a proper age, they would, uſed with moderation, be a comfortable and wholeſome beverage; but while they continue to be drunk under every circumſtance oppoſite to ſalubrity, the effects they produce muſt be more injurious than beneficial to health.

Whatever kind of drink is uſed, it ought, as well as food, to be taken always in a juſt and moderate quantity. Sufficient drink, beſides its uſe in digeſtion, prevents the blood from becoming too thick, and the ſmaller veſſels from being obſtructed. It likewiſe tends to mitigate any acrimony in the blood, and promotes the neceſſary ſecretions, ſuch as the bile, and the gaſtric juice of the ſtomach.

Were we to be governed by the dictates of nature, we ought to drink only when ſolicited by thirſt, and to deſiſt when that was ſatisfied; but as many of our liquors ſtimulate the palate, this is ſeldom the caſe. Pure water is, on this account, an ineſtimable beverage, as it will not induce us to drink more than is neceſſary. The proportion of drink, however, ought in general to be greater than that of food; for the quantity of our fluids by far exceeds that of the ſolids, and conſequently the waſte of them muſt be more conſiderable. It is by ſome regarded as a general rule, that the quantity of liquid ſhould be double that of the dry food; but this cannot be accurately obſerved, nor is it applicable in all caſes. The ſeaſon of the year, the ſtate of the weather, and the nature of our food, with the greater or leſs degree of our exerciſe, all contribute to render the proportion of drink indeterminate. Thirſt, however, is a more certain guide for its own gratification than hunger; and he who is accuſtomed to drink water only, will be in little danger of tranſgreſſing the proper meaſure, if he drinks as often as the calls of nature demand. Perſons of a phlegmatic conſtitution have both leſs inclination and occaſion to drink than thoſe of a warm temperament; while the laborious, or thoſe who take much exerciſe, ought to drink more than the ſedentary, and ſtill more in summer than in winter.

To drink immediately before a meal is a practice not to be commended: becauſe the ſtomach is thereby ſtretched, and rendered leſs fit for performing its office. Beſides, the gaſtric juice is by this mean too much diluted; and digeſtion, of conſequence, is much obſtructed. To drink much during a meal is alſo liable to objection; the ſtomach being thus rendered incapable of receiving the due portion of aliment. In the hot weather of ſummer it is ſcarce poſſible to delay drinking till the dinner be finiſhed, and it is leſs hurtful, if not more neceſſary, at this time, as the bile, which ſerves to prepare the chyle, then requires greater dilution. When the drink is water, a moderate quantity of wine may be uſed with advantage; but in thoſe whoſe ſtomach and bowels are weak, the mixture of wine and malt-liquors is apt to produce flatulence; as likewiſe, indeed, does the mixture of malt-liquors and water.

Freſh meat is the moſt wholeſome and nouriſhing. But to preſerve theſe qualities, it ought to be dreſſed in ſuch a manner as to remain tender and juicy. The fleſh of tame animals is, upon the whole, preferable to game: for though the latter be in general more mellow and eaſier of digeſtion, it does not contain the ſweet jelly and mild juices with which the former is commonly impregnated.

Some vegetables are not ſo eaſily digeſted as even hard and tough animal ſubſtances; but the fleſh of young animals, with a full proportion of wholeſome vegetables, the ſort which leaſt diſagrees with the ſtomach, is the diet moſt ſuitable to our frame. The fleſh of cattle fattened in the ſtall is by no means ſo wholeſome as that of animals ſuffered to go at large; for, uſing no motion, and their food being often of a bad kind, not to mention the putrid air of the places in which they are confined, their fleſh is little adapted to afford ſalutary juices.

Fat, though more nouriſhing than lean, is not ſo eaſy of digeſtion. On this account it is proper to uſe with it a ſufficient quantity of ſalt, which conduces greatly to diſſolve the fat of meat, and render it more eaſy of digeſtion.

In ſummer, at which ſeaſon the blood is much diſpoſed to putreſcency, it is adviſable to increaſe the proportion of vegetable food, and to make uſe of acids, ſuch as vinegar, lemons, oranges, and the like, provided that they do not diſagree with the ſtomach and bowels which is the caſe in thoſe conſtitutions where too much acid is generated in the ſtomach. This may frequently be known from feeling the ſenſation of hunger in a painful degree. In ſuch conſtitutions cold proviſion as well as cold drink is often preferable to hot.

I ſhall now give a general account of the qualities of the different kinds of animal and vegetable food moſt commonly uſed in diet; firſt, of animal food.

*Beef.* When this is the fleſh of a bullock of middle age it affords good and ſtrong nouriſhment, and is peculiarly well adapted to thoſe who labour, or take much exerciſe. It will often ſit eaſy upon ſtomachs that can digeſt no other kind of food; and it's fat is almoſt as eaſily digeſted as that of *veal.*

*Veal* is a proper food for perſons recovering from an indiſpoſition, and may even be given to febrile patients in a very weak ſtate, but it affords leſs nouriſhment than the fleſh of the ſame animal in a ſtate of maturity. The fat of it is lighter than that of any other animal, and ſhows the leaſt diſpoſition to putreſcency. *Veal* is a very ſuitable food in coſtive habits; but of all meat it is the leaſt calculated for removing an acid from the ſtomach.

*Mutton,* from the age of four to ſix years, and fed on dry paſture, is an excellent meat. It is of a middle kind between the firmneſs of beef and the tenderneſs of veal. The lean part of mutton, however, is the moſt nouriſhing, and conducive to health; the fat being hard of digeſtion. The head of the ſheep, eſpecially when diveſted of the ſkin, is very tender; and the feet, on account of the jelly they contain, highly nutritive.

*Lamb* is not ſo nouriſhing as mutton; but it is light, and extremely ſuitable to delicate ſtomachs.

*Houſe-lamb,* though much eſteemed by many, poſſeſſes the bad qualities common to the fleſh of all animals reared in an unnatural way.

*Pork* affords rich and ſubſtantial nouriſhment; and its juices are wholeſome when properly fed, and when the animal enjoys pure air and exerciſe. But the fleſh of hogs reared in towns is both hard of digeſtion and unwholeſome. Pork is particularly improper for thoſe who are liable to any foulneſs of the ſkin. It is almoſt proverbial, that a dram is good for promoting its digeſtion: but this is an erroneous notion: for, though a dram may give a momentary ſtimulus to the coats of the ſtomach, it tends to harden the fleſh, and of courſe to make it more indigeſtible.

*Smoked-hams* are a ſtrong kind of meat, and rather fit for a reliſh than for diet. It is the quality of all ſalted meat that the fibres become rigid, and therefore more difficult of digeſtion; and when to this is added ſmoking, the heat of the chimney occaſions the ſalt to concentrate, and the fat between the muſcles to become rancid,

*Bacon* is alſo of an indigeſtible quality, and is apt to turn rancid on weak ſtomachs.

The fleſh of *goats* is hard and indigeſtible; but that of kids is tender, as well as delicious, and affords good nouriſhment.

*Veniſon*, or the fleſh of *deer*, and that of *hares*, is of a nouriſhing quality, but is liable to one inconvenience; which is, that though much diſpoſed to putreſcency of itſelf, it muſt be kept for a little time before it becomes tender.

The *blood* of animals is uſed as aliment by the common people; but they could not long ſubſiſt upon it unleſs mixed with oatmeal, &c. for it is not ſoluble alone by the digeſtive powers of the human ſtomach, and therefore cannot prove nouriſhing.

*Milk* is of very different conſiſtence in different animals; but that of cows being the kind uſed in diet, is at preſent the object of our attention. Milk, where it agrees with the ſtomach, affords excellent nouriſhment for thoſe who are weak, and cannot digeſt other aliments. Though an animal production, it does not readily become putrid, as being poſſeſſed of the properties of vegetable aliment; but it is apt to become ſour on the ſtomach, and thence to produce flatulence, the heart-burn, or gripes, and, in ſome conſtitutions, a looſeneſs. The beſt milk is from a cow at three or four years of age, about two months after producing a calf. It is lighter, but more watery, than the milk of ſheep and goats; while, on the other hand, it is more thick and heavy than the milk of aſſes and mares, which are the next in conſiſtence to human milk.

On account of the acid which is generated after digeſtion, milk coagulates in all ſtomachs; but the caſeous or cheeſy part is again diſſolved by the digeſtive juices, and rendered fit for the purpoſe of nutrition. It is, however, improper to eat acid ſubſtances with milk, as theſe would tend to prevent the due digeſtion of it.

*Cream* is very nouriſhing, but, on account of its fatneſs is difficult to be digeſted in weak ſtomachs. Violent exerciſe, after eating it, will in a little time convert it into butter.

Some writers inveigh againſt the uſe of *Butter* as univerſally pernicious; but they might with equal reaſon condemn all vegetable oils, which form a conſiderable part of diet in the ſouthern climates, and ſeem to have been beneficently intended by nature for that purpoſe. Butter, like every other oily ſubſtance, has doubtleſs a relaxing quality, and, if long retained in the ſtomach, is liable to become rancid; but, if eaten in moderation, it will not produce thoſe effects in any hurtful degree. It is, however, improper in bilious conſtitutions. The worſt conſequence produced by butter, when eaten with bread, is, that it obſtructs the diſcharge of the ſaliva in the act of maſtication or chewing; by which means the food is not ſo readily digeſted. To obviate this effect, it would be a commendable practice at breakfaſt, firſt to eat ſome dry bread, and chew it well, till the ſalivary glands were exhauſted, and afterwards to eat it with butter. By theſe means ſuch a quantity of ſaliva might be carried into the ſtomach as would be ſufficient for the purpoſe of digeſtion.

*Cheeſe* is likewiſe reprobated by many as extremely unwholeſome. It is doubtleſs not eaſy of digeſtion; and, when eaten in a great quantity, may load the ſtomach; but, if taken ſparingly, its tenacity may be diſſolved by the digeſtive juices, and it may yield a wholeſome, though not very nouriſhing chyle. Toaſted cheeſe is agreeable to moſt palates, but is rendered more indigeſtible by that proceſs.

The fleſh of *Birds* differs in quality according to the food on which they live. Such as feed upon grain and berries afford, in general, good nouriſhment, if we except *geeſe* and *ducks*, which are hard of digeſtion. A young *hen* or chicken is tender and delicate food, and extremely well adapted where the digeſtive powers are weak. But of all tame fowls, the *capon* is the moſt nutritious.

*Turkeys*, as well as Guinea or India fowls, afford a ſubſtantial aliment, but are not ſo eaſy of digeſtion as the common domeſtic fowls. In all birds thoſe parts are the moſt firm which are moſt exerciſed: in the ſmall birds, therefore, the wings, and in the larger kinds the legs, are commonly the moſt difficult of digeſtion.

The fleſh of *wild birds*, in general, though more eaſily digeſted, is leſs nouriſhing than that of quadrupeds, as being more dry, on account of their almoſt conſtant exerciſe. Thoſe birds are not wholeſome which ſubſiſt upon worms, inſects, and fiſhes.

*Eggs*. In the laſt claſs of terreſtrial animal food we may rank the eggs of birds, which are a ſimple and wholeſome aliment. Thoſe of the turkey are ſuperior in all the qualifications of food. The white of eggs is diſſolved in a warm temperature, but by much heat it is rendered tough and hard. The yolk contains much oil, and is highly nouriſhing, but has a ſtrong tendency to putrefaction; on which account eggs are improper for people of weak ſtomachs, eſpecially when they are not quite freſh. Eggs hard boiled or fried are difficult of digeſtion, and are rendered ſtill more indigeſtible by the addition of butter. All eggs require a ſufficient quantity of ſalt, to promote their ſolution in the ſtomach.

*Fiſh*, though ſome of them be light, and eaſy of digeſtion, afford leſs nouriſhment than vegetables or the fleſh of quadrupeds, and are of all the animal tribes the moſt diſpoſed to putrefaction. Salt-water fiſh are, in general, the beſt; but when ſalted, though leſs diſpoſed to putreſcency, they become more difficult of digeſtion.

Whitings and flounders are the most easily digested. Acid sauces and pickles, by resisting putrefaction, are a proper addition to fish, both as they retard putrescency, and correct the relaxing tendency of butter, so generally used with this kind of aliment.

*Oysters* are eaten both raw and dressed; but in the former state they are preferable: because heat dissipates considerably their nutritious parts, as well as the salt-water, which promotes their digestion in the stomach: if not eaten very sparingly, they generally prove laxative.

*Muscles* are far inferior to oysters, both in point of digestion and nutriment. Sea muscles are by some supposed to be of a poisonous nature; but though this opinion is not much countenanced by experience, the safest way is to eat them with vinegar, or some other vegetable acid.

*Bread.* At the head of the vegetable class stands bread, that article of diet which, from general use, has received the name of *the staff of life*. Wheat is the grain chiefly used for the purpose in this country, and is among the most nutritive of all the farinaceous kinds, as it contains a great deal of mucilage. Bread is very properly eaten with animal food, to correct the disposition to putrescency; but is most expedient with such articles in diet as contain much nourishment in a small bulk, because it then serves to give the stomach a proper degree of expansion. But as it produces a slimy chyle, and disposes to costiveness, it ought not to be eaten in a large quantity. To render bread easy of digestion, it ought to be well fermented and baked; and it never should be used till it has stood twenty-four hours after being taken out of the oven, otherwise it is apt to occasion various complaints in those who have weak bowels; such as flatulence, the heart-burn, watchfulness, and the like. The custom of eating butter with bread hot from the oven is compatible only with strong digestive powers.

*Pastry*, especially when hot, has all the disadvantages of hot bread and butter; and even buttered toast, though the bread be stale, is scarcely inferior in its effects on a weak stomach. Dry toast with butter is by far the wholesomest breakfast. Brown wheaten bread in which there is a good deal of rye, though not so nourishing as that made of fine flour, is both palatable and wholesome, but apt to become sour on weak stomachs, and to produce all the effects of acidity.

*Oats*, when deprived of the husk, and particularly *barley*, when properly prepared, are each of them softening, and afford wholesome and cooling nourishment. *Rice* likewise contains a nutritious mucilage, and is less used in this country than it deserves, both on account of its wholesomeness and economical utility. The notion of its being hurtful to the sight is a vulgar error. In some constitutions it tends to make them coſtive; but this ſeems to be owing chiefly to flatulence, and may be corrected by the addition of ſome ſpice, ſuch as caraway, aniſe ſeed, and the like.

*Potatoes* are an agreeable and wholeſome food, and yield as much nouriſhment as any of the roots used in diet. The farinaceous or mealy kind is in general the moſt eaſy of digeſtion; and they are much improved by being roaſted.

*Green peaſe*, and *Turkey beans*, boiled in their freſh ſtate, are both agreeable to the taſte, and wholeſome; being neither near ſo flatulent, nor difficult of digeſtion, as in their ripe ſtate; in which they reſemble the other leguminous vegetables. *French beans* poſſeſs much the ſame qualities; but yield a more watery juice, and have a greater diſpoſition to produce flatulence. The leguminous vegetables in general ought to be eaten with ſome ſpice.

*Salads*, being eaten raw, require good digeſtive powers, eſpecially thoſe of the cooling kind; and the addition of oil and vinegar, though qualified with muſtard, hardly renders the free uſe of them conſiſtent with a weak ſtomach.

*Spinage* affords a ſoft lubricating aliment, but contains little nouriſhment. In weak ſtomachs it is apt to produce acidity, and frequently a looſeneſs. To obviate theſe effects, it ought always to be well beaten, and but little butter mixed with it.

*Aſparagus* is a nouriſhing article in diet, and promotes urine; but, in common with the vegetable claſs, diſpoſes a little to flatulence.

*Artichokes* reſemble aſparagus in their qualities, but ſeem to be more nutritive, and leſs diuretic.

*White cabbage* is one of the moſt conſpicuous plants in the garden. It does not afford much nouriſhment, but is an agreeable addition to animal food, and not quite ſo flatulent as the common greens. It is likewiſe diuretic, and ſomewhat laxative. Cabbage has a ſtronger tendency to putrefaction than moſt other vegetable ſubſtances; and, during their putrefying ſtate, ſends forth an offenſive ſmell, much reſembling that of putrefying animal bodies. So far, however, from promoting a putrid diſpoſition in the human body, it is, on the contrary, a wholeſome aliment in the true putrid ſcurvy.

*Turnips* are a nutritious article of vegetable food, but not very eaſy of digeſtion, and are flatulent. This effect is, in a great meaſure, obviated by preſſing the water out of them before they are eaten.

*Carrots* contain a conſiderable quantity of nutritious juice, but are among the moſt flatulent of vegetable productions.

*Parſnips* are more nouriſhing and leſs flatulent than carrots, which they alſo exceed in the ſweetneſs of their mucilage. By boiling them in two different waters, they are rendered leſs flatulent, but their other qualities are thereby diminiſhed in proportion.

*Parſley* is of a ſtimulating and aromatic nature, well calculated to make agreeable ſauces. It is alſo a gentle diuretic, but preferable in all its qualities when boiled.

*Celery* affords a root both wholeſome and fragrant, but is difficult of digeſtion in its raw ſtate. It gives an agreeable taſte to ſoups, as well as renders them diuretic.

*Onions, garlic,* and *ſhallot,* are all of a ſtimulating nature, by which they aſſiſt digeſtion, diſſolve ſlimy humours, and expel flatulency. They are, however, moſt ſuitable to perſons of a cold and phlegmatic conſtitution.

*Radiſhes* of all kinds, particularly the horſe-radiſh, agree with the three preceding articles in powerfully diſſolving ſlimy humours. They excite the diſcharge of air lodged in the inteſtines; but this proceeds from the expulſion of the air contained in themſelves.

*Apples* are a wholeſome vegetable aliment, and in many caſes medicinal, particularly in diſeaſes of the breaſt and complaints ariſing from phlegm. But, in general, they agree beſt with the ſtomach when eaten either roaſted or boiled. The more aromatic kinds of apples are the fitteſt for eating raw.

*Pears* reſemble much in their effects the ſweet kind of apples, but have more of a laxative quality, and a greater tendency to flatulence.

*Cherries* are, in general, a wholeſome fruit, when they agree with the ſtomach, and they are beneficial in many diſeaſes, eſpecially thoſe of the putrid kind.

*Plums* are nouriſhing, and have beſides an attenuating, as well as a laxative, quality; but are apt to produce flatulence. If eaten freſh, and before they are quite ripe, eſpecially in large quantities, they occaſion colics and other complaints of the bowels.

*Peaches* are not of a very nouriſhing quality, but they abound in juice, and are ſerviceable in bilious complaints.

*Apricots* are more pulpy than peaches, but are apt to ferment, and produce acidities in weak ſtomachs. Where they do not diſagree they are cooling, and tend likewiſe to correct a diſpoſition to putreſcency.

*Gooſeberries,* as well as *currants,* when ripe, are ſimilar in their qualities to *cherries,* and, when uſed in a green ſtate, they are agreeably cooling.

*Strawberries* are an agreeable, cooling aliment, and are accounted good againſt the gravel.

*Cucumbers* are cooling, and agreeable to the palate in hot weather; but to prevent them from proving hurtful to the ſtomach the juice ought to be ſqueezed out after they are ſliced, and vinegar, pepper, and ſalt, afterwards added.

*Tea.* By ſome the uſe of this exotic is condemned in terms the moſt vehement and unqualified, while others have either aſſerted its innocence, or gone ſo far as to aſcribe to it ſalubrious and even extraordinary virtues. The truth ſeems to lie between theſe extremes: there is however an eſſential difference in the effects of green tea and of black, or bohea; the former of which is much more apt to effect the nerves of the ſtomach than the latter, eſpecially when drunk without cream and likewiſe without bread and butter. That when taken in a large quantity, or at a later hour than uſual, it often produces watchfulneſs, is a point which cannot be denied; but if uſed in moderation, and accompanied with the addition juſt now mentioned, it does not ſenſibly diſcover any hurtful effects, but greatly relieves an oppreſſion of the ſtomach, and abates a pain of the head. It ought always to be made of a moderate degree of ſtrength: for if too weak it certainly relaxes the ſtomach. As it has an aſtringent taſte, which ſeems not very conſiſtent with a relaxing power, there is ground for aſcribing this effect not ſo much to the herb itſelf as to the hot water, which not being impregnated with a ſufficient quantity of tea to correct its own emollient tendency, produces a relaxation unjuſtly imputed to ſome noxious quality of the plant. But tea, like every other commodity, is liable to damage, and when this happens it may produce effects not neceſſarily connected with its original qualities.

*Coffee.* It is allowed that coffee promotes digeſtion, and exhilarates the animal ſpirits; beſides which, various other qualities are aſcribed to it, ſuch as diſpelling flatulency, removing dizzineſs of the head, attenuating viſcid humours, increaſing the circulation of the blood, and conſequently perſpiration; but if drunk too ſtrong it affects the nerves, occaſions watchfulneſs, and tremor of the hands; though in ſome phlegmatic conſtitutions it is apt to produce ſleep. Indeed it is to perſons of that habit that coffee is well accommodated: for to people of a thin and dry habit of body it ſeems to be injurious. Turkey coffee is greatly preferable in flavour to that of the Weſt-Indies. Drunk only in the quantity of one diſh after dinner to promote digeſtion, it anſwers beſt without either ſugar or milk: but if taken at other times it ſhould have both, or in place of the latter rather cream, which not only improves the beverage but tends to mitigate the effect of coffee upon the nerves.

*Chocolate* is a nutritive and wholeſome compoſition if taken in ſmall quantity, and not repeated too often; but is generally hurtful to the ſtomach of thoſe with whom a vegetable diet diſagrees. By the addition of vanilla and other ingredients it is made too heating, and ſo much affects particular conſtitutions as to excite nervous ſymptoms, eſpecially complaints of the head.

## CHAP. VI.

### *Of the Paſſions.*

NOTWITHSTANDING the univerſal condemnation of the paſſions by the ſtoical ſect of philoſophers, they are a natural and neceſſary part of the human conſtitution, and were implanted in it by the Great Creator for wiſe and uſeful purpoſes. Indeed without them we could have no motive to action, the mind muſt become utterly torpid, and, there being no foundation for morality or religion, virtue and vice would be nothing more than indiſcriminate and unintelligible terms. The paſſions are only prejudicial when allowed to exceed their proper bounds; and to preſerve them within thoſe limits, we are furniſhed, not only with reaſon and the light of nature, but likewiſe that of revelation.

From the intimate though myſterious connection between the mind and body, they reciprocally affect each other, and thence the paſſions exert a powerful influence both in the production and cure of diſeaſes. The two great ſources of the paſſions reſpectively are deſire and averſion; thoſe of the former claſs tending in general to excite, and the others to depreſs, the powers of the animal ſyſtem. The chief paſſions which ariſe from deſire are joy, hope, and love; and the moſt eminent in the train of averſion are fear, grief, and anger.

Joy is a paſſion in which the mind feels a ſudden and extraordinary pleaſure; the eyes ſparkle, a flood of animation overſpreads the countenance, the action of the heart and arteries is increaſed, and the circulation of the blood becomes vigorous. Inſtances are not wanting where this paſſion, when unexpectedly excited and violent, has produced immediate death; but if moderate, and exiſting only in the form of cheerfulneſs, it has a beneficial effect in preſerving health, as well as in the cure of diſeaſes.

Of all the paſſions hope is the mildeſt; and, though it operates without any commotion of the mind or any viſible ſymptom of the body, it has a moſt powerful influence on the health of one and the ſerenity of the other: it contributes indeed ſo much to the welfare of both, that if it were extinguiſhed we could neither enjoy any pleaſure in this life nor any proſpect of happineſs in the life to come; but by the beneficent will of Providence it is the laſt of the paſſions that forſakes us.

Love is one of the ſtrongeſt paſſions with which the mind is affected, and has at its commencement a favourable influence on the functions of the body; but being often in its progress attended with other passions, such as fear and jealousy, it is liable to become the source of infinite disquietude: no passion undermines the constitution so insidiously as this; for, while the whole soul is occupied with the thoughts of a pleasing attachment, both the mind and body become languid from the continuance of vehement desire; and should there arise any prospect, real or imaginary, of being frustrated in its pursuit, the person is agitated with all the horrors and pernicious effects of despair. Love when violent and unsuccessful frequently produces a wasting of the flesh, called nervous consumption, which terminates in death.

Fear has its origin in the apprehension of danger or evil, and is placed as it were a sentinel for the purpose of self-preservation; it retards the motion of the blood, obstructs respiration, and when in a moderate degree relaxes the body; but if it rise to the height of terror it puts all the springs of life into disordered action, and produces the most violent efforts in every muscle of the body. By weakening the energy of the heart this passion disposes greatly to infection during the prevalence of contagious diseases: in some instances it has produced palsy, loss of speech, epilepsy, and even madness.

There is no passion more destructive than grief when it sinks deep into the mind: by enfeebling the whole nervous system it depresses the motion of the heart, and retards the circulation of the blood with that of all the other fluids; it commonly debilitates both the stomach and bowels, producing indigestion, obstructions, obstinate watchfulness, and disposing to every disease that may arise from extreme relaxation; it preys upon the mind as well as the body, and is nourished by indulgence to the utmost degree of excess: during the violence of its earlier period it spurns at all the consolations either of philosophy or religion; but if life can subsist till the passion be alleviated by time, and submit to the cheering influence of company, exercise, and amusement, there is a prospect of recovery; though grief long continued often gives a shock to the constitution in a manner that nothing can retrieve.

Anger is a passion suddenly excited, and which often no less suddenly subsides. Equally furious and ungovernable in its nature, it may justly be considered as a transient fit of madness. The face, for the most part, becomes red, the eyes sparkle with fury, an outrageous commotion is visible in the countenance, and pervades the whole body. The animal spirits flow with rapidity, the pulsation of the heart and arteries, and with them the motion of the blood, are sometimes so much increased as to occasion the bursting of vessels. This passion being most frequent among persons of a choleric temperament, it is particularly hurtful to the liver and its ducts, which it seems to affect with spasmodic and irregular agitations, sometimes productive of the jaundice. But it operates likewise towards the production of fevers, inflammations, spitting of blood, apoplexy, and other disorders. As anger is liable to be spent by its own violence, it is commonly of short duration; but when existing in a more moderate degree, and combined with sadness or regret it gives rise to fretting, which is extremely pernicious to the health. A person ought never to eat or drink immediately after a violent fit of anger; and those who are constitutionally exposed to its influence should make every effort to restrain such an odious ebullition of the temper. Some have supposed that in a violent fit of anger the saliva possesses a slightly poisonous quality; but perhaps this opinion is founded more on analogy and conjecture than on real and accurate observation.

From the general view which has been taken of the principal passions, it appears that there are two of them which have a particular claim to the attention of the medical faculty. These are hope and fear. By encouraging the former, and obviating the disposition to the latter, the most important assistance may be given in the treatment of many diseases not otherwise curable. In the whole compass of medicine there is not a more enlivening and salutary cordial than the passion of hope, nor any which can be compared to it in point of permanent operation.

It is natural to persons who have any dangerous complaint, to entertain fear and anxiety with respect to its termination. Such a state of mind never fails to aggravate any disorder; and the physician ought to exert himself all in his power to counteract the effects of the passion; for nothing can prove effectual for removing the disease, if baneful despondency support it.

## CHAP. VII.

### *Of Sleep.*

SUCH is the general constitution of animal bodies, that with all the aid of aliment they cannot long subsist unless refreshed by the natural vicissitudes of waking and sleep. These periodical changes in the state of our existence are as necessary to health and life as the alternate returns of day and night to the regularity of the solar system. In what proportion they ought to divide our time, is a question worthy of consideration; and for this purpose it is proper to aſcertain the end for which mankind was created. Both reaſon and ſcripture aſſure us that we are placed here in a ſtate of probation, to exercife our natural faculties according to the laws of morality; and, by improving ourſelves in habits of virtue, to be rendered fit for the enjoyment of a nobler and eternal ſtate of exiſtence.

Such being the caſe, it follows, that the proper cultivation of the mind ought always to be our principal object: and as this duty can be performed only when awake, we may juſtly conclude that the ſmalleſt portion of our time ſhould be devoted to the repoſe of the bed. In this, however, we are left entirely to be guided by our own diſcretion: but it happens fortunately, that the dictates of reaſon coincide with the beſt phyſical rules for the preſervation of health. In moſt conſtitutions, ſix hours will be found a ſufficient time for the indulgence of ſleep; and if protracted beyond eight it proves rather injurious than beneficial; though in reſpect of children a greater latitude is allowed.

The proper time for the periodical return of ſleep is pointed out by nature herſelf, when the light of the day gives place to night, and when thoſe who have laboured from the morning ſtand in need of repoſe. I would not, however, be underſtood to fix the commencement of ſleep preciſely to the approach of darkneſs, ſince in winter, unleſs for thoſe who intend to riſe early, ſuch a practice would lead to the prolongation of ſleep beyond the period which has been mentioned as the moſt ſalutary; beſides that this would interfere with the innocent gratifications of ſociety, than which nothing is more agreeable, or more beneficial to health.

To ſecure ſound ſleep, the beſt expedient is to take ſufficient exerciſe in the open air, to eat no heavy ſupper, and to lie down in bed in perfect tranquility of mind, and without the attention being fixed on any ſubject connected with abſtruſe inquiry. It ought likewiſe to be obſerved, that a perſon ſhould not go to bed till an hour and a half after ſupper.

It is a general opinion that ſleep is moſt refreſhing in the fore part of the night; but perhaps this notion aroſe originally from a preſumption, that the perſon who goes to bed at a moderate hour will of courſe riſe ſooner in the morning. It is certain, however, that the hour of going to bed ought not to be ſo late as to protract the time of waking till the morning is far advanced: for the cuſtom of early riſing is extremely conducive to health.

When the muſcles are fatigued by the labours or exerciſe of the day, and the ſenſes have for ſome time been active, we ſtand in need of the viciſſitude of reſt, particularly that of ſleep, which is as it were a periodical ſuſpenſion of our exiſtence; and the ordinance of this expedient, ſo neceſſary for the ſupport of animal life, is one of the wonders that excite our admiration in ſurveying the works of the Creator. During a ſound ſleep, the ſenſes, and the voluntary muſcular motions, are not exerciſed; but the vital functions, ſuch as reſpiration, and the circulation of the blood, as well as digeſtion, and the other natural functions, are regularly though more ſlowly performed. While we are aſleep, the motion of the heart and the blood veſſels, even the action of the brain and the nervous ſyſtem, as likewiſe the peculiar motion of the ſtomach and inteſtines, and the ſecretion of the fluids, are performed in an uniform and ſteady manner. Previous to ſleep, we perceive a languor of the ſenſes, of the muſcles which are ſubject to our will, and of thoſe alſo which keep the body in an erect poſture. The head inclines downwards, the upper eye-lid and the lower jaw-bone likewiſe ſink; the blood in the veins accumulates towards the heart, and compels us to yawn, in order to facilitate the tranſition of the blood into the lungs by the deep breathing. The brain itſelf, as the organ of the mind, appears to be fatigued: hence our ideas become irregular, and there ariſes a ſlight imbecility of the underſtanding. That the motions of the heart are ſtronger during ſleep, and that perſpiration is more abundant, muſt be aſcribed to the warmth of the bed-clothes, by which the inſenſible perſpiration ſoftens and relaxes the ſkin.

As the ſenſes are inactive during ſleep; as the nervous energy is leſs expended, and its ſecretion continued, a new ſupply of it is collected, and the organs of ſenſe, as well as the muſcles, receive additional vigour. This occaſions us to awake, particularly if rouſed by any ſtimulus. While we are aſleep, the nutritive particles of the blood can more eaſily attach themſelves to the fibres, and fat alſo is more eaſily generated, from the ſlower circulation of the blood. After we have ſlept ſufficiently, we are apt on awaking to ſtretch the limbs and joints, and ſometimes to yawn; the former of theſe to reſtore the equilibrium of the muſcles, which had been affected during ſleep; and the latter from an inſtinctive deſire of promoting the circulation of the blood through the lungs, which was retarded during ſleep. Such is the proceſs of nature in conducting the tranſition from waking to ſleep and back again, and thence reſtoring both the body and mind to the grateful viciſſitudes of ſenſe and action.

To explain one remarkable phenomenon, which frequently occurs during ſleep, namely, that of dreams, is a ſubject which has exerciſed the ingenuity of many phyſiological enquirers. Theſe ſportive fancies are evidently vagaries of the imagination, and take place only when our ſleep is unſound. We ſeldom dream during the firſt hours of ſleep; perhaps becauſe the nervous fluid is then too much exhauſted; but dreams moſtly occur towards the morning, when this fluid has been in ſome meaſure reſtored. Every thing capable of interrupting the tranquillity of the mind or body may produce dreams. Such are affections, passions, and exertions of the mind, crude and undigested food, &c. Those ideas which have lately occupied our mind, or made a lively impression upon us, generally constitute the principal subject of a dream, and more or less employ our imagination when we are asleep. Dreams are, as it were, a middle state between sleeping and waking; and when accompanied with startings, abrupt and incoherent speeches, and a frequent change of posture, they are often either the effect or the forerunner of some indisposition. In general, however, they proceed from the irritation of the stomach, or intestinal canal. Sleep without dreams, of whatever kind they be, is more healthful than when attended with these fancies. Yet dreams of an agreeable kind promote the free circulation of the blood, the digestion of the food, and a due state of perspiration.

To continue awake beyond a proper time consumes the vital spirits, hurts the nerves, and causes many uneasy sensations. The fluids of the body become more acrid or sharp, the fat is consumed, and there comes on at length a tendency to giddiness, head-ach, and anxiety. Those who indulge themselves in much sleep are seldom liable to very strong passions. Excess of sleep, however, is prejudicial. The body sinks gradually into a complete state of inactivity, the solid parts become relaxed, the blood circulates slowly, and remains particularly long in the head. Perspiration is disordered, the body increases in fat and thick humours, the memory is enfeebled, and the person falls into such a state that his sensibility is, in a great measure, destroyed.

## CHAP. VIII.

### *Of Intemperance.*

TEMPERANCE being one of the cardinal virtues, the character of its opposite must be vice; and there is no vice of a sensual nature that is not prejudicial to health. Such is the effect of intemperance, that it disorders the whole animal economy. It relaxes the nerves, greatly injures digestion, renders all the secretions irregular; and, thence, vitiating all the fluids, gives rise to various diseases.

To explain at length the effects of intemperance on the body, would comprise an account of almost every disease to which mankind is liable. It is, therefore, sufficient to observe, in general, that this odious vice is no leſs hurtful to the individual, than pernicious to the interests of ſociety and diſgraceful to human nature. What ruinous effects are the conſequence of drunkenneſs alone! and how often do we behold whole families reduced to miſery from this cauſe!

Every act of intoxication excites commotion in the blood by which nature endeavours to throw off the baneful load that oppreſſes her; and when the exceſs becomes habitual, it is eaſy to conceive what ravages it muſt neceſſarily make in the conſtitution. Fevers occaſioned by drinking do not always ſubſide in a day; but frequently terminate in inflammations, which ſoon put a period to life. If the drunkard, however, ſhould not fall by an acute diſorder, he is generally overtaken by one or other of a chronic kind, under which he may drag for ſome time a miſerable life, embittered by the thoughts of his folly, and the fatal effects it has produced. Of the ſlow diſeaſes moſt commonly induced by frequent intoxication, are obſtructions of ſome of the viſcera (bowels), dropſies, nervous atrophies, and conſumptions of the lungs; and when theſe diſeaſes are the conſequence of hard drinking, they prove, for the moſt part, equally obſtinate and fatal.

Another abuſe of liquors is a habit of ſoaking, as it is called; by which many are injured, without ever drinking to ſuch a degree as to produce intoxication. This practice, though not attended with ſuch violent effects as the former, is equally deſtructive. For the veſſels, by being conſtantly kept upon the ſtretch, ſoon looſe their elaſticity; digeſtion is impaired, and a vitiated ſtate of the humours of conſequence enſues. The uſual effects of this habit are conſumptions, ulcerous ſore legs, a diſpoſition to the gout, and frequently likewiſe the gravel. The two laſt-mentioned diſorders, as well as the dropſy, are likewiſe, in general, the portion of the epicure who indulges in exceſs; while another claſs of voluptuaries, the debauchees, or votaries to Venus, are commonly cut off by a nervous atrophy, or other conſumption.

## CHAP. IX.

### *Of Evacuations.*

EVACUATIONS, as well as ſupplies, are neceſſary for the preſervation of life and health. Without ſupplies, we ſhould die of famine; and without evacuations we ſhould periſh by a ſuperabundance of fluids become acrimonious and hurtful. The food, likewiſe, which we conſume every day, neceſſarily depoſits uſeleſs matter, which, if long retained in the bowels, would prove extremely injurious. To free the body from theſe incumbrances, nature has eſtabliſhed three principal evacuations, which are thoſe by ſtool, urine, and inſenſible perſpiration.

## *Of the Evacuation by Stool.*

A regularity and moderation in this diſcharge is of great importance to health; for, if the fæces be expelled too ſoon, they deprive the body of its nouriſhment; and if too long retained, they communicate a noxious quality to the fluids. Once in the day, if the ſtool correſpond to the quantity of the food, is the beſt ſtandard of frequency in this evacuation; but the diſcharge is variable in different perſons, and even in the ſame at different times, according to any incidental deviation from regularity in diet, exerciſe and ſleep. It is liable to be affected either by eating too much or too little; the former frequently producing a looſeneſs, and the latter the oppoſite extreme. Eating much ſalt, or muſtard, tends likewiſe to promote it, while, on the other hand, it is retarded by the uſe of hard and dry meat. Some perſons are naturally ſo conſtipated as not to go to ſtool for ſeveral days; and there occur extraordinary inſtances of the diſcharge having been withheld for ſome weeks. But theſe degrees of coſtiveneſs, though not ſenſibly injurious, muſt neceſſarily taint the fluids with a ſcorbutic acrimony, which may in time produce obſtinate complaints.

Lying late in bed is unfavourable to this diſcharge, not only by the warmth, which, increaſing perſpiration, diminiſhes all the other diſcharges; but likewiſe by the inactivity, and even the poſture of the body. Thoſe are ſeldom ſubject to coſtiveneſs who riſe early, and paſs ſome time abroad in the open air. The method recommended by Mr. Locke, for procuring regularity in this diſcharge, is founded in juſt conception—"to ſolicit nature, by going regularly to ſtool every morning, whether one has a call or not." Such a practice induces a habit which in time becomes natural.

The province of phyſic furniſhes a variety of gentle laxatives for obviating a coſtive diſpoſition; but the frequent uſe of purgatives, however mild, tends to weaken the bowels, and conſequently to vitiate digeſtion; by which effects the coſtive habit is increaſed, and with it the neceſſity of repeating the medicines, till, in the end, they become more hurtful than the original complaint. It is, therefore, more ſafe to obviate coſtiveneſs by means of diet than medicine. But this ſubject will afterwards be more particularly conſidered under the article Coſtiveneſs (Obſtipatio), which is ranked among the diſeaſes. At preſent I ſhall only obſerve, that perſons of this habit ought not to keep the body too warm, nor allow themſelves the free uſe of any thing in diet that is of a binding nature; ſuch as cruſt of bread, hard cheeſe, port, claret, &c. Thoſe, on the contrary, who have an habitual diſpoſition to looſeneſs will receive benefit from uſing a diet the counterpart of the former; for example, ſuch as eggs, cheeſe, rice-milk, rice-puddings, &c. Red wine and water, or water mixed with a little brandy, is the drink moſt ſuitable to ſuch perſons. A defect of perſpiration is frequently the cauſe of an habitual looſeneſs; on which account the wearing a flannel waiſtcoat next the ſkin is found to be of great advantage; as is, likewiſe, in particular, the keeping the feet warm; beſides every other means of ſupporting a due perſpiration. More explicit directions relative to this complaint ſhall be given in the treatment of Looſeneſs (Diarrhoea).

## *Of Urine.*

The diſcharge by urine is more frequent than that by ſtool, and is alſo more variable in quantity; on account of its being greatly influenced by the nature of the aliments, the ſtate of perſpiration, and the temperature of the air. As the urine is ſtrongly impregnated with ſalts and oils, which, if too long retained in the body, would prove the cauſe of many diſorders, the free diſcharge of it is highly conducive to health. So much regard was paid by the antients to the appearances of urine, that phyſicians predicted from them the different ſtates of health and diſeaſe; but more accurate obſervation, and a more intimate acquaintance with the animal economy, have taught that theſe appearances are extremely fallacious; and that though the urine, in conjunction with other circumſtances, may lead to the knowledge of the preſent ſtate of the body, it never can, in any degree, tend to aſcertain its future affections, in reſpect either of health or diſeaſe. Such pretenſions to knowledge, therefore, are founded only in prejudice or impoſture; and it is much to be regretted, that popular credulity ſtill continues to ſanction, by an amazing attachment, the falſe claims of thoſe who attempt to delude the public with ſo ſtale and palpable an artifice.

The quantity of the urine, as well as of the other evacuations, may be either too copious or defective. In the former caſe, it conſtitutes the diſeaſe named Diabetes, which ſhall be treated under its reſpective head; and in the latter (Iſchuria), when proceeding from a ſtoppage of ſecretion, it will fall under the Obſtruction of the Kidneys, from gravel, or ſome other cauſe. Many inſtances occur, where persons, by too long retaining their urine, from motives of false delicacy, have lost the power of discharging it. The bladder, being too much distended, has become paralytic; and every effort to cure it has proved abortive. Such dreadful examples ought to serve as a warning against ever permitting a preposterous delicacy to operate, when the consequence must be fatal.

A free discharge of urine not only prevents but actually cures many diseases, and ought, on this account, to be promoted; at the same time that every thing should be carefully avoided that tends to obstruct it. Food of a heating quality, and sleeping on beds that are too soft and warm, are in this case hurtful. When a deficiency of urine is perceived the person ought to take moderate exercise, and to eat of those herbs and fruits which naturally increase this discharge; such as parsley, asparagus, celery, strawberries, cherries, juniper-berries, and the like; using also light thin drinks, rendered gently acid by juice of lemons, or something else of that nature.

## *Of Insensible Perspiration.*

Of all the natural evacuations that of insensible perspiration is the most important; and on the proper state of this function the health of man chiefly depends. Nor ought it to be thought surprising that so great are the effects of an evacuation not perceptible to the senses, when we know that it exceeds in quantity every other discharge, and that the fluid discharged by it is of an acrimonious quality. According to the calculation of some physiologists, a person of a middle stature, and in perfect health, perspires from three to four pounds weight, according to others, about five pounds, within twenty-four hours. But it varies in different seasons, climates, and constitutions, and likewise in proportion to the casual diversities in exercise and food. In general, however, it is most copious during the night, on account of the warmth of the bed, and the greater uniformity of the surrounding atmosphere. Rheumatisms, agues, and most of the acute fevers, with various other disorders, arise from a suppressed perspiration.

Insensible perspiration is weaker after a plentiful meal, which accounts for the chillness often felt on that occasion. But as soon as the food is digested the discharge returns with increased energy; the chyle, then changed into blood, imparting additional force to the vital powers, as well as to the circulation of the blood itself. According to the experiments made by different inquirers into the nature of insensible perspiration, this process is most forcibly affected, and sometimes totally suppressed, by the following circumstances; 1. By violent pain, which in a remarkable degree consumes the fluids of the body, or propels them to other parts. 2. By obstructions of the vessels of the skin, which are frequently occasioned by the use of salves, ointments, and cosmetics. One of the most celebrated beauties of the present age lost her life by this practice. 3. By severe colds, especially those contracted at night, and during sleep. 4. When nature is either weak, or endeavours to promote any other species of evacuation; or, as was before observed, during the time of concoction, particularly after using food that is difficult to be digested.

Perspiration, on the contrary, is promoted by moderate exercise, the warm bath, and mild sudorific medicines; to which may be added cleanliness, and the exhilarating passions, hope and joy.

Too plentiful a perspiration indicates great weakness of the body, or a laxity of the vessels of the skin, which may frequently be removed by cold bathing or washing.

In this country, one of the most frequent causes of obstructed perspiration is the variable state of the atmosphere, producing sudden changes of the weather; to counteract the influence of which, and fortify the body against them, nothing is so efficacious as being abroad every day; for the habit of keeping much within doors renders a person extremely susceptible of cold on going into the open air.

The perspiration, even in summer, is often obstructed by night air; and this is more hurtful when accompanied by dews, which fall most plentifully after the hottest day. People, therefore, even in this climate, those especially who have been much heated by day, ought to avoid as much as possible being abroad in the night. In marshy countries, where, on account of the great daily exhalations, the dews are more copious, labourers are often seized with agues, quinseys, and other dangerous diseases, from an imprudent neglect of this caution.

Perspiration is liable to be greatly obstructed by wet clothes, which are prejudicial not only by their coldness, but by the moisture absorbed from them into the body. Fevers, rheumatisms, and a multiplicity of diseases, derive their source from this cause. The bad consequences of getting wet might generally be prevented by changing the clothes soon, or at least by keeping in motion till they are dry; but so regardless are many of this precaution, that they often sit or lie down in the fields with their clothes wet, and frequently sleep even whole nights in this condition; an act of imprudence liable to produce the most fatal effects.

Wet feet, by stopping the perspiration, are likewise often the cause of diseases, particularly colics, inflammation of the bowels, &c. Nothing sooner induces a fit of the gout in people subject to that complaint. The best preservative against the danger of wet feet is to wear thick shoes in walking over damp grounds, and to avoid the morning dews.

Damp houses have a strong tendency to suppress perspiration, especially in those who live in sunk stories, which ought never to be in any house not built in a dry situation. The same bad effect is produced by inhabiting a house too soon after the walls have been plastered or painted. To dampness, in this case, is added the noxious smell of the materials used in painting, the unwholesomeness of which is evident from the frequency of consumptions of the lungs among the people who work in those articles.

Damp beds have generally been considered as a fruitful source of diseases; and that the opinion is founded in more than prejudice would seem to be confirmed by experience. Fevers, consumptions, rheumatisms, and other disorders, have been confidently imputed to this cause. A physician of great eminence,* however, maintains the opposite opinion; but, in a disputed point of this nature, it is difficult to ascertain the fact, as the great danger supposed to result from damp sheets must deter all who have a regard for health from submitting to make a personal experiment on the subject. It is certain that opinions long held sacred have, in the end, been found to be vulgar errors: nor is it less certain, that, in particular constitutions, and perhaps in many in particular circumstances, a powerful cause of disease may exist without producing any effect. The contagion of the plague itself is resisted by many constitutions. If we examine the question respecting damp sheets by the balance of impartial judgment, the authority in one scale is great and venerable; but the united weight of general prescriptive opinion and analogy would seem to preponderate in the other.

Nothing more frequently obstructs perspiration than sudden transitions from heat to cold. The bad effects of this practice are generally known, but the prevention of them too much neglected. Heat, by expanding the blood, and rendering its motion more quick, increases perspiration, which being suddenly checked is apt to produce dangerous consequences. To sit in a warm room, and drink hot liquors till the pores become open, and immediately go into the cold air, is an act of imprudence by which thousands have forfeited their lives. The same bad effects are apt to ensue, when people, to relieve themselves from the inconveniences of a hot room, throw open a window and sit near it: for, the current of air being thus directed against one particular part of the body, there is much greater danger of catching cold in such a situation than in sitting

* Dr. Heberden.

without doors; and the caſe will prove ſtill more hazardous if the people ſo placed be thinly clothed. Similar to this, in effects, is the practice of ſleeping with open windows too near the bed, even in the hotteſt ſeaſon.

The foregoing obſervations relative to air are applicable likewiſe to drinking too freely of cold water, or ſmall liquors, when a perſon is hot. In ſuch a caſe a mouthful of brandy, or other ſpirits, where it can be procured, is preferable to any thing elſe; but ſhould water be the only thing at hand, thirſt may be quenched without drinking a large quantity of it. Water kept in the mouth for a little time, and ſpit out again, if frequently repeated, has a powerful effect in abating thirſt; and if a bit of bread be eaten with a few mouthfuls of water, the expedient is ſtill more ſucceſsful: but if, regardleſs of bad conſequences, a man has imprudently when hot drunk freely of cold liquor, he ought to continue his exerciſe till what he drank be thoroughly warmed upon his ſtomach, and thereby prevent the hurtful effects of the chillneſs which would otherwiſe enſue.

So numerous are the inſtances of fatal effects produced by drinking cold liquors when the body is hot, that people ought to avoid that indulgence with the utmoſt precaution. The uſual conſequences of acting otherwiſe are hoarſeneſs, quinſeys, and fevers of various kinds; but, in ſome inſtances, immediate death has enſued. Though to eat freely of raw fruits, or ſalads, when a perſon is hot, be not ſo dangerous as the error committed in cold liquors, it is by no means void of danger, and ſhould therefore be guarded againſt.

## *Of the Saliva.*

The ſaliva is a fluid ſeparated in the glands of the mouth, for the purpoſe of mixing with the food in the act of maſtication or chewing, and is entirely different from the mucus, or ſlime, collected in conſequence of cold. The ſaliva being of great importance in preparing the food for the ſtomach, it ought not to be unneceſſarily waſted by frequent ſpitting: the cuſtom of ſmoking tobacco, therefore, is in many caſes prejudicial, as by depriving the body of this uſeful fluid it greatly weakens digeſtion. Frequent ſmoking makes the teeth yellow and black; white clay pipes are apt to canker the enamel to ſuch a degree as to infect the breath, and produce putrid ulcers in the gums. To perſons of a middle age, or thoſe of full growth, particularly the corpulent, the phlegmatic, and ſuch as are ſubject to defluxions of the head and throat, it may occaſionally be of ſervice, if uſed with moderation, eſpecially in damp, cold, and hazy weather. Such perſons, however, ought never to ſmoke immediately before or after a meal, as the saliva is essentially requisite to assist the digestion of the food. They ought to smoke slowly; frequently take small draughts of beer, ale, tea, or other diluting liquors, but neither spirits nor wine. Lastly, they ought to use a clean pipe with a long tube; for the oil of tobacco, settling on the sides of the pipe, is one of the most acrimonious and hurtful substances, and may thus be absorbed, and mixed with the fluids of the body.

### *Of the Mucus of the Nose.*

This humour is intended by nature to protect the olfactory nerves, or those nerves which are destined for smelling: hence every artificial method of increasing that discharge is hurtful, unless required by some particular indisposition of the body. By the discharge now mentioned, I do not mean the slime that is secreted in colds of the head, and is rejected as useless. The effect of snuff is to stimulate the mucous membrane of the nose, and sympathetically the whole body. If used as a medicine only, and on occasions which require such a stimulus, it may be productive of some advantage; but a liquid for this purpose is preferable to a powder, which, in the end, always obstructs the nostrils.

In several disorders of the head, eyes, and ears, the taking of snuff may occasionally supply the place of an artificial issue; though an immoderate use of it is liable to be followed with a contrary effect, viz. bleeding of the nose, and other complaints. Snuff-taking would be particularly injurious to persons of a consumptive disposition, or those who are afflicted with internal ulcers, and subject to a spitting of blood; as, by the violent sneezing it at first occasions, they might be exposed to imminent danger.

## CHAP. X.

### *Of Cleanliness.*

CLEANLINESS is not only a moral virtue, but has an extensive influence on the preservation of health: the neglect of it is indeed so hurtful, that to that cause is owing a variety of diseases, and some of the most dangerous kind. Putrid fevers frequently have their origin in this source; and of cutaneous diseases, or those of the skin, it is of every cause the most prevalent. Uninterrupted perspiration is indispensible for the security of health;

but it cannot long be maintained without an uniform attention to cleanlineſs. Thoſe parts of our apparel which are in contact with the ſkin muſt neceſſarily be impregnated, in a ſhort time, with the vapours which continually exhale through the channels of perſpiration; and when not frequently changed they prove extremely hurtful, both by obſtructing that diſcharge, and by acting in effect as a putrid fomentation to the body.

But the conſequences that reſult from want of cleanlineſs are not confined to the individual. From this baneful origin a whole community may be infected, and in a manner ſo violent and pernicious as often to prove fatal. On this account, cleanlineſs becomes an object of public attention: yet ſorry am I to ſay, that inſtead of being enforced in great towns by thoſe who have the charge of the police, violations of it, even in the ſtreets, are tolerated to a degree that merits the ſevereſt reprehenſion Beſides the nuiſance from ſlaughter-houſes, frequently in the very centre of great towns, how often do we behold dung-hills, dead animals putrefying, and naſtineſs of every kind! In fact the importance of general cleanlineſs, towards the preſervation of health, ſeems not to be ſufficiently underſtood by the magiſtrates of moſt great towns in this country; and while we pretend to civilization, politeneſs, and delicacy, we tolerate ſuch abuſes as place us almoſt upon a level with the Hottentots themſelves.

Perſonal cleanlineſs is not only an amiable virtue, but a ſource of comfort to the individual. For example, after waſhing our feet we feel ourſelves conſiderably refreſhed; and this ſenſation would be ſtill more perceptible, if the wholeſome cuſtom where introduced of frequently waſhing the whole body. In this point of cleanlineſs we are certainly far too deficient. Bathing or waſhing in cold water would not only clear the ſkin from impurities, but greatly ſtrengthen the body. Thoſe who have an averſion to cold water, or for whom the uſe of it would be unſafe, might waſh themſelves in tepid or lukewarm water, by which they might reap the benefit of purification without any injury to their health.

Bathing, whether in tepid or cold water, produces the moſt ſalutary effect on the abſorbent veſſels (thoſe which take up any fluid from the ſkin, and carry it into the body). Theſe would otherwiſe carry back the impurities of the ſkin through the pores, to the no ſmall injury of the health. To perſons in a perfect ſtate of vigour, the frequent uſe of the bath is leſs neceſſary than to the infirm; as the former poſſeſs a greater power to reſiſt impurities, by means of more abundant perſpiration. But in the infirm, the ſlowneſs of circulation, the clammineſs of the fluids, with the conſtant efforts of nature to propel the impurities towards the skin, render the frequent washing of their bodies of essential importance to their health.

The tepid or luke-warm bath, commonly called the *warm* bath, which is about the same temperature with the blood, between 96 and 98 degrees of Fahrenheit's thermometer, has usually been considered as apt to weaken the body; but this is an ill-founded notion. It is only when its heat exceeds that of the human body that the warm bath produces any debilitating effect. The tepid bath from 85 to 96 degrees is always safe; and is so far from relaxing the solids, that in fact it powerfully strengthens them. Instead of heating the body, it has a cooling effect. It diminishes the quickness of the pulse, and reduces it in a greater proportion, corresponding to its former quickness, and the time the bath is continued. Hence tepid baths are of great service where a person has been overheated, from whatever cause, whether after fatigue from travelling, severe exercise, or after violent exertion and perturbation of mind; as they allay the tempestuous and irregular movements thence produced, and consequently, in the strictest sense, give new vigour to the constitution. By their softening and moistening power they greatly contribute to the formation and growth of young persons, and are of singular benefit to those in whom is perceived a tendency to arrive too early at the consistence of a settled age; so that the warm bath is particularly adapted to prolong the state of youth, and retard in proportion the approach of full manhood.

The tepid bath, as well as the cold, considerably increases the pressure on the body from without; hence breathing, particularly on entering the bath, is frequently somewhat difficult, till the muscles have by practice been inured to a greater degree of resistance. Yet this effect, which in most instances is of little importance, requires the greatest caution in some particular cases, so far as to prevent the use of the bath altogether. This happens in persons of a full habit, who are in danger of bursting some of the internal blood-vessels by the precipitate use of the bath, whether warm or cold.

Bathing in rivers, as well as in the sea, is effectual for every purpose of clearing the body. It washes away impurities from the surface, opens the cutaneous vessels for a due perspiration, and increases the circulation of the blood. The apprehension of bad consequences from the coldness of the water is entirely chimerical: for, besides that it produces a strengthening effect, the cold sensation is not of itself hurtful. Precaution, however, is requisite in the use of the cold as well as in that of the tepid bath. Going into it when the body is over-heated might prove instantly fatal, by inducing an apoplexy. The plethoric, or those of a full habit of body, the aſthmatic, and all thoſe who perceive a great determination of the blood to the head, ought to be very circumſpect in the uſe of it. For, though the conſequence may not prove immediately fatal, yet, from the ſudden force and preſſure of the water, ſome of the ſmaller blood-veſſels of the head and breaſt may eaſily burſt, and thereby lay the foundation of an incurable diſorder.

The ſenſible properties of the cold bath, in general, conſiſt in its power of contracting the ſolid parts, and rendering the fluids more thick. Any part of the body which is expoſed to the ſudden contact of cold water experiences at the ſame inſtant a degree of tenſion and contraction, and becomes narrower and ſmaller. Hence it happens, that by the cold bath all the blood-veſſels of the ſkin, and of the muſcles in immediate contact with it, are ſo conſtricted, that, at the time of this violent exertion, they are unable to receive the uſual quantity of blood. The ſmaller veſſels of the ſkin are likewiſe cloſed, and preſs upon the humours contained in them, ſo as to prevent all perſpiration during this preſſure. Thus all the fibres of the ſkin and muſcles are brought into cloſe contact; and if the humours contained in theſe tubes had no other outlets, by which to diſcharge themſelves, they would become thick, and loſe their natural warmth. Were this to take place, it would be attended with dangerous ſtagnations and obſtructions. That it does not, however, produce theſe fatal effects, may be aſcribed to the following cauſe: as ſoon as the preſſure is made againſt the external veſſels, the blood retreats from them into places where it finds leſs reſiſtance. All the great veſſels within the body afford receptacles into which it now flows, till, the principal arteries and the veins of the inteſtines being entirely filled, it riſes to the heart. Though the effect conſequent on the cold bath may be conſidered as purely mechanical, yet this ſimple operation is frequently productive of the moſt important and beneficial effects.

The ſudden changes ariſing from the application of the cold bath contribute in various ways to brace the human body. The relaxed fibres of the ſkin and the muſcles acquire more ſolidity and compactneſs from contraction. Their elaſticity is increaſed, and thus a conſiderable defect removed. The nerves are ſtimulated and excited to thoſe powerful exertions, on which the vigour of the body ſo much depends. The blood, which by external preſſure is driven into the internal veſſels, extends and enlarges them, without diminiſhing that contractile force or tendency which is peculiar to every artery. At the moment when the external preſſure ceaſes, all the internal veſſels exert their inherent power of contracting more forcibly than uſual, as they are more ſtrongly extended, and consequently enabled to exercise a greater force. The blood, returned to the cutaneous and muscular vessels, finds its reservoirs contracted and invigorated; and it flows through muscles the fibres of which have acquired greater elasticity and power of resistance. It is now accelerated in its motion by these improved fibres and veins, and the result of the collective powers is a fresh impulse and rapidity given to its circulation.

It has already been observed, that to go into the cold bath when a person is overheated is dangerous; but the popular opinion that it is hest to enter the water perfectly cool is a mistaken notion; and when put into practice it will render the use of the bath ineffectual. To use the bath without any danger, and, on the contrary, with great advantage, is to dip into the water when the heat of the body has been a little increased by exercise. In this way only is the plunge productive of a shock, without which not the smallest benefit arises from cold bathing. As a corroborant, or strengthener, however, the cold bath, when properly used, is found of incomparable efficacy. All other strenthening remedies, operating in generally only on the fluid parts of the body, require to be previously dissolved, and undergo we know not what changes, before they be conducted with the mass of blood to the solid parts. The cold bath, on the contrary, acts almost instantaneously on the solid parts themselves, and produces its bracing effect, without the necessary intervention of any other precarious aid.

The external use of cold water is of a singular benefit, when applied to particular parts of the body, where its use may be much longer continued without danger, and where we may, in a manner, by compulsion and perseverance, accomplish the intended effects. Of all the parts of the body the head receives most benefit from the affusion of cold water. This is a simple and effectual remedy against too great an impulse of the blood towards the head, where persons are threatened with an apoplexy; in disorders likewise of the brain and skull; as well as in wounds and other complaints to which the head is subject. In these instances, its efficacy may be improved by the addition of common or any other cooling salt.

In cases where the cold bath may be of service, it should be used according to the following directions: Every cold bath applied to the whole body ought to be of short duration; for its efficacy depends upon the sudden impression of the cold upon the skin and nerves. The head should be always first wetted by immersion, by pouring water upon it, or the application of wet cloths, and when plunging over head into the bath. The immersion ought always to be sudden, not only because it is less felt than when we enter the bath slowly and timorously, but likewise because the effect of the first impression is uniform all over the body, and the blood in this manner is not propelled from the lower to the upper parts. Hence the ſhower bath poſſeſſes great advantages, as it pours the water ſuddenly upon the whole body, and thus perfectly fulfils the three rules above ſpecified. Gentle exerciſe, as was before obſerved, ought to precede the cold bath; for neither complete reſt nor violent exerciſe is proper previous to the uſe of this remedy. The morning or forenoon is the moſt proper time for cold bathing; either when the ſtomach is empty, or two hours after a light breakfaſt. While in the water the perſon ought to move about, in order to promote the circulation of the blood from the inward parts of the body to the extremities. After immerſion the whole body ought to be rubbed dry as quickly as poſſible, with a dry and ſomewhat rough cloth. Moderate exerciſe out of doors, if convenient, is adviſeable, and indeed neceſſary.

It may here be proper briefly to enumetate certain caſes in which the cold bath muſt not be uſed: theſe are in a general plethora, or full habit of body; in hæmorrhages, or fluxes of blood, and in every kind of inflammation; in conſtipations, or obſtructions of the inteſtines; in diſeaſes of the breaſt, difficult breathing, and ſhort and dry coughs; in an acrimonious or ſharp taſte of the fluids, bad colour of the face, difficult healing of the fleſh, and the ſcurvy, properly ſo called; in fits of the gout; in cutaneous diſeaſes, or thoſe of the ſkin; in a ſtate of pregnancy.

The beſt mode of cold bathing is in the ſea; but when this cannot be procured, in a river, or ſpring water. Should bathing in the houſe be preferred, the moſt eligible method is by the *ſhower bath*, a proper apparatus for which is to be had at the tin-ſhops. Where the ſaving of expence is an object, it may be effectually ſupplied by the following eaſy expedient: fill a common watering-pot with cold water, let the patient ſit down undreſſed upon a ſtool, which may be placed in a large tub; and let the hair, if not cut ſhort, be ſpread over the ſhoulders as looſely as poſſible; then pour the water from the pot over the patients head, face, neck, ſhoulders, and all parts of the body progreſſively down to the feet, till the whole has been thoroughly bathed; let him then be rubbed dry, and take gentle exerciſe, as has been already recommended, till the ſenſatiou of cold be ſucceeded by a moderate glow all over him. On firſt reſorting to this kind of bath it may be uſed gently, and with water in a ſmall degree warm, ſo as not to make the ſhock too great; but, as the patient becomes accuſtomed to it, the degree of cold may be increaſed, the water may be allowed to fall from a greater height, and the holes in the pot may be made larger, to render the ſhower more heavy. A large ſponge may, in ſome meaſure, be ſubſtituted for a watering pot.

Though the ſhower bath does not cover the ſurface of the body ſo univerſally as the cold baths, this circumſtance is rather favourable than otherwiſe; for thoſe parts which the water has not touched feel the impreſſion by ſympathy, as much as thoſe in actual contact with it. This bath, for the following reaſons, poſſeſſes advantages ſuperior to all others: the ſudden contact of the water, which in the common bath is only momentary, may here be prolonged, repeated, and modified at pleaſure. The head and breaſt, which are expoſed to ſome inconvenience and danger in the common bath, are here effectually ſecured, by receiving the firſt ſhock of the water: the blood is conſequently impelled to the lower parts of the body, and the patient feels no obſtruction in breathing, nor any tendency of the blood towards the head. The heavy preſſure on the body occaſioned by the weight of the water, and the free circulation of the blood in the parts touched by it, being for ſome time at leaſt interrupted, make the uſual manner of bathing often more detrimental than uſeful. The ſhower bath, on the contrary, deſcends in ſingle drops, which are at once more ſtimulating and pleaſant than the immerſion into cold water, and it can be more readily procured, and more eaſily modified and adapted to the circumſtances of the patient.

I have been led into this digreſſion on the cold bath, in conſideration of the utility of waſhing the body for the purpoſe of cleanlineſs; and indeed cleanlineſs is ſo conducive to health, ſo amiable in itſelf, as well as ſo productive of comfort, and ſo inſeparable from decency, that too much cannot be ſaid in recommendation of it; nor can its oppoſite, the abominable vice of naſtineſs, be ſtigmatiſed with ſufficient ſeverity.

## CHAP. XI.

### *Of Clothing.*

CLOTHING, though not abſolutely neceſſary for the preſervation of health in extremely hot and dry climates, is indiſpenſible in thoſe where the temperature of the air is remarkably different; and it ought to be progreſſively varied in thickneſs and warmth, from the equator to the poles. A dreſs, therefore, which is ſufficiently well adapted to ſummer, in northern latitudes, is by no means calculated to withſtand the inclemency of winter, nor even the ſudden incidental changes in the atmoſphere which occur at all ſeaſons, in countries where the weather is naturally variable. To this circumſtance we may juſtly aſcribe the greater part of the diseases which prevail in Great-Britain. To adapt the dress with a scrupulous nicety to the fluctuations of temperature every day, would indeed require such minute attention as hardly any person can bestow; but every person may comply with the general rules of clothing, as far as not to lay aside too early the dress of the winter, nor to retain that of the summer too late; from a neglect of which precaution thousands of lives are every year sacrificed to mortality. The perfection of dress, considered merely as such, is to fit without fettering the body.

One of the chief considerations respecting dress is, What ought to be worn next the skin? as the several articles so employed affect the perspiration very differently. In most parts of Europe linen is commonly used for this purpose: by diminishing the elasticity of the skin it increases the internal warmth; while, from its compactness, it is more apt than wool to retain the matter perspired. Shirts, therefore, when wore longer than a day or two, are not only liable to excite a sensation of coolness, but to obstruct perspiration, which effect linen produces in proportion to the thickness of its texture. Silk attracts less humidity from the atmosphere than linen; but, though it occasions a gentle stimulus, it is not very favourable to perspiration. Wool, on account of the gentle friction it occasions on the skin, produces a moderate warmth, and promotes perspiration; at the same time that, on account of the porous nature of its substance, the matter which it absorbs from the skin is easily evaporated. Cotton is an intermediate substance between linen and wool: it increases warmth and perspiration; but, having the quality of retaining the perspired humours, it affords opportunity for their being taken again into the blood, and by that means tainting the fluids.

From the above concise view of the different substances worn next the skin, it would appear that wool has greatly the advantage over the others. Flannel, by its gentle stimulus on the skin, has the beneficial effect of keeping the pores in a state the most favourable to perspiration. In flannel, the discharge by perspiration proceeds uniformly; but not so in linen, when soiled with the moisture of the skin. The different effects of flannel and linen are particularly perceptible during brisk exercise. When the body is covered with the former, though perspiration be necessarily increased, the perspired matter passes off through flannel into the atmosphere or air, and the skin remains dry and warm. If the same exercise be taken in linen shirts, perspiration, as in the former case, is indeed also increased, but the perspired matter, instead of being dispersed into the atmosphere, remains upon the linen, and not only clogs the pores, but gives a very disagreeable sensation.

Flannel has another advantage which merits attention. As it does not retain the humours discharged from the skin, people who perspire profusely in flannel shirts will not easily catch cold on going into the open air. But the same is not the case in respect of linen shirts, which, by retaining the perspired matter, will occasion a sensation of chillness, often followed by a violent cold, and sometimes even fatal effects.

The prejudices of people have been much excited, both in favour of flannel and against it. It has been objected, that flannel worn next the skin occasions weakness, by too much increasing perspiration: but this objection seems not to be founded in truth, since perspiration scarcely ever can be immoderate or hurtful, as long as the skin remains dry.

Flannel when first used, is apt to cause an uneasy sensation, but this soon goes off. In those who wear flannel, the skin, on being much rubbed, will become red and inflamed; but we ought not, on that account, to infer that flannel produces cutaneous eruption; on the contrary, by preserving the pores open, and increasing perspiration, it tends greatly to remove the cause of cutaneous eruptions, which arise chiefly from an irregular state of that discharge through the pores of the skin.

The prejudice against the use of flannel next the skin seems to be owing, in great measure, to the effects which ensue from not changing it sufficiently often; but this objection is to be imputed to the wearer, not to the flannel itself.

It must be acknowledged, that the advantages above mentioned strongly recommend the use of flannel as a preservative of health, particularly to those who are exposed to all kinds of weather. It has the additional advantage of being suitable to all seasons, and of compensating a deficiency of upper dress. Extraordinary beneficial effects have been experienced from flannel in a variety of cases. In gouty, and particularly, rheumatic habits, it has operated with singular advantage. In obstinate coughs, where symptoms of consumption were apparent, it has proved highly serviceable; and, upon the whole, it merits, both as a preventive and remedy of various diseases, a more general and extensive application than it has ever yet obtained.

Cotton stockings, though not generally worn, are far from conducing to the preservation of health. For, when once filled with perspirable matter, they do not admit any more to pass through them; but there accumulates a glutinous substance which obstructs the pores of the skin. Silk stockings, likewise, unless worsted be worn under them, retard perspiration. The same may be said of thread stockings. In fact, no kind of stockings is equal to woollen, in regard to ſupporting perſpiration; but taſte and faſhion cannot readily adopt what common uſe has depreciated.

Whatever be the form of clothes, all tight bandages ſhould be avoided, as they retard the circulation, and are likewiſe injurious to the muſcles of the parts to which they are applied.

In reſpect of clothing, it is a matter of no ſmall importance to keep the feet warm; without which the blood accumulates towards the head, and there is a ſenſation of coldneſs over the whole body extremely prejudicial to perſpiration.

The general voice of antiquity is in favour of the precept that the head ſhould be lightly covered; and, indeed, the covering which nature has given, ſeems alone ſufficient for its protection, except where the hair is extremely thin, or the head bald. By going uncovered in the open air, if dry, the head is ſtrengthened; but, to render the practice perfectly ſafe, it ſhould be begun at an early age. At no age, however, ought a perſon to go uncovered in ſunſhine, when the weather is hot, as the conſequence may be an inflammation, or ſome other affection of the brain. Againſt ſuch accidents black hats afford little defence; for, inſtead of reflecting the heat, they admit the ſolar rays to act more ſtrongly upon the head. For people who are much in the open air, hats of a white or any other colour would be preferable.

Having ſaid thus much of the quality of clothes, we muſt leave the quantity to the determination of individuals, as being a point which can be ſettled only by perſonal experience. But it may be proper to impreſs the caution, that all ſudden changes ought to be carefully avoided; and that no perſon ſhould either anticipate the ſummer dreſs too early, or poſtpone that of the winter to too late a period; both theſe errors being productive of the moſt pernicious effects.

## CHAP. XII.

### *Of the Means of attaining Long Life.*

THE deſire of long life may be regarded as an affection natural to the human mind, and is connected with the ſtrongeſt and moſt univerſal principle in the animal kingdom, that of ſelf-preſervation. Whether long life be an object really deſirable in itſelf, may admit of ſome doubt, as extreme old age is liable to many infirmities: but, confidered in a moral point of view, we muft acknowledge it to be an object of great importance. It carries man forward to a period when the tumultuous paffions have fubfided, and all temptations to irregular gratification have loft their influence on the heart: by which means it not only weans the affections of the foul from this tranfitory world, but affords opportunity of preparing it for the attainment of eternal happinefs in that which is to come. Thefe certainly are fuch effects as may juftly recommend longevity to particular attention, and ought to excite a degree of folicitude concerning the means to obtain it.

If we inquire into the habits of thofe who have lived to the greateft extent, we do not find, fo far as our information reaches, that they paid any particular regard to their method of living: fome of them have even been addicted to propenfities which have, in general, a tendency to fhorten the duration of life. But we can infer from this nothing more than that thofe perfons have had good conftitutions; and there is reafon to think, that, had they lived more conformably to the rules of temperance, they might have protracted life to a ftill greater extent.

Were we to draw up a fyftem of rules for the prolongation of life, they would be founded in a ftrict attention to the obfervations contained in the preceding chapters; but we know that thefe rules, however falutary, are not always practicable.

In the firft place, it may be laid down as a principle, that to be a candidate for long life, one ought to be defcended of healthy parents, and poffefs the rudiments of a good conftitution by inheritance. To this muft be added good nurfing; for the right management of infancy is of great importance in the fubfequent ftages of life.

To live in a pure and wholefome air is another effential circumftance towards procuring longevity. There are, in moft countries, particular fituations celebrated for the falubrious quality of the air; but, in general, it may be healthful in places where the ground is not wet and fwampy, where there are no ftagnant waters, and where the dwelling is perfectly dry. If the fituation be elevated, or fuch as has a free ventilation by the winds, it is an additional advantage; and, if near the fea, ftill more healthful. In fuch fituations, it is common for many to live to a great age, who enjoy no other benefits conducive to longevity.

Much depends on wholefome diet for the prefervation of health, and confequently for the attainment of long life. It is, however, not neceffary to obferve great ftrictnefs in this article. A mixture of animal and vegetable food is the moft proper; but there are many inftances of people living to a great age, who confine themfelves to the latter. But a diet entirely of vegetables does not agree with every constitution, especially the weak and delicate; and those who use it are generally incapable of bearing great exertion, or violent exercise.

Temperance in eating and drinking is doubtless advantageous to the prolongation of life: I do not mean a scrupulous exactness in point of quantity, but a general mediocrity in both, and an abstinence from habitual excess. Voluptuousness, however, and luxury are extremely prejudicial.

There is another kind of temperance of the utmost importance in determining the limits of human life; namely, that which relates to the commerce of the sexes. Nothing seems adequate to secure the prospect of longevity, where there is a too early and immoderate propensity to this baneful indulgence. In the state of wedlock, the passion may be sustained without injury to a constitution not previously enfeebled; but in illicit connections it operates to general ruin of health and morality.

Daily exercise, or labour not immoderate, is highly conducive towards the lengthening of life; for, besides their immediate effects on the body, they tend to secure sleep in the night, which is also an essential requisite for the preservation of health. Early rising is a habit generally found amongst those who have attained to a great age. It lays in a fresh stock of health for the consumption of the day; on the transactions of which it appears likewise to have a salutary influence.

To these observations which relate to the body, I have only to add, that the constitution best disposed to longevity is that in which the passions are moderate, and where life is spent in the enjoyment of tranquillity of mind.

Many are the nostrums and arcanums which extravagance or imposture has fabricated, and superstition implicitly received, for the prolongation of life; but it is a privilege which cannot be purchased, though indeed it is too often and profusely bartered for pernicious enjoyments.

From the extraordinary age to which many have attained, it is evident that the human constitution is susceptible of long existence; and where its strength is not exhausted by hard labour, there is reason to believe, that, by a proper government of the appetites and passions, it might frequently be extended to a period even beyond any instance recorded in natural history.

In cold climates men in general become older than in warm; because vital consumption is increased in the latter, and restrained in the former. This, however, is the case only in a certain degree. By the highest cold, such as that of Greenland, Nova Zembla, &c. the duration of life is shortened

Uniformity in the ſtate of the atmoſphere, particularly in regard to heat, cold, gravity, and lightneſs, contributes in a very conſiderable degree to the duration of life. Countries, therefore, where ſudden and great variations in the barometer and thermometer are uſual cannot be favourable to longevity.

Upon the whole, it appears, that moderation in every thing, the *aurea mediocritas*, ſo deſervedly extolled, is the means of greateſt efficacy in prolonging life; which leads to the concluſion, that longevity is intimately connected with habits of virtue; and ſeems, as it were, an emblem of that immortality which moral perfection ſhall obtain.

The true preſcription for procuring length of days is to be careful of health, but without being too anxious; and in every viciſſitude of life, to endeavour, as much as poſſible, to preſerve tranquillity of mind.

---

END OF THE PRELIMINARY MATTER.

---

# BOOK II.

## *OF CHILDREN:*

### *THEIR MANAGEMENT AND DISEASES.*

## CHAP. I.

### *Of the Treatment of Infants.*

THE conſtitution of children, as depending much on that of the parents, is often hereditary; and perhaps incapable, in moſt caſes, of being altered for the better, by any kind of treatment after birth. There are happily, however, many inſtances which contradict this general remark: and it is found, by repeated obſervation, that the offspring of weakly if not even diſeaſed parents are ſometimes conducted through childhood in ſo healthy a ſtate, as not only to enjoy the ſame bleſſing in the ſubſequent periods of life, but to acquire a habit of body both hardy and vigorous. If ſuch be the caſe under the circumſtances now mentioned, how much more ought the children of healthy parents to enjoy the happineſs which nature has intailed on their deſcent? But that in general they do not, is a truth unfortunately evinced by the moſt undeniable evidence. It appears from the annual regiſters, that nearly one-half of the children born in Great-Britain die under twelve years of age. Impartial reaſon will not juſtify the ſuppoſition that ſo great a mortality can be owing either to the climate of the country, which is in general temperate and ſalubrious, or to all the uſual diſeaſes of childhood; eſpecially conſidering that one of the moſt fatal of theſe has been for many years reſtrained in its ravages by the practice of inoculation. We muſt ſeek for the ſource of this lamentable evil in other cauſes; and whoever takes a view of the nurſery will find them there in abundance. Let us firſt direct our attention to the clothing of children.

## *Of the Clothing of Children.*

It is certainly conformable both to nature and common ſenſe, that the clothing of infants ſhould be, as much as poſſible, eaſy, and free from all preſſure or incumbrance. Nothing more is requiſite than to keep the child ſufficiently guarded againſt the inclemency of the air; but nurſes, not content with the ſimple expedients required for this purpoſe, exert all their induſtry in ſo fettering the tender body entruſted to their care, that, through their miſtaken prejudices, they often render it, in a very ſhort time, not only weak and ſickly, but, perhaps, likewiſe deformed. The abſurd practice of rolling children in a load of bandages is now in a great meaſure diſuſed; but the pernicious principle ſtill continues of moleſting them with a preſſure, undoubtedly painful to the ſenſibility of their delicate feelings, and certainly injurious, in an extreme degree, to their health. Many inſtances might be mentioned of children dying of convulſions ſoon after birth, in conſequence of the tightneſs of their clothing. Nor is ſuch an effect to be wondered at, when we conſider how much the circulation of the blood muſt be obſtructed in the tender bodies of infauts, either by a general or partial preſſure from without. In the former caſe, the whole frame is affected with oppreſſion; in the latter, a complaint may be engendered which nothing can afterwards remove. The cheſt and belly are the parts that ſuffer particularly from ſuch treatment; and in theſe are contained the bowels, moſt eſſential to health, as well as to life itſelf. But even ſuppoſing that the practice ſhould be confined to the limbs, the bones of an infant are ſo ſoft and flexible, that they readily yield to the ſlighteſt preſſure, and are eaſily diſtorted. On every account, therefore, the practice of tight ſwaddling is highly pernicious, and ought to be univerſally exploded.

But it is not the tightneſs only of clothes that is prejudicial to children; they are likewiſe overloaded with quantity, which, by encumbering and too much heating their tender bodies, increaſes a feveriſh diſpoſition that commences at their birth, and continues for ſome time after. Nor is this the only way in which the ſame effect is produced. From the natural affection of the parent, the child is commonly laid in bed with the mother, who is herſelf often feveriſh. To this may be added the unwholeſome heat of the bed-chamber, the fumes of hot-candle, and the effects of wine, which is often imprudently given to infants, even ſoon after birth. From all theſe cauſes combined, it is not ſurpriſing if, at this period, there ſhould be laid the foundation of complaints which will affect the conſtitution during life.

Eaſe and warmth are the only objects which require the attention of thoſe who have the management of children; but they have hitherto been generally ſacrificed to the dictates of prepoſterous vanity and fantaſtic caprice. It may be affirmed, with great probability, that more children have been deſtroyed by the baneful uſe of ſtays, than ever, in ancient times, were paſſed through the fire unto Moloch.

But whatever be the faſhion in which children are clothed, cleanlineſs of their garments is an indiſpenſable object. Children, from the moiſture of their bodies, and the openneſs of the pores, perſpire, comparitively, more than perſons in the prime of their age; and unleſs their clothes be frequently changed, they muſt ſoon become foul and hurtful; not only by fretting the ſkin, and occaſioning noxious ſmells, but by producing vermin, and cutaneous diſeaſes, ariſing from impurity.

There is another operation practiſed by nurſes which deſerves ſevere reprehenſion, that is, forcing out the milk from the breaſts of the new born infant. Some children, a day or two after birth, have the breaſts much enlarged, hard, and painful, containing ſomething like milk; and nurſes are extremely ready to milk it out, as they call it. The fact is, that the child's breaſts are already in a ſtate of inflammation; notwithſtanding which the officious and miſguided attendant continues ſqueezing the parts for ſome time, though the cries of the infant might convince her that ſhe is putting it to pain.

In the caſe of inflammation, the moſt proper remedy is a poultice of bread and milk; but if the part be really not inflamed, every application is ſuperfluous. If, however, ſomething muſt be done, a little oil, with a drop or two of brandy, may be gently rubbed in; or ſmall bits of the litharge plaſter may be applied, and lie on the parts till they fall off themſelves. Indeed it is ſufficiently aſcertained, in reſpect even to a conſiderable tumefaction and hardneſs of the breaſts, that when no violence is offered to the parts, the application of a bread and milk poultice will always prevent either ſuppuration or other unpleaſant conſequences.

### *Of the Food of Children, and other Particulars.*

With reſpect to the proper food for children, in the early ſtate of infancy, one ſhould think it was impoſſible for a rational inquirer to entertain any doubt: yet ſuch is the caprice of human ſentiments that there have been found men who condemn not only the aliment itſelf which nature has ordained for their ſupport, but likewiſe the common manner of giving it, in direct contradicton to the united voice both of reaſon and inſtinct. It would be in vain to contend with argument where the underſtanding is ſo inſenſible to conviction; and I shall therefore assume it as a self-evident proposition, that the milk of the mother, or, in case of her incapacity of suckling, that of some other healthy woman, of suitable endowments for the office, is the wholesomest and most proper food for children in the state of infancy.

Some are of opinion that the child ought not to be put to the breast till many hours after its birth; but such practice seems to be destitute of any just foundation. The infant, while in the womb, was receiving from its mother a constant supply of blood, without the smallest intermission; and after it is once put to the breast, the calls of its appetite are frequent; for what good reason, then, I would ask, should the child be denied the benefit of the law of nature for a considerable time after its birth? Even a man in the vigour of life would find himself weak and faintish, after an abstinence from meat and drink for forty-eight hours; and is it reasonable to suppose, as some maintain, that a tender infant can suffer no hurt from a total privation of aliment during so long a period? If we are not to renounce every dictate of reason on the subject, we must implicitly admit that the infant ought to be put to the breast as soon after birth as the circumstances of the mother will allow.

But here a crowd of absurdities, sanctioned both by custom and authority, open upon us at once. If the mæconium or fæces of the child be not discharged almost as soon as born, of which there is no immediate necessity, the nurses instantly have recourse to syrups, oils, and other favourite laxatives, with which they stuff the infant's stomach, at the hazard of producing sickness, if not some more dangerous complaint. But this is perhaps the least hurtful manner in which their preposterous officiousness operates. From a fallacious idea that a new born infant stands in need of cordials, they almost universally mix wine, and perhaps spiceries, with the first food it takes—a practice which tends to heat the blood, already too much agitated by the recent birth, and a sudden transition from a close and warm receptacle into a new, and, in respect of its feelings, a painful state of existence. A small quantity of wine is sufficient to inflame the body of an infant; and, instead of such liquor, it properly admits of nothing but what is weak, light, and of a cooling quality. If the mother or nurse has enough of milk, the child will require little or no other food before the third or fourth month; when it may be proper to give it once or twice a-day a little of some food that is easy of digestion, such as milk-pottage, water-pap, weak broth with bread in it, and the like. This will not only ease the mother, but accustom the child by degrees to take food, and will render the weaning both less difficult and less dangerous. Milk, however, ought to be the chief part of the diet of infants for a certain time, whether it be breaſt-milk or any other; and next to this natural food is good light bread, which may be given to a child as ſoon as it has an inclination to chew. Indeed it will not only ſerve as food, but will promote the cutting of the teeth; and is preferable to the hard ſubſtances generally uſed for this purpoſe. It is alſo of advantage by promoting the diſcharge of the ſaliva, and carrying it down into the ſtomach, where it is of great uſe in digeſtion.

Bread, beſides being uſed dry, may be many ways prepared into food for children. A very good way is to boil a piece of roll, together with the upper cruſt, in a good deal of water, till it becomes very ſoft, by which means the bread will part with ſome of its aceſcent quality: the water ſhould then be ſtrained off, and the bread mixed up with the milk, which ought to be boiled, if the child is very young, or inclined to a purging. Bread is at all times a proper food for children, provided it be made of wholeſome grain, and well fermented; but it ought never to be mixed with fruits, ſugars, or other ingredients, unleſs indeed it were ſome carminative ſeeds, ſuch as aniſe or carraway, eſpecially if they be troubled with any flatulency in the ſtomach or bowels.

Children ought never to be allowed any animal food till after they are weaned, and even then it ſhould be ſparingly uſed. It muſt be owned, that when children live wholly on vegetable food, it is apt to ſour on the ſtomach; but, on the other hand, too much fleſh heats the body, and is ready to occaſion fevers and other inflammatory diſeaſes. The ſafeſt way, therefore, is to uſe a due mixture of animal and vegetable food.

Strong liquors of every kind are injurious to the health of children; and ſuch as are encouraged to uſe them become generally liable, in a higher degree than others, to the violence of the uſual diſeaſes of childhood, as well as to inflammatory fevers. The moſt proper drinks for children are thoſe of the ſimpleſt kinds, ſuch as water, milk, butter-milk, or whey. The ſtrongeſt ought to be only ſmall-beer, or a little wine mixed with water. Children require no ſtimulants to aſſiſt digeſtion; and being naturally hot, as well as eaſily affected by whatever is endowed with that quality, they ſuffer from the uſe of ſuch liquors.

Fruit is an article of which children in general are particularly fond; and this natural taſte may ſafely be indulged in moderation when the fruit is ripe. But all unripe fruits are highly prejudicial to their ſtomachs, and ought to be kept as much as poſſible out of their way. Many children likewiſe hurt themſelves by eating immoderately of raw carrots. Nor ought they to eat much of roots which have a viſcid juice, even though prepared in the kitchen. Butter, as it relaxes the ſtomach, and tends to produce groſs humours, is an article of diet not the moſt proper for children; and its place might be well ſupplied by honey, where this proves not griping or purgative.

The cuſtom of ſweetening the food of children is extremely prejudicial, as it entices them to eat more than is proper; by which means they grow fat and bloated. On the other hand, children may be hurt by too little as well as too much food. After a child is weaned, it ought to be fed four or five times a day; but never have too much at a time: neither ſhould it be accuſtomed to eat in the night. To theſe cautions it may be added, that infants ought not to be fed lying on their backs, but ſitting upright; for in this poſition they will not only ſwallow their food more eaſily, but will more readily perceive when they have had enough.

If milk be the proper food for infants brought up by hand, it becomes an object of inquiry, what milk is the moſt ſuitable? The queſtion ſeems to be moſt generally decided in favour of cow's milk, in preference to all others, as being the moſt nouriſhing, and therefore in general the moſt proper. To the milk ſhould be added a little thin gruel or barley-water, which forms a very ſmooth and pleaſant nouriſhment. A few weeks after birth, and indeed the ſooner the better, inſtead of the barley-water or gruel, there ſhould be mixed with the milk a ſmall quantity of thin jelly of hartſhorn, made to the conſiſtence that veal-broth acquires when it has ſtood to be cold. The jelly renders the food more nutritive, as well as corrects, in ſome meaſure, the aceſcency of the milk. To this compound of jelly and milk, a little Liſbon or raw ſugar may be added, if the child be not inclined to a purging, or, in that caſe, a little loaf-ſugar; but the leſs of either the better. At firſt, the milk ought to be boiled, to render it leſs opening; but when the child is ſeveral months old, or may chance to be coſtive, the milk need only be warmed. If it be freſh from the cow, and very rich, a portion of water may be added to it, whilſt the infant is very young. It ought likewiſe to be as new as poſſible; ſince milk, as an animal juice, probably contains ſome fine ſubtile particles which evaporate upon its being long out of the body.

When it was ſaid that cow's milk is preferable to any other, it was underſtood to be for infants who are ſtrong and healthy. But aſſes' milk is more ſuitable for many tender infants during the firſt three or four weeks, or perhaps for a longer time, as well as for children who are much purged; for, being thinner, and having far leſs curd than any other milk, it ſits much lighter on the ſtomach.

It is obſerved that children brought up at the breaſt do not require a thicker kind of food ſo early as thoſe who are brought up by hand, breaſt-milk being more nouriſhing than any other. It is recommended upon good authority, that the firſt addition of this kind ought to be beef-tea or broth, with a little bread beat up in it in the form of panada. A very wholeſome and nouriſhing broth for the purpoſe is the gravy of beef or mutton, not over-roaſted, and without fat, properly diluted with water. But as this cannot be given oftener than two or three times a-day, a little bread and milk may be allowed them every morning and evening, as their ſtrength and circumſtances may require.

It has been already obſerved, that children may be hurt by too little as well as too much food; and this remark is more worthy of attention, as ſome parents, running into that error, keep their children too long upon a thin and ſlender diet, which diſpoſes them much to the rickets. For when they have reached the period of going alone, not only ought a little light meat and ſome of the mild vegetables to be allowed them once a-day, or alternately, with broths, puddings, and different preparations of milk, but even a little red wine is beneficial to many conſtitutions. This diet will not only promote digeſtion, and obviate in a great meaſure a diſpoſition to worms, but, by ſtrengthening the habit, will alſo render children leſs liable to become rickety, at the very period when they are much diſpoſed to that diſorder. This plan deſerves the more to be enforced, becauſe ſome parents, from a miſtaken opinion of doing right, keep their children too low; allowing animal food only every other day to thoſe of four or five years of age. This practice, unleſs in very particular habits, is ſurely an error, at leaſt in the climate of this country, and diſpoſes to ſcrofula.

When a child is unwell, of whatever kind the diſorder may be, the lighteſt diet poſſible ſhould be uſed. If a fever accompanies it, the child will require ſtill leſs food than in any other complaint, but a larger portion of drinks. Theſe may alſo be ſo calculated as to furniſh nearly as much nouriſhment as the infant will require, and may in the ſummer-time be given cold. Of this kind are, barley-water, water in which a cruſt of bread has been boiled or ſteeped, and thin tapioca: or, if a purging attends, rice-water, and a drink made of hartſhorn ſhavings, with a little baked flour in it. In this complaint, in which more nouriſhment is required to ſupport the child than under moſt others (if not attended with fever), baked flour mixed up with boiled milk is admirably calculated both as a proper diet and medicine; and if the flour be kept in a dry place, it may be preſerved fit for uſe for a conſiderable time. Should this diſagree with the child, on account of the great acidity in the firſt paſſages, good beef-broth, thickened with baked flour inſtead of bread, ought to be made trial of. It makes a very pleaſant diet, as well as corrects the acidity in the ſtomach and bowels.

Much has been ſaid of acidity by all who have written on the diſeaſes of children. When it has riſen to the height of being injurious, it is probably often an effect rather than the cause of the disorders of infants. It seems indeed to be natural to them; arising both from the weakness of their organs of digestion, and the nature of their food. But till the body be disordered, and digestion impaired from one cause or other, the acescent quality of their food is not likely to prove very injurious to them, and probably far less so than food of a very alcaline nature would be, with a like weak digestion. The most obvious inconvenience which it produces is flatulence or wind in the stomach and bowels. This symptom may be relieved by mixing, now and then, with their food, some carminative seeds, or the waters distilled from them; such as sweet fennel, or cardamom-seeds, bruised very fine; or a little of the water of dill-seed. But though such an occasional addition to their food is often extremely useful, it ought not to be used habitually; otherwise it loses its effect. Children, however, become less subject to wind and hurtful acidities as they grow older, and the stomach acquires more strength. But if these complaints continue obstinate, a little fine powder of chamomile flowers, or a few drops of the tincture of columbo mixed in water, and warmed with a little ginger, will prove very bracing to the stomach and bowels, and render them less disposed to acidity. Exercise also, according to the age and strength, is a great preservative and remedy.

When milk is frequently thrown up curdled, a little of prepared crabs claws or oyster-shell powder may be added to it: or a very small quantity of almond soap, or of common salt, which will not at all injure the flavour, and will prevent this change from happening too soon in the stomach.

It may not now be improper to make some observations on wet-nurses and weaning.

The chief and essential quality of a wet-nurse is, doubtless, that her milk be good: to which end it is necessary that she should be healthy and young, not of weak nerves, nor disposed to menstruate whilst she gives suck; and that her body be rather costive than otherwise. Her nipples should be small, but not short, and the breast prominent, and rather oblong than large; such distention being rather from fat than from milk. The chief marks of good milk are its being thin, of a blueish colour, rather sweet, and in great quantity; and if under six months old, it is an advantage: for after this time it generally becomes too thick for a new-born infant, and is not easily digested. A wet-nurse ought to have good teeth; at least her gums should be sound, and of a florid colour. She must be perfectly sober, and rather averse to strong liquors; which are seldom necessary to young and healthy people for making them have plenty of milk. She should be cleanly in her perſon, good tempered, careful, fond of children, and watchful in the night; or at leaſt not liable to ſuffer in her health from being robbed of her ſleep.

The diet proper for wet-nurſes is likewiſe worthy of attention. And here a ſtrict regard ſhould be paid to natural conſtitution and habit. Due allowance being made for theſe conſiderations, the proper diet for a ſuckling woman ſhould conſiſt of milk, broth, and plain white ſoups: plain puddings, fleſh meats of eaſy digeſtion, and a due mixture of vegetables; with plenty of diluting drinks, and ſuch a proportion of more generous liquors (ſpirits excepted) as the caſual variety of circumſtances ſhall be found to ſuggeſt. Reſpecting vegetables in particular, the moſt ſcrupulous regard ſhould be had to conſtitution and habit. Wherever vegetables, or even acids, uniformly agree with the ſuckling parent or nurſe, healthy children will rarely ſuffer by her partaking of them; but, on the contrary, the milk being rendered thereby thin and cooling, will prove more nouriſhing and ſalutary, on account of its being eaſier of digeſtion. Beſides theſe regulations, there ſhould be added an attention to exerciſe, and frequent walks in the open air; to both which hired wet-nurſes have been previouſly accuſtomed, and are therefore ſure to ſuffer by confinement to warm rooms, to the detriment both of their own health and that of the infants whom they ſuckle.

The weaning of children is a period which alſo demands particular attention; and the proper age for it will greatly depend upon accidental circumſtances. To undergo this change, a child ought to be in good health, eſpecially in regard to its bowels; and doubtleſs ought firſt to have cut at leaſt four of its teeth. This ſeldom takes place till it is near a twelvemonth old; and it may be obſerved, that healthy women who ſuckle their own children, and take proper exerciſe, ſeldom become pregnant again in leſs time. Aſtruc adviſes children to be ſuckled till they are two years old: but for this he gives no ſufficient reaſon; and indeed ſuch a practice would, in many caſes, be ſacrificing the health, if not the life, of the mother or nurſe, without procuring to the child any advantage which might not be otherwiſe obtained. From nine months to a twelvemonth ſeems to be the period which, excluſive of any urgent motives, either to anticipation or delay, may be fixed upon as the moſt proper time for the weaning of children. Small and weakly infants, if rather feeble than ill, are ſometimes benefited by being weaned. They ſhould, therefore, about this age, be taken from the breaſt, inſtead of being, on account of weakneſs, nouriſhed much longer in that way. At leaſt, in moſt caſes, it is adviſeable to make a trial of ſuch a change. Any preparation for weaning is in general ſuperfluous, and eſpecially that of feeding children before-hand; though this is made a common excuſe for ſtuffing them, whilſt at the breaſt, with indigeſtible food.

When the weaning is once entered upon, a great part of the child's food ought ſtill to be of milk, with puddings, broths, and but little meat; and every kind of food and even drink, ſhould be prohibited in the night, even from the firſt, ſuppoſing them to be weaned at a proper age. The mere giving drink, even for a few nights, creates the pain and trouble of two weanings inſtead of one; and if the practice be continued much longer, it not only breaks the reſt, but the child will acquire a pernicious habit of being fond of drinking; the conſequence of which is very often a large belly, weak bowels, general debility, infirm joints, and all the ſymptoms of rickets. The child need only be fed the laſt thing before the nurſe goes to bed, which may generally be done without waking it; and whilſt the child ſeems to enjoy this ſleepy meal, it becomes a moſt pleaſant employment to the mother or nurſe, from obſerving how greedily the child takes its food, and how ſatisfied it will lie for many hours on the ſtrength of this meal.

Healthy children ſleep a great deal for the firſt three or four days after they are born, probably from having been accuſtomed to it in the womb. They ought not however, to be ſuffered to continue this habit in the day time, to the degree ſome children are permitted, but ſhould be gradually broken of it. Indeed, if not indulged, they will not be ſo much diſpoſed to ſleep as is generally imagined, and will therefore take more reſt in the night. This is equally beneficial to the child and the mother, if ſhe be in the ſame room, who, eſpecially if ſhe ſuckles, will be leſs diſturbed at a time when ſhe particularly requires the refreſhment of ſleep.

When infants ſleep badly in the night, they ſhould be kept more awake, and have as much exerciſe as poſſible in the day time, which, though they be ever ſo young, may be pretty conſiderable, by playing with them, dandling on the knee, and otherwiſe amuſing them; and when older, by every kind of exerciſe they can bear.

The child, if healthy, will ſoon contract a habit of being very much awake while it is light, through that lively and reſtleſs ſpirit peculiar to infancy: and by this means another evil will be very much avoided, that of often laying a child down to ſleep in the day time, for hours together, loaded with a thick dreſs, and covered beſides with heavy clothes in a ſoft cradle, or bed; all which, beſides being heating, are extremely injurious, to the circulation of the blood.

It is certain, at the ſame time, that many children have much leſs ſleep than they require; but this deficiency is chiefly in the night, and is often the conſequence of ſome complaints which the child labours under.

It deſerves to be remarked, that the cuſtom of conſtantly placing infants on their backs, whether in the cradle or bed, is extremely improper: for by this means the ſuperfluous humour ſecreted in the mouth, which, in the time of teething eſpecially, is very conſiderable, cannot be freely diſcharged, and muſt fall down into the ſtomach, where its too great quantity gives riſe to various diſorders. Infants ſhould therefore be frequently laid on their ſides, partieularly the right, as favourable to the ſtomach getting eaſily rid of its contents; to which ſide alſo children, when ſtrong enough, will inſtinctively turn, if not prevented by the weight or confinement of their own clothes or thoſe of the cradle or bed. The reaſon aſſigned for all which is a fear of the infant's falling or turning on its face: but this is rather an apology for the neglect of that neceſſary attention to children, which, when it can be commended ſhould never be ſpared them.

Infants ought ſcarcely ever to be in a quieſcent ſtate except when aſleep; and happily for them, that active diſpoſition with which nature has endowed them correſponds to this obſervation. Exerciſe, like air, is indeed of ſo much importance to children, that they cannot be healthy without it: care only ſhould be taken that it be properly ſuited to their age. The firſt kind of exerciſe conſiſts in dandling, as it is called; patting the back after feeding, and gently moving the child up and down in the arms; taking care at firſt not to toſs it very high, infants being very early ſuſceptible of fear, even to the degree of being thrown into fits by it. Another exerciſe adapted to this tender age, and of the utmoſt advantage, is rubbing them with the hand. This ſhould be done all over, at leaſt twice a day, when they are dreſſed and undreſſed, and eſpecially along the whole courſe of the ſpine or back-bone. It ought alſo to be continued for ſome time, being peculiarly ageeable to the child; as it conſtantly teſtifies by ſtretching out its little limbs, and puſhing them againſt the hand, with a ſmile expreſſive of the ſatisfaction which it enjoys. Such gentle exerciſe may be partially repeated, every time the child's clothes are changed, by rubbing the lower limbs and every other part within reach. Theſe frictions not only promote the circulation of the blood, but excite a lively ſenſation in the parts, and tend greatly to ſtrengthen the body.

When children are older, they ought never to be carried in an indolent poſture, but the arm that ſupports them ſhould be conſtantly in ſuch motion as the nurſe is able to continue. The manner of carrying an infant is of more importance than is generally imagined: for by it the child will contract a habit, good or bad, that it will not readily give up; and may be as much disposed to become rickety by improper management in the arms, as if it were lying wet in the cradle, than which nothing is more pernicious to the constitution of an infant. In recommendation of proper exercise to children, I shall just mention the great advantages of which it is known to be productive. Besides strengthening the digestive powers, and indeed the whole body, it tends to push forward the blood through the small vessels, and to unfold these in the manner in which nature designed them to be extended, for promoting the growth of the infant. At the same time it preserves the blood in a proper state of fluidity, and promotes both the secretions and excretions, so indispensable to the preservation of health.

## CHAP. II.

### *Diseases of Infants and Children.*

HOWEVER extraordinary the remark may appear, it is beyond a doubt, that the infant offspring of the human race are more liable to diseases and early death than those of all the other animal tribes. A variety of causes concur to produce this effect: the weakly constitution of many parents, whether hereditary or acquired, the incapacity of some mothers to nurse their own children, and the disinclination of others to that natural duty, with the carelessness of mercenery nurses in performing the task, and theamismanagement usually practised, all conspire to injure the tender frame, and increase the mortality of children. It therefore becomes a subject of great importance to the interests of society to point out in as clear a manner as possible the most rational method of treating those complaints to which the infant generation is peculiarly liable.

Some writers have regarded any inquiry into this subject as fruitless and unnecessary, because, infants being incapable of giving any information concerning their complaints, the physician can only form his opinion by the help of conjecture; while others, ascribing all diseases to one general principle in the constitution of children, have paid little or no attention to examining into the variety of causes which may occasionally produce disorders in their delicate frame. The consequence is, that the diseases of infants have only latesy begun to be studied with any suitable degree of application; and old women and nurses have in general assumed to themselves the sole right of practising even in the most dangerous circumstances of the infant state. This blameable remissness on one hand, and unwarrantable officiousness on the other, are objects of the most serions regret; and every effort should be made by the friends of humanity to rescue a helpless generation from so fatal an evil, and prevent them from daily falling a sacrifice, in thousands of instances, to the pernicious and lamentable effects of ignorance and error. To remedy therefore this grievous abuse, I shall deliver, as concisely as possible, the method of discovering and curing the disorders of children, upon principles not only agreeable to rational theory, but confirmed by the observations of men the most attentive to, and most experienced in, the diseases of infants.

## *Of the Retention of the Meconium.*

The meconium is a black, thick matter, lodged in the intestines, and which is generally discharged by stool, for the two or three first days after birth. To answer this purpose nature has wisely ordained that the milk of the mother, during the earlier part of this period, should be endowed with a purgative quality: but through a mistaken opinion, too common among nurses, the infant is debarred from this wholesome aliment, and not permitted to suck till the breasts have been drawn, when the milk has no longer the quality which it originally possessed; and there arises a necessity of having recourse to other means for unloading the bowels, at this time oppressed with the quantity of what they contain. In general, very little medicine will suffice for the purpose: it may be answered, for the most part, by a little syrup of roses, along with some thin gruel, and given from time to time in the quantity of a tea-spoonful: but if this should fail, a tea-spoonful of castor oil will commonly be found effectual.

It is observed, however, that the meconium does not always yield to the use of the common purgative medicines; and therefore, if the child has had no stool during twelve or fourteen hours after birth, it will be advisable to give immediately a clyster, such as the following, which, if necessary, may be repeated a few hours after.

Take of milk, or water-gruel, or an infusion of linseed, four table-spoonfuls; brown sugar, and sweet oil, each a table-spoonful; common salt, a tea-spoonful. Mix them together.

It is always proper to begin with gentle remedies: but if these still prove unsuccessful, which is sometimes the case, and that the discharge of the meconium is not accomplished in two or three days, there is reason to suspect a deficiency of nervous influence, and more powerful means must be made use of. The dose of castor oil should be increased, or the quantity formerly given be repeated as occaſion requires; and the clyſter be rendered ſtronger, by doubling the quantity of ſalt.

Even after the meconium is diſcharged children are frequently ſubject to coſtiveneſs, either conſtitutional or accidental; and this circumſtance proving the cauſe of wind and pains in the bowels ſhould always be remedied by the uſe of opening medicines. Beſides what have been already mentioned, the powder of rhubarb, given occaſionally, in the quantity of four or five grains, will be found extremely beneficial, as it not only diſcharges any matter that irritates the bowels, but likewiſe tends greatly to ſtrengthen them. Where the mother is very much conſtipated her children are generally the ſame.

## *Of the Jaundice, or Yellow-Gum.*

This diſeaſe is not to be confounded with the yellowneſs of the ſkin that appears about the third day after birth, termed by ſome the yellow gum, and which is too trifling to be mentioned as a diſeaſe. The true jaundice, accompanied with a yellowneſs of the eyes, is a diſeaſe by no means frequent among infants, though it ſometimes does occur. It proceeds from ſome viſcid or thick matter ſtopping up the gall-ducts, to remove which it is neceſſary to give a gentle emetic, or vomit. The beſt thing for this purpoſe, as being moſt certain in its operation, is the powder of ipecacuanha, given in the quantity of three or four grains; and next morning four or five grains of rhubarb. Should the diſorder continue, the emetic ought to be repeated after two or three days, and the rhubarb every other day, giving, on the intermediate days, eight or ten grains of tartariſed kali, diſſolved in ſome water. In many caſes, one grain of calomel, mixed with three or four grains of rhubarb, and repeated two or three times, will effect a cure.

Sometimes this diſeaſe ariſes from a ſpaſm or cramp of the gall-duct. In ſuch a caſe the infant ſhould be put into the warm bath, and continue in it about ten minutes. The following medicine likewiſe will then be of ſervice: Take of tincture of caſtor, a tea-ſpoonful; tincture of opium or laudanum, twenty drops. Mix them, and give ſix or eight drops two or three times a day, out of a ſpoonful of mint tea, or any other liquid.

It is obſerved that women afflicted with the jaundice, during any part of their pregnancy, and even actually brought to bed in that ſtate, do not affect their children, unleſs they alſo ſuckle them; but in that way they are capable of communicating the true jaundice to a great degree; and the diſeaſe cannot be removed by medicine, without the ſuckling mother or nurſe is firſt cured, or the infant is weaned.

### *Of Wind in the Bowels.*

This complaint is almoſt always attended with coſtiveneſs, from which it commonly ariſes. If the coſtiveneſs be conſtitutional, there is required a ſtronger doſe of the purgative to open the body than in other caſes. Inſtead of five grains, therefore, of the powder of rhubarb, eight or ten may be given; and this ſhould be accompanied with a little calcined magneſia, as coſtiveneſs is uſually productive of acid or ſour humours in the bowels of young children. If the child be ſo habitually coſtive as to require the frequent uſe of purging medicines it will be better to have recourſe to other means of opening the body, as the conſtitution might be impaired by adminiſtering ſuch remedies too freely. A clyſter, therefore, occaſionally, will be more adviſable; or in the room of it a ſuppoſitory; which may be made of the end of a very ſmall candle. If ſuch a thing ſhould not be at hand, a little ſlip of paper or linen cloth twiſted up and dipt in oil may be ſufficient for the purpoſe. Theſe means will be aſſiſted by rubbing the belly morning and evening with a warm hand or a piece of flannel, moved in a circular direction, correſponding to the ſituation of the bowels.

### *Of the Looſeneſs.*

Children are often ſubject to a diarrhœa, or looſeneſs; but this is not always a diſeaſe: for ſuch a diſcharge may either prevent or remove other complaints, and is hurtful only when it continues ſo long as to occaſion weakneſs.

Causes.—Both vomiting and purging frequently ariſe from unwholeſome milk or other food, and from a moiſt cold air, as well as from the ſudden diſappearance of ſome eruption on the ſkin. The diſcharge therefore ought not to be ſtopped till the cauſe is removed and the offenſive matter carried off.

Cure.—A doſe or two of the powder of rhubarb ſhould firſt be given, and afterwards abſorbent medicines. The following julep is highly advantageous in ſuch a caſe:

Take of crabs claws prepared, two drachms; gum Arabic a drachm and a half; cinnamon-water and mint-water each four table ſpoonfuls; loaf ſugar two drachms. Mix.

Two or three tea-ſpoonfuls of this mixture may be given frequently in the day, firſt ſhaking the glaſs. Should the diſcharge ſtill continue, on account of the great irritability of infants, three or four drops of the tincture of opium or laudanum may be added to each doſe; or inſtead of it two tea-ſpoonfuls of the ſyrup of white poppies.

When the ſtools appear very ſlimy, ſour, or curdled, or when the child is much disposed to hiccup, the absorbent medicines have great effect, and ought never to be omitted. If to the above quantity of crabs claws and gum Arabic there be added one scruple of ginger or nutmeg, and two drachms of sugar, it will make an excellent powder, which may be divided into six or eight doses, to be taken two or three times a day in a little tea or pure water.

## *Of the Lientery, or Watery Gripes.*

In most of the loosenesses of children the stools are thin and watery when the disorder has continued a few days; but in the true watery gripes they are of that consistence from the beginning, or at least very early in the disease: the child looks extremely indisposed, and every thing it takes runs almost immediately through it, as in the lientery of adults. The cure of this disorder should begin with a vomit, which may be repeated with advantage, especially if the stools are of a dark colour and foetid, or of an offensive smell, as they frequently are in the earlier periods of the complaint. The emetic in this case should be pretty strong, and given in divided doses at the distance of about a quarter of an hour, till it has produced a proper effect.

Take of the powder of ipecacuanha one scruple; pure water one ounce; loaf sugar one dram. Mix.

Two tea-spoonfuls may be taken immediately, and one every hour after till it begins to work, when some thin water gruel should be given to promote its operation. Next day a purge ought to be administered, consisting of six, eight or ten grains of the powder of senua, according to the circumstances of the child, with a few grains of powdered ginger or cardamom-seeds, a table-spoonful of water, and a small bit of sugar. When the stomach and bowels are cleansed, recourse may be had to the julep mentioned in the preceding article, to which it will be proper to add two scruples of the aromatic confection. In the more advanced stage of the watery gripes, and where the child has reached the age of six or seven years, the following medicine has often been attended with good effect:

Take of Locatellus' balsam half an ounce; conserve of red roses an ounce. Mix them together with a little simple syrup or syrup of sugar.

Of this from the quantity of a horse-bean to that of a nutmeg may be given three or four times a day.

When outward applications can be used with advantage they ought never to be neglected in the diseases of young children; not only because such patients are most incapable of taking medicines by the mouth, but likewise because, their pores being more open than those of others, they are more readily affected by the influence of any thing applied to the skin. For these reasons three or four drachms of the compound plaster of ladanum, spread upon leather, and applied to the belly, will prove a very suitable assistant in the cure of the disorder.

As long as the stools continue remarkably sour it would not be safe to give opium or strong astringents: for the acid humours must first be corrected by absorbents, such as the crabs claws before mentioned, and carried off by warm purges. The absorbents may be given in pretty large and repeated doses, and for the purge make use of the following:

Take of senna leaves one drachm, cardamom-seeds half a drachm. Infuse them for an hour in something less than a gill of boiling water; then strain and add to the infusion two drachms of the tincture of rhubarb, and a tea-spoonful of the compound spirit of lavender.

Give four tea-spoonfuls immediately, and repeat the dose every hour till the sour smell of the stools appears to be gone. When this happens, have recourse to the prescription next mentioned.

Take of cinnamon-water and mint-water, each four table-spoonfuls; aromatic confection two scruples;* tincture of opium twenty drops; syrup of saffron a table-spoonful. Mix them.

Give three or four tea-spoonfuls every two hours, first shaking the vial, till the discharge ceases.

In the advanced stage of watery gripes, or where the disorder is accompanied with great weakness, such a medicine, consisting of aromatics and an opiate, is absolutely necessary.

Complaints of the bowels are frequently owing to improper food, which on this account always demands particular attention. Cow's milk is often found to disagree with children when their bowels are too open; at which times a little mutton-broth deprived of the fat, or beef-tea, is greatly to be preferred. A physician of much experience in the complaints of young children affirms, that he knows of no diet so proper for infants who do not suck, or who cannot have enough of the breast, as flour slowly baked for a long time till it breaks into a soft greyish coloured powder, and afterwards mixed with cow's milk boiled, the scum being first taken off: the flour and milk should then be boiled a little together till the whole appears like a thin custard. This is a very light and soft food, and sufficiently binding; and he has often known more good from it, than from all the absorbent medicines ever devised. The powder of arrow-root boiled in water, and then mixed with milk, is an admirable remedy when it can be procured genuine.

* For scruples, see *Appendix.*

When the watery gripes, or indeed any violent purging, attacks infants at the breaſt, the wet-nurſe ought to be changed, if the diſcharge of ſour humours continue many days, and medicines do not ſeem to take a proper effect; which they cannot if any offenſive matter be continually taken into the ſtomach. In all complaints of the bowels it is obſerved that infants are expoſed to eruptions on the ſkin. By this they are ſo frequently benefited, that, if any kind of raſh appears during long or ſevere purging, a recovery may almoſt with certainty be prognoſticated. On the other hand, likewiſe, good effects have often been obſerved from a purging taking place in ſome obſtinate eruptions of the ſkin.

## *Of Worms.*

Worms in the ſtomach and bowels are a frequent complaint of young children; but all are not equally affected by the preſence of this cauſe; ſome infants diſcharging great numbers without any ſign of indiſpoſition, whilſt others who have apparently very few worms ſuffer greatly on the occaſion. In ſuch a caſe it is probable that the pains and other complaints ariſe from ſome other ſource. Worms are chiefly of four kinds: the large round worm; the very ſmall maw-worm, or aſcarides, reſembling bits of thread; the ſhort, flat worm, or cucurbitina; and the jointed, called the tape-worm, or tænia, which is ſometimes many yards long. The laſt kind, however, is rarely found in children. Theſe animals are hurtful in various ways; but principally by ſucking up the chyle deſigned for the nouriſhment of the child, and by the irritation they occaſion. They ſometimes likewiſe have been known to eat their way through the inteſtines; but this is a very extraordinary occurence.

Symptoms.—The ſymptoms of worms are various, and ſome of them may proceed from other cauſes. The moſt certain ſigns are a fœtid breath, eſpecially in the morning; itching of the noſe, and of the anus, eſpecially from the aſcarides; a very irregular appetite; a large, hard belly; pains in the ſtomach or belly; ſometimes vomiting, but more frequently coſtiveneſs or purging, with ſlimy ſtools; ſtartings in the ſleep, and grinding of the teeth; to which may be added an unhealthy and bloated countenance, with a dark hollow circle round the eyes. Beſides theſe ſymptoms there is ſometimes a ſlow fever, with a ſmall irregular pulſe, pale urine, a ſhort and dry cough; which laſt ſymptom is almoſt conſtant where the complaint is of long ſtanding, and has injured the health. In ſome caſes there happen convulſions, epilepſies, and partial pallies of the lower extremities. When convulſions enſue, if the pulſe be ſmall attended with a hiccup, it is almoſt a certain ſign that the complaint is occasioned by worms. The same may be said of a pain at the stomach if it be very violent, sudden, attended with great anxiety, and a hardness and soreness of the parts about the navel. According to Dr. Home, a whitish swelling of the upper lip, and of the nostrils, is a certain token of worms.

CURE.—When worms exist in the bowels they are to be carried off by purgative medicines, to which other remedies are joined, or the latter are given during the intervals of purging. By many the male fern has been extolled as a specific against these vermin. Olive oil likewise has been strongly recommended as being destructive to worms, but castor oil is certainly preferable; because by its purgative quality it also carries them off by stool. Oil, however, of any kind can have very little effect upon them, as they are defended from it by the moisture and slime of the intestines; and the same is the case with lime-water. A very large dose of alcaline or other salt will destroy both the slime or mucus, and the worms together; but it is apt to hurt and inflame the stomach and intestines, and thus produce worse disorders than that which it was intended to cure. Two remedies highly useful in this complaint are worm-seed and cowhage, or cow-itch. Ten or fifteen grains of the former may be given with a little treacle twice a day. With regard to the cowhage, it is the hairy part scraped off from the pods that is to be used. It may be made up with common syrup into the consistence of thin honey, and given in the quantity of a tea-spoonful twice a day. In separating the hairy part of this herb from the pods care must be taken to prevent their penetrating the skin; for they cause an intolerable itching. The best way to perform the separation is to shake the pods in a box.

As a purgative against worms, calomel either alone or joined with the powder of rhubarb is advantageous. Thus for a child of two or three years old, Take of rhubarb six grains, calomel one grain, mix them and give the dose in a spoonful of water, or milk.

For preventing the breeding of worms in the stomach and bowels, nothing is better than stomachic bitter medicines, such as the following: Take of Peruvian bark grossly powdered, one drachm and a half; gentian root one drachm; the fresh outer rind of Seville oranges, two drachms; boiling water, one pint. Infuse for twenty-four hours, and strain them through a linen cloth. Two or three tea-spoonfuls of this infusion may be given twice a day.

Instead of water, the same quantity of materials may be infused in a pint of white wine, or brandy, for two or three days, and then filtered through brown paper. The dose of this tincture may be the same as that of the infusion; only, if the tincture be made with brandy, the dose must be weakened, by adding at least an equal quantity of water.

The following outward application, for killing and expelling worms, has been found advantageous.

Take of the powder of dried rue, and Socotorine aloes, each half an ounce—mix, and make them into a plaster with Venice treacle; which apply to the belly, first covering the navel with a little cotton.

For children troubled with worms, fat and greasy aliments are improper. The best diet is broth, with meat of easy digestion; and toasted bread and honey should be used instead of butter, which is extremely pernicious.

## *Convulsions.*

Convulsions consist in an involuntary and alternate contraction of the muscles.

CAUSES.—They are caused by irritation in some particular part of the body, and are chiefly occasioned by teething; wind pent up; some indigested matter in the stomach or bowels; and by a rash imprudently repelled. Among the various causes may likewise be mentioned that of foul air, and want of cleanliness in the dress and other accommodations of infants.

CURE.—The cure of convulsions, like that of all other diseases, consists, principally, in removing the exciting causes. When they arise from improper food and indigestion, a gentle vomit should be given. If the irritation be in the bowels, the acrid matter must be discharged by purgatives; and generally the first thing given should be a clyster. Rhubarb and calomel, as prescribed in the case of worms, will here also be proper. But if the disposition to convulsions continues, after the bowels have been properly cleansed, recourse should be had to the medicines of the anti-spasmodic class, or those that are good against cramps.

Take of tincture of assafœtida, half an ounce*; tincture of castor, two drachms; tincture of opium, forty drops. Mix them. Fifteen or twenty drops of this mixture may be taken occasionally in a little mint-tea.

When the convulsions arise from the disappearance of a rash, a little weak wine whey should be given with the mixture, and the child kept warm, to promote perspiration. If they proceed from the stoppage of a discharge behind the ears, it should be recalled by the immediate application of blisters. During the continuance of convulsions, the warm bath is of great service; but for curing a disposition to this complaint nothing is more powerful than sea-bathing, or, in want of it, the cold bath; either of them to be used every other morning for a considerable time.

* See *Appendix*.

When convulsions arise from teething, the only effectual remedy is lancing the gums. But it is not sufficient once to set free all the teeth that are evidently making their way; for the divided parts soon heal up again, and give rise to fresh irritation. The cutting therefore ought to be repeated for several days successively, if the convulsions do not ecase.

If the convulsions do not arise from any of the causes mentioned above, there is reason for supposing the complaint to be a primary disease, and to proceed immediately from the brain. In this case, an attempt should be made to procure a derivation from the head; which is best effected by putting the feet and legs into warm water. Some blood, if the child is able to bear it, ought likewise to be taken away; or leeches may be applied behind the ears, or on the temples. Blisters ought also to be laid on the legs or thighs, and a clyster be given; which, if the convulsions continue, should be followed by a gentle purge. Blistering may be thought harsh treatment in the disorders of infants; but it ought to be remembered that their life is now at stake, and that the temporary pain of blisters is not so intolerable as a violent fit of convulsions.

If children of two or three years old are subject to slight and frequent fits of convulsions, issues or setons should be made between the shoulders, or in the neck, and be kept open for a length of time.

Convulsions arising from any of the causes above mentioned, will sometimes disappear of themselves as the infant gets older. At other times, the appearance of some other complaint has put an end to the convulsions; and sometimes the disorder has been removed even by weaning children, when six or eight months old. In some of the worst cases of convulsions, after all the usual remedies have been tried without success, musk, freely given, has perfectly cured the disorder. Five or six grains of it powdered may be given in a little mint-tea, and repeated two or three times a day.

Though all convulsion-fits are, indeed, in their appearance, extremely alarming, yet experience warrants the conclusion, that under proper treatment they are much less frequently fatal than is generally imagined. Neither is the frequency of their returns during infancy, nor the long continuance of such a disposition, any real indication of future evils. But where the intervals are short, though the fit itself be not long, nor violent, the disease is more dangerous than when severe fits are attended with long intervals.

### *Dentition, or Teething.*

Teething is an important period in the constitution of infants, notwithstanding some writers entertain the contrary opinion. The body, during teething, is much difpofed to inflammation; and lufty, ftrong children often fall into a fever at this time, while thofe who are weak and delicate cut their teeth eafily, though frequently later than the others. It is obferved by Hippocrates, "That infants cut their teeth more readily in winter than in fummer; that fuch as are rather inclined to be lean cut them more eafily than thofe that are very fat; and children who are loofe in their belly the moft fafely of all." This period commonly begins between the fifth and tenth months; and the firft teething continues, for the moft part, to the fixteenth at leaft, and fometimes much longer.

Symptoms.—Various fymptoms ufually precede and accompany its progrefs. The child drivels, the gums fwell, and become hot; there is often a rednefs in the cheeks, and eruptions on the fkin, efpecially on the face and head. There is alfo a loofenefs, and griping, and the ftools are green or pale. The urine, fometimes of a milky colour, is frequently made in lefs or greater quantity than ufual, and accompanied with pain. Thefe fymptoms are often followed by a cough, difficult breathing, convulfions, fever, fcrofula, and fometimes by water in the head.

Cure.—When teething is difficult, it muft be treated nearly as other acute difeafes where there is an inflammation of any part. If the child be any way bound, fome opening medicine fhould be given; and if much fever attends, the lofs of a little blood, either by the lancet, or by leeches behind the ears, will be neceffary; though children do not bear bleeding fo well as other evacuations. Clyfters are alfo highly ufeful, efpecially if the urine be fparingly made; in which cafe, the ufe of the warm bath will be likewife advifable. Some gentle medicine to promote perfpiration fhould be given. This purpofe may be anfwered by antimonial wine, in the quantity of from fix to ten drops, or upwards, according to the age and other circumftances of the child. This remedy has befides the advantage of opening the belly. It may be given in a little balm or mint-tea. If there be any difpofition to fits, a blifter fhould be applied between the fhoulders; or, inftead of this, a Burgundy-pitch-plafter will fometimes fuffice, and ought to be removed every ten days till the fymptoms difappear, or the teeth come into fight.

But if this fhould not fucceed, and the child be feized with convulfions, a bliftering-plafter ought to be applied between the fhoulders, or one behind each ear.

Teething almoft invariably begins with the fore-teeth of the lower jaw. After two teeth in each jaw have appeared, it is, in fome inftances, a confiderable time before they are followed by thofe which are next them; but fometimes, though not often, fix or eight are cut in hasty succession. The fore-teeth, or *cutters*, are succeded by the four *grinders*; then come the *dog-teeth*, as they are called; and, last of all, of an infant's first teeth, their antagonists or the *eye-teeth*; making in all sixteen.

This is the usual number of children's first teeth; though some infants cut four double teeth in each jaw, instead of two; making the whole number twenty. But an infant has sometimes been known to cut twenty-four teeth.

A symptom less common than any of those above mentioned, and appearing only in certain habits, is a swelling of the tops of the feet and hands. It seems, however, to be of no importance, and goes away upon the appearance of the teeth; though, in some instances, this symptom is accompanied with considerable fever. A transient palsy of the arms or legs has also sometimes been observed during the progress of teething. Those symptoms are often followed by a cough, difficult breathing, convulsions, fever, and scrofula, and sometimes by water in the head.

It is observable, that the extremes of high health, and a sickly disposition, are both dangerous: the former being exposed to acute fever, or convulsions; the other to a slow hectic and consumption. Pure air, therefore, exercise, wholesome food, an open belly, with every thing that has a tendency to promote general health, and to keep off a fever, will greatly contribute to the safety of teething, and to children's passing quickly through this hazardous period.

A purging is found to be of advantage during the progress of teething; and it is surprising how considerable a looseness children will bear on this occasion, as well as how bad the stools will be for many weeks together. The looseness, therefore, is to be cautiously treated, and rather to be encouraged than suppressed.

For the fever accompanying teething, besides bleeding, the absorbent powders, such as crabs claws prepared, are eminently useful, and are, in various respects, calculated to afford relief. To these, sometimes, a grain or two of Dr. James's powder may be added at bed-time. One, two, or three grains of nitre are very often useful, joined with the powders just now mentioned, in the quantity of eight or ten grains; or with four or five grains of the compound powder of contrayerva. Sydenham directs two, three, or four drops of the spirit of hartshorn to be given in a simple water, every four hours. Nor is a drop or two of laudanum to be feared, if the bowels have been opened, the pain be very great, and the breathing not difficult. A free discharge of the bowels, however, must, above all, be preserved, when teething is attended with a fever. The state of their gums must also be carefully attended to, or it is a chance that their fevers may be mistaken, and imputed to cold, or other caufes, when the fource of the diforder is entirely in the pain of the gums.

It is admitted that the lungs is one of thofe parts which are apt to be affected by the pain of teething ; and, when this happens to be the cafe, the fymptoms have an alarming appearance. A precife acquaintance with their true caufe is, therefore, of the greateft importance ; otherwife, an unfuccefsful plan of cure will moft probably be adopted.

In fuch cafes, we fometimes meet with the moft alarming fymptoms of an inflammation of the lungs ; forenefs of the breaft, or fides ; cough ; great difficulty of breathing, with lofs of appetite, continual fever, and the appearance of general decay. In this ftate, purging the bowels, and properly lancing all the fufpected parts of the gums, have given immediate relief ; and, by keeping up the purging for three or four days, every threatening fymptom has fo thoroughly abated, that, in a fortnight's time, a child, expected from day to day to die of inflammation, or fall into a confumption, has been reftored to its former health and fpirits.

It ought to be a general rule, during the time of teething, to abate a little of the ufual quantity of food, and to increafe the quantity of drink, unlefs the child is very weakly, or every thing goes on perfectly well. If the child be at the breaft, a regard of the fame kind ought to be paid to the diet of the nurfe.

Children will fometimes have ulcerated gums in teething, and more frequently where they have not been lanced ; which are eafily cured by keeping the body open, and touching them with a little white vitriol, or roche alum. As much as will give a moderate roughnefs to a little honey is commonly fufficient for this purpofe.

## *Hydrocephalus, or Water in the Head.*

This complaint is diftinguifhed into two kinds ; namely the external and internal : in the former, the water lies upon the furface of the brain, but in the latter it is feated much deeper.

SYMPTOMS.—In both kinds, he difeafe commonly begins with the appearance of a flow fever, a weaknefs of the arms, and pains in the limbs ; as alfo frequently, in the upper part of the neck. In fome time after, the child is fuddenly feized with pain in the head, generally in the fore-part : it becomes heavy and dull, and can bear no pofture but that of lying horizontally, or flat. The pulfe becomes irregular, but commonly very flow. As the difeafe advances, the faculties and fenfes are impaired, and the eyes are offended by the light ; the patient fees objects double, and becomes delirious. In the further progrefs of the difeafe, the pulfe grows frequent, the cheeks become flufhed, the pupils of the eyes are enlarged, the ftools and urine come away involuntarily, and the child lies sleeping, or is convulsed.

Cause.—This disease commonly takes place between two and ten years of age, but it is not universally confined within that period. It may arise from falls and blows on the head, from tumours within the skull, and from a watery state of the blood, and a lingering illness. This is sometimes a very short disease, and, at others, continues many months; but, in either case, ending for the most part fatally.

Cure.—Whatever may be the immediate cause of the hydrocephalus, in attempting to cure it, practitioners have chiefly depended on repeated bleedings; purges with jalap, or calomel; blisters to the neck, or head, with medicines to promote the discharge of urine, and the outward use of mercurial ointment. Some have, from experience, recommended the use of sternutatories, or sneezing-remedies; such as the compound powder of asarum, or white hellebore. To these means may be added, the application of a narrow caustic upon the head, along the whole course of the longitudinal sinus, instead of a small blister to the crown, as some have advised.

## *Aptha or the Thrush.*

Symptoms.—This disorder generally appears first in the angles of the lips, and then on the tongue and the inside of the checks, in the form of little white specks; which sometimes extend to the stomach, and along the whole length of the intestines. If the specks are of a pale colour, superficial, and easily fall off, they are reckoned not dangerous; but the contrary is the case when they are thick, brown, or black, and run much together.

Causes.—This complaint seems to be occasioned originally by indigestion. Some ascribe it to the taking of victuals either too hot in themselves or of too heating a quality, especially when made very sweet. When the thrush attacks strong infants of a costive habit of body, it is easily cured, and requires little more than keeping the bowels sufficiently open; for which purpose, the daily use of castor oil is very advisable. But the complaint is not void of danger in delicate infants, whose bowels are weak.

Cure.—When the thrush is not attended with any fever, or other uncommon symptom, the testaceous powders, such as that of crabs claws, are the best and safest remedy. To this may be joined a little calcined magnesia, if the child be costive: but if, on the contrary, it is loose in the belly, and weakly, two or three grains of the compound powder of contrayerva may be added instead of the magnesia. This medicine should be given for three or four days ſucceſſively, and afterwards ſomething more purgative, to carry down the ſloughs as they fall off. Rhubarb, to which a grain of calomel may be joined, is generally the beſt for this purpoſe. In delicate and weak infants, where the diſeaſe is of a bad kind, a decoction of Peruvian bark with aromatic confection, is found the beſt remedy. It may be made as follows:

Take of Peruvian bark, half an ounce. Boil it in a pint of water to a gill and a half; and, after ſtraining, add of aromatic confection, one drachm and a half.

The quantity of four tea-ſpoonfuls to be given every four or five hours.

If the inſide of the cheeks and tongue are thickly covered with ſloughs, it may be convenient to clean the mouth two or three times a day, with a little roſe water, in which ſome honey and a little borax is diſſolved; but any raſh application is in general improper, till the ſloughs are diſpoſed to fall off, and the parts underneath inclined to heal. When a gangrene is apprehended, ſome ſpirit of ſalt, or vitriol, ſhould be added to thoſe applications, and the uſe of the Peruvian bark be perſiſted in.

## *Of the Hooping-Cough, or Chin-Cough.*

Symptoms.—This diſorder often begins as a common cold, but in its progreſs ſoon becomes more ſevere. From the beginning it is accompanied with a greater difficulty of breathing than is common in a cold; and there is a remarkable affection of the eyes, as if they were ſwelled, and a little puſhed out of their ſockets. The fits of coughing become gradually more violent, till at laſt they are plainly convulſive. The diſeaſe is tedious, and ſometimes continues many months, but not commonly attended with a fever, though an infectious diſorder. Like other contagious diſeaſes, occuring to a perſon only once it may naturally be expected to be more frequent in childhood than in any other period of life. In general, whatever weakens the body promotes a diſpoſition to this complaint. It is often obſerved to be more dangerous in one ſeaſon than at another. Its effects are commonly worſt in children under two years of age, whom, if it continues long, it is apt to render ſcrofulous or rickety.

Cure.—The diſeaſe proves moſt favourable when the fit ends by vomiting; which ſeems to point out the benefit of promoting ſuch a diſcharge. Bleeding, however, when the cough is violent, and the child in danger of being ſuffocated, ought certainly to be performed, eſpecially if there be a fever attended with a hard full pulſe. The next object in the cure is to give a gentle vomit for cleanſing the ſtomach, which is here generally loaded with tough phlegm. The belly is next to be kept gently open with rhubarb; and both the vomit and purge must be repeated as occasion requires, but always by the gentlest means. It is of great advantage to bathe the feet every day in warm water, and to keep a Burgundy-pitch-plaster constantly applied between the shoulders: but instead of the latter, when the disease is violent, recourse should be had to a blistering-plaster, and the part be kept open for some time by means of issue ointment. Eight or ten drops of antimonial wine, given two or three times a day, is frequently of great service.

The practice has hitherto been common to give oily and balsamic medicines in this disease; but they certainly are extremely hurtful by loading the stomach and bowels, which are already too much oppressed with phlegm. A far more suitable remedy is Peruvian bark, and castor.

Take of the powder of Peruvian bark, two drachms; of castor, two scruples; spearmint-water, half a pint; syrup of sugar, two table-spoonfuls. Mix them.

To a child about four years of age, three tea-spoonfuls may be given every four or five hours; and the dose proportionably increased, or diminished, to those of a less or greater age. A change of air is of great advantage in the decline of the hooping-cough, and even after its first seizure, when the child can be conveniently removed. It would seem as if the disease was supported by its own infectious air, when the child is kept long in the same place. The diet, in this disorder, ought to be of the lightest kind. Little more than milk and broths should be given to children even of five or six years of age; and no greater quantity than a tea-cupful taken at a time.

### *The Croup.*

The Croup has never been noticed in Great-Britain before the present age, and there is yet a difference of opinion respecting both its real nature and the method of cure. According to the most prevailing opinion, however, it consists of an inflammation of the upper part of the trachea, or wind-pipe, accompanied with an uncommon secretion of mucus or phlegm from that part. It seldom attacks infants till after they have been weaned, and becomes less frequent as children advance in years; hardly ever appearing in any who have reached ten or twelve years of age. It is more frequent in winter than in summer, and more common upon the sea coast than in the midland counties.

Symptoms.—It generally comes on with a hoarseness, a pain about the top of the wind-pipe, and a difficulty of breathing, attended with a peculiar kind of croaking noiſe, that may be heard at a conſiderable diſtance. The pulſe is quick, with much heat, and the patient is reſtleſs.

CURE.—If the patient be of a full habit of body, as is commonly the caſe in this diſorder, and the fever runs high, or the breathing be very difficult, it is proper to bleed, and apply leeches to the pained part: after which a bliſter ſhould be laid over it; and if the difficulty of breathing continues, another bliſter between the ſhoulders.

Upon the firſt attack of the diſeaſe, it is often of great advantage to give a vomit, immediately after bleeding; which has ſometimes ſo good an effect, as almoſt immediately to remove the complaint. If this ſhould not happen, the vomit muſt, nevertheleſs, be repeated; and this as often as the continuance of the difficulty of breathing ſhall give reaſon to think that a freſh accumulation of phlegm has taken place in the wind-pipe. This frequent repetition of emetics is abſolutely neceſſary while the ſymptoms continue violent. The body, in the mean time, is to be kept open by laxative clyſters; and the feet and legs ought to be put twice a day into warm water.

Though this diſeaſe be of the inflammatory kind, it ſeldom ends either in a ſuppuration or gangrene. Its common effect, when fatal, is to ſuffocate the patient by the violent diſorder in the wind-pipe. But if it terminates favourably, the inflammation is reſolved; as is likewiſe the ſpaſm, or cramp, at the top of the wind-pipe; ſometimes with a conſiderable diſcharge of phlegm from the throat, and at other times with little more than what happens in a common cold.

Such is the treatment of the diſeaſe, when purely inflammatory; but in other caſes, where it is almoſt entirely ſpaſmodic, proceeding as it were from a cramp of the throat, the method of cure is very different. Here the remedy moſt generally recommended is aſafœtida, two drachms of which may be diſſolved in four table ſpoonfuls of mint-water, and the ſame quantity of penny-royal-water. A table ſpoonful of this mixture may be given every hour, or oftener, if the patient's ſtomach can bear it. Some children are extremely averſe to it, while others take it not only without diſguſt, but even with great pleaſure. But where they cannot be prevailed upon to take it by the mouth, it ought to be given in a ſmall clyſter, in the quantity of two drachms at a time.

The tincture of opium may be given with the ſame intention, in the quantity of ſix or eight drops every two hours, until ſleep, or a remiſſion of the conſtriction, take place.

To prevent a return of this diſorder, a ſeton between the ſhoulders, or an iſſue in the arm, is adviſable. Children who are diſpoſed to it, ſhould be guarded as much as poſſible againſt catching cold, and likewiſe againſt the uſe of ſuch aliments as are crude, or of difficult digeſtion.

### *Rickets.*

CAUSES.—The Rickets is ſaid to have been unknown in this country, till about the year 1628, when, upon the advancement of manufactures, people left their occupations in the country to ſettle in large towns. There wanting that exerciſe, and pure air, which they had formerly enjoyed, their ſtrength declined, and of conſequence they produced a weak and ſickly offspring. It is certain that the diſorder ariſes frequently from unhealthy parents, eſpecially from mothers who paſs too ſedentary a life in a bad air, and uſe a crude and watery diet. The ſame unwholeſome air and diet affect ſtill more the tender bodies of their children; on which account it is obſerved that the children of poor people are particularly liable to the rickets. From improper food and weak digeſtion, their ſtomach and bowels are loaded with undigeſted juices; an univerſal thickneſs of the fluids prevails in the extreme veſſels, eſpecially of the joints; from too languid a circulation the humours become depraved, and an almoſt general obſtruction takes place in the fibres of the muſcles.

SYMPTOMS.—The rickets ſeldom attacks children under nine months; from which period to two years old the diſorder uſually breaks forth, and ſhows itſelf chiefly by the following ſigns: The child's fleſh becomes ſoft and flabby; the face appears full, and the head and belly increaſe in a proportion beyond the other parts of the body. The bones next begin to be affected, the knees, wriſts and ancles become thicker than uſual; the bones of the arms and legs become crooked; the ſpine or back bone is altered from its natural ſhape, as is likewiſe the appearance of the breaſt.

Such are in general the ſymptoms, but they vary in different children according to the violence of the diſeaſe. The appetite and digeſtion are commonly bad; the teething is ſlow and difficult; and after the teeth have appeared, they are ſeized with rottenneſs, and fall out. Rickety children uſually diſcover a degree of underſtanding beyond their years.

The cure of this diſorder ought to be begun with cleanſing the ſtomach and bowels by gentle vomits of ipecacuanha, and purges of rhubarb and calomel, ſuch as have been repeatedly mentioned above: after which the conſtitution is to be ſtrengthened by ſtomachic bitters, the Peruvian bark and ſteel medicines, compounded in the following manner:

Take of the root of the ſweet-ſcented flag, and gentian-root, each three drachms; Peruvian bark, in powder, half an ounce; iron filings, tied up in a linen bag, ſix drachms; Spaniſh white wine, or Liſbon, one quart. Digeſt for the ſpace of three days, and then filter the tincture. Four tea-ſpoonfuls of this tincture may be given twice a day.

Nothing is more effectual in this diſeaſe than the cold bath, but it ought not to be uſed at the ſame time with the Peruvian bark and ſteel; and the winter is not the moſt proper ſeaſon for it. Rubbing the back and belly, in particular, with flannel and aromatic powders, or the fumes of frankincenſe, maſtic and myrrh, will tend greatly to promote the cure, by ſtrengthening the body.

The diet ought to be nouriſhing, and rather of a dry than moiſt kind. For drink, wine mixed with water is preferable to malt liquors: but of the latter, good porter is the beſt.—Dry air, and exerciſe, eſpecially riding on horſeback, are highly advantageous.

## *Scrofula, or King's Evil.*

Symptoms.—This diſeaſe is one of the moſt obſtinate that affects the human frame, and of all others it is the moſt generally handed down by parents to their offspring. Sometimes, however, it will lie concealed for one or two generations, and afterwards appear with redoubled violence. It is originally a diſorder of thoſe parts of the body called glands, but in proceſs of time ſeizes others. It is often preceded by a peculiar look about the eyes, which are generally large, and a thickneſs of the upper lip. The belly is ſometimes obſerved to be hard and enlarged, and there is a remarkable ſoftneſs of the ſkin. The diſeaſe is not uſually fatal at an early period, but may prove the cauſe of bad health even to the end of life. It often diſappears, however, about the age of fourteen or fifteen, and ſometimes ſooner, eſpecially in females. On the other hand, after diſappearing for ſeveral years, during which the health has been perfectly good, the humour has unexpectedly fallen upon ſome inward part, occaſioning various complaints, often aſcribed to other cauſes, and has in the end produced a conſumption of the lungs or ſome other fatal diſorder.

Cure.—This diſeaſe has ſuch an affinity to the rickets in the cauſes which commonly produce it, namely, bad diet, and a weakneſs of conſtitution, that it requires in great meaſure the ſame method of treatment, ſo far as relates to a diet of eaſy digeſtion, and to medicines for ſtrengthening the body, as well as to keeping always the ſtomach and bowels free from impurities. Bark and steel are also excellent remedies, but nothing is better than sea bathing. In children of a gross habit of body a glassful or more of sea-water drunk in a morning has often produced good effects; as has also lime water* used for common drink.

The use of hemlock in this disease both inwardly and outwardly used has been much recommended by some writers, but the most extraordinary instances that we meet with of success are some cases in which the inhaling of vital or superoxygenated air has performed a perfect cure, after all the usual remedies had been tried to no purpose. This unexpected discovery is of singular importance; and if fully ascertained by a greater number of trials will serve to extirpate a disease, which has hitherto generally baffled the utmost efforts of medicine.

The Moffat and Harrowgate waters are likewise highly serviceable in the scrofula, when used for a considerable time; but they ought only to be taken in such a quantity as to keep the body gently open.

The method too frequently practised of plying the patient with strong purgative medicines, from a notion of discharging the humours, deserves to be severely condemned, as it weakens the constitution, and thereby increases the disease. That the body ought indeed to be kept open has been already observed; but for this purpose the gentlest means only are advisable. Dr. Underwood very properly recommends one drachm of cathartic salt dissolved in a pint of water, to be taken every day as common drink. This quantity of salt will give very little taste to the water, and we are told that in some instances it has alone had a good effect in subduing the disease, especially in stronger children, and such as are otherwise healthy. In those, however, of a delicate and spare habit of body, remedies that warm and strengthen the constitution, such as aromatics, with the bark and steel as before mentioned, are chiefly to be employed. But while these are used, and still more if the use of them be interrupted, the strictest attention should be given to the diet of a scrofulous patient, as otherwise no medicines, however well suited to the disease, can produce the desired effect. Let all meats, therefore, that are hard of digestion be avoided, and the diet be wholesome, generous and nourishing; for more depends upon a proper regulation in this respect than is commonly imagined: but sea-bathing in this disorder can never be enough recommended.

* Lime-water is made in the following manner: Take of quick-lime one pound, boiling water a pint and a half; pour the water gradually upon the lime, and stir them together; then let the water be filtered through paper, and kept in a vessel closely stopped.

## *Small-Pox.*

Though the ſmall-pox ſometimes ſeizes perſons at a late time of life, it is however chiefly incident to children, and is one of the moſt fatal diſorders to which they are liable. It appears generally in the ſpring, from which time through the ſummer it increaſes in frequeney, till autumn advancing it begins to decline, and in winter either entirely diſappears or ſpreads its contagion more ſlowly.

There are, beſides ſome inferior diviſions, two principal kinds of this diſeaſe; namely, the diſtinct and the confluent, the latter of which is always attended with danger.

Symptoms.—On the approach of the diſeaſe children generally diſcover a drowſineſs, after which come on the ſymptoms of an inflammatory fever, accompanied with fits of cold and heat by turns. There is a pain in the head and back, ſickneſs and pain at the ſtomach, and ſometimes vomiting; coſtiveneſs generally prevails; and ſometimes the patients are attacked with convulſive fits, which in this diſorder is always conſidered as a good ſign. A fever is now formed, accompanied with a great heat of the ſkin and reſtleſſneſs: the child wakes out of his ſleep with a ſudden ſtart, which, as well as convulſive fits, is a ſign that the eruption is on the point of making its appearance. This generally happens about the third or fourth day from the time of ſickening: ſometimes they appear ſooner, but the diſeaſe is then judged to be of an unfavourable kind. They are firſt diſcovered like flea-bites on the face, arms, and legs, extending ſucceſſively over the body to the feet, and are accompanied with pains and ſoreneſs of the throat, which is commouly in three, or four days.

As ſoon as the eruption is completed the fever diſappears or abates. The moſt favourable kind of puſtules are thoſe which are diſtinct, with a florid red baſe, and which fill with a thick, purulent matter, firſt of a whitiſh, and afterwards of a yellowiſh colour. Pox of a livid brown colour, or which are ſmall and flat, with black ſpecks in the middle, are unfavourable; and ſuch as contain a thin, watery humour, yet worſe. It is a bad ſign when they run into one another; and a great number of pox on the face is accounted a dangerous ſymptom: but the moſt unfavourable circumſtance of all is when purple, brown, or black ſpots are interſperſed among the puſtules, as they afford a ſign that the blood is in a putrid ſtate. Other bad ſymptoms are bloody ſtools or urine, with a ſwelled belly. Pale urine, accompanied with a violent throbbing of the arteries of the neck, are ſigns of an approaching delirium, or of convulſion fits. When the face does not ſwell, or falls before the pox comes to maturity, it gives juſt ground for apprehending an unfavourable event; but when at the ſame time that the face falls, which is about the eleventh or twelfth day, the hands and feet begin to swell, the disease proceeds well. Cold shivering fits coming on at the height of the disorder, with a brown crust on the tongue, are both unfavourable symptoms; as is likewise a grinding of the teeth, when this proceeds from an affection of the nervous system, and is not occasioned by worms or any disorder of the stomach. About the seventh day from the eruption, sometimes the ninth, the pustules dry, or *turn* as it is called; and, sealing off, leave red marks, and sometimes pits, behind them.

Cure.—During the eruptive fever the patient ought to be kept cool and easy, and allowed to drink freely of barley-water, balm-tea, gruel, or other diluting liquors; his food should be very light; he ought not to be confined to bed, but sit up as much as he is able, and should have his feet and legs bathed frequently in water agreeably warm.

It is a common prejudice among the lower class of people, that the linen of the children should not be shifted through the course of the disease, lest they catch cold: but this is a most pernicious as well as loathsome practice; for the linen being hardened by the moisture which it absorbs frets the tender skin, and creates much uneasiness, at the same time that the vapours rising from the dirty linen again enter into the body, and increase the disease. Shifting at this period is highly necessary, but doubtless care ought to be taken that the linen be thoroughly dry; with which caution, and shifting likewise when the patient is most cool, no danger needs to be apprehended.

When this disease proceeds in a favourable manner, it would only be disturbing the salutary efforts of nature to ply the patient with medicines. Bleeding is seldom necessary in infants, though it is sometimes proper and requisite in those who have passed the age of childhood. During the first three or four days of the disease a cool treatment is to be carefully observed, to prevent too great an eruption; but after the pox have made their appearance, the physician's business is to promote the suppuration by light food, and such diluting drinks as have been already recommended; and should nature flag in this important process, her efforts must be assisted by suitable cordials; such as wine made into negus, and sharpened with the jelly of currants, the juice of orange, or the like. Wine-whey is also proper in this case; but care must be taken not to over-heat the patient by those cordial remedies; for such conduct, instead of promoting, would actually retard the eruption, and might be productive of dangerous consequences.

The same cautions are to be observed during the maturation or ripening of the small-pox. The chamber ought to be kept cool;

the patient be lightly covered when in bed, and be likewife occafionally taken out of it. The filling of the pox is often prevented by great reftleffnefs; and when this happens gentle opiates are neceffary. A tea-fpoonful of the fyrup of poppies may be given to an infant every four or five hours, till the fymptom is removed.

It often happens in the fmall-pox that the patient is troubled with a ftrangury, or fuppreffion of urine. In this cafe he fhould be frequently taken out of bed, and if he be able, it is found of advantage to walk acrofs the room with his feet bare. When this cannot be done, he ought frequently to be raifed on his knees in bed, and fhould endeavour to pafs his urine in that fituation. A plentiful difcharge of urine is highly beneficial in the fmall-pox; and when it does not enfue naturally, a tea-fpoonful of the fweet fpirits of nitre fhould be mixed with his drink occafionally.

During the rifing of the fmall-pox the patient is generally coftive, to fuch a degree as not to have a ftool for eight or ten days. It may well be imagined, that this extreme conftipation, in a feverifh diforder, muft prove highly prejudicial. It not only tends to heat and inflame the blood, but from the fharp and putrid nature of what is thus unduly retained in the bowels very bad effects may enfue. In fuch circumftances a foftening clyfter fhould be given, every fecond or third day through the whole courfe of the difeafe; by which means the patient will be cooled, and otherwife greatly relieved.

When purple or black fpots appear among the fmall-pox, the Peruvian bark muft immediately be given in as large dofes as the patient's ftomach can bear, and be likewife frequently repeated; by which the happieft effects may be produced.

Take of the powder of bark two drachms; pure water fix table-fpoonfuls; cinnamon-water half a gill; fyrup of orange, or lemon, two table fpoonfuls. Mix them.

This may be fharpened with the fpirits of vitriol, and a table-fpoonful of it given to an infant every hour. Spirit of vitriol, or inftead of it vinegar, the juice of lemon, or currant-jelly, ought alfo to be mixed with the patient's drink, which, in this cafe, fhould be wine or ftrong negus. The diet muft confift of fruits of an acid nature, fuch as apples, roafted or boiled, preferved cherries, plums, and the like.

The fame method of treatment with refpect to the bark and acids, is likewife to be purfued in what is called the lymphatic or cryftalline fmall-pox, where the matter is thin and watery; for they render the confiftence thicker, and promote a kindly maturation. When the fmall-pox ftrike in, as it is called, or the puftules fuddenly fink and become flat before they have arrived at maturity, the cafe is extremely dangerous. As foon as this happens, blisters ought to be applied to the wrists and ancles, and the patient be supported by cordials: sharp poultices likewise, composed of mustard-seed, oat-meal, and vinegar, may be applied to the feet and hands, to promote the swelling of those parts, and draw the humours towards the extremities.

The most dangerous period of the small-pox is what is called the secondary fever, which generally comes on when the pustules begin to blacken or turn on the face; and most of those who die of the small-pox are carried off by this fever. At this critical period nature frequently attempts to relieve the patient by loose stools; and this salutary effort ought by all means to be assisted; supporting the patient, at the same time, by food and drink of a nourishing and cordial nature.

On the approach of the secondary fever, if the pulse be very quick, hard, and strong, the heat very great, and the breathing laborious, accompanied with other symptoms of an inflammation of the breast or lungs, blood must immediately be drawn, in a quantity suitable to the urgency of the case, and the strength and age of the patient: but if, on the other hand, the sick be faintish, the pox become suddenly pale, and there be great coldness of the extremities, blisters must be applied, and the patient supported with generous cordials. In such cases, wine, and even spirits, have sometimes been given with the best effect. The secondary fever arising, in a great measure, from the matter of the pox being absorbed into the body, it would be extremely advisable to open the pustules, and let the matter out; by which the danger might at this period be lessened, if not entirely removed. Very little art is necessary for such an operation; and it ought to be done when the pox begin to be of a yellow colour. It may be performed either with a lancet or needle, and the matter cleared away with a little dry lint. As the pustules are generally first ripe on the face, it will be proper to begin in that part, and afterwards to proceed regularly downward: but once to perform the operation is not sufficient; for the pustules generally fill again a second or even a third time. Besides the beneficial effects of this practice in diminishing the fever, it tends to prevent the pitting, which is an object of some consideration.

After the small-pox it is proper to give a gentle purge two or three times, at the distance of a few days between each; but if, notwithstanding this precaution to carry off the dregs of the disease, it should be succeeded by a cough, a difficulty of breathing, or other signs of a consumption, the patient must be put upon a course of asses milk, with such exercise as he can bear; and it is of importance that he should be sent to a place where the air is dry and wholesome.

It often happens that imposthumes or swellings are formed in some part of the body after the small-pox. In such a case the swelling, if the means employed to discuss it fail, must be brought to a head as soon as possible, by means of poultices; and when it has been opened, or has broke of itself, the patient must be purged. In these circumstances, the Peruvian bark and a milk diet are highly advisable.

## *Inoculation.*

The method of communicating the small-pox by inoculation has been practised from time immemorial in the eastern countries, where it is regarded as so simple an operation that in many parts the women perform it. Various prejudices have hitherto concurred to obstruct its progress in this country, but they now appear to be diminishing; and there is reason to expect, from the example of those who are more liberal in their opinions, that in the course of some years the practice, if not universally adopted, will at least become very general. Could the minds of people be influenced by the force of reason alone, they could not hesitate a moment to determine on embracing the practice of inoculation. So evidently great is the advantage of it in saving the lives of children, that while in the natural small-pox not more than one patient out of four survives the disease, it is a chance if one in five hundred be cut off in consequence of inoculation. This fact is of itself a sufficient argument to establish the usefulness of the practice.

With regard to the manner of inoculating, nothing can be conceived as more easy. In some parts of the world it is performed by rubbing the variolous matter upon the skin; and this is generally successful in communicating the disease. But the method of inoculating at present in this country is, to take a little matter from a pustule when the pox are fully ripened, on the point of a lancet, and insert it in the arm, by making one or two small incisions between the true and scarf skin, which may afterwards be pressed down with the flat side of the lancet. In three or four days after the part appears inflamed, and in about three days more the symptoms of infection come on. But if fresh matter be applied long enough to the skin, there is no occasion for making any puncture at all. Let a bit of thread, about half an inch long, wet with the matter, be applied to the arm, mid-way between the shoulder and the elbow, and covered with a bit of common sticking plaster. In eight or ten days this method will seldom fail of communicating the disease.

The most proper season for inoculation is when the weather is temperate and healthy; and the fittest age between three and five years. Many approve of inoculating even on the breast; but children are more liable to convulsions at this time than afterwards; and if the child should seem to be in any danger, the anxiety of the mother or nurse, by spoiling the milk, could not fail to heighten the disease.

Very little preparation of the body is necessary previous to inoculation. In children who have been fed on simple and light diet, such as milk, panada, weak broths, bread-pudding, mild roots, and white meats, no change of diet is necessary. But those who have been accustomed to richer food, and are of a gross habit of body, or abound with bad humours, ought to be put upon a spare diet, for a fortnight or three weeks before inoculation. Their food should be light, and not of a heating quality; and their drink whey, butter-milk, milk and water, or the like. There is no occasion for the use of medicines before inoculation; but two or three mild purges, suited to the age and strength of the patient, should be given. When the signs of infection have begun to appear, the proper management is to keep the patients cool, and their bodies gently open; by which means the fever is kept low, and the eruption greatly lessened. The fever proceeds very moderately when the pustules are few, and their number is generally in proportion to the degree of fever which precedes or attends the eruption. The food and drink during the disease are to be regulated in the same manner as in the natural small-pox; and the same is to be said respecting medicines should any bad symptoms appear, which is seldom the case. Purging, when the disease has ceased, is here likewise no less necessary than in the former kind of disease.

### *Of the Cow-Pox, and its Inoculation.*

In the preceding article, I have given place to the method of inoculating for the small-pox, as having hitherto been successfully practised during a number of years; but, by a fortunate discovery, it is now found, that the infection may be introduced in a manner equally successful, and the disease rendered still less considerable than by the former kind of inoculation. This is done by inoculating with matter either taken from a cow affected with the disease, or from some person who had received the infection originally derived from that animal. It may be proper here to give a general account of the manner in which so surprising a discovery has been made.

In several parts of England, where cows are kept for the purposes of the dairy, a peculiar eruptive disease has been occasionally observed among the herd, and which affects in particular the udders and teats of thoſe animals. It has, therefore, pretty generally obtained the name of the *cow-pox*, (*vaccinia*, or *vacciola*.)

Till within theſe laſt two years, the knowledge of this diſtemper has been chiefly confined to the people employed in the dairies, and to farriers and cow-doctors in the neighbourhood; but, by the latter, it appears to have been obſerved with particular accuracy, and they have even employed means for its removal.

It farther appears, that wherever the exiſtence of this diſeaſe was known, the fact was likewiſe aſcertained, that the diſorder is communicated by the touch to the milkers who handle the teats of the diſeaſed cows, and from them again is often ſpread through a numerous herd: that, when affecting the human ſpecies, it is not merely confined to the local diſeaſe of the hands and arms, but alſo occaſions a general indiſpoſition, often ſevere, but never fatal, which runs a regular courſe; and that the perſon who has once undergone the diſeaſe ſo communicated is ever after ſecure againſt the infection of the ſmall-pox, either in the natural way by contagion, or by inoculation.

All theſe circumſtances, however, though known, as we are told, from time immemorial in certain parts of the kingdom, ſtill remained in obſcurity till within theſe three years, when Dr. Jenner, of Berkley, in Glouceſterſhire, conceived the important idea of employing the cow-pox to annihilate the ſmall-pox, and publiſhed ſeveral intereſting particulars concerning this diſeaſe, which works have now made it known to the public in general.

It appears, from obſervations made by thoſe who are moſt converſant with cows, that ſeveral cauſes may produce ſores upon the udder and teats of this animal, eſpecially ſuch as excite any irritation in thoſe parts, during the ſeaſon when the cows abound moſt in milk. The ſtinging of flies, or rough handling while milking, and other ſuch external irritations, will often occaſion ſmall white bliſters on the parts; which, however, never extend more than ſkin-deep, and are generally eaſy of cure.

Another, and a more ſerions diſorder in thoſe parts, is ſaid to be ſometimes produced by ſuffering a cow, while in full milking, to remain for a day or two unmilked; in order to diſtend the udder when naturally ſmall. This, it appears, is a common artifice practiſed at fairs and cattle-markets, with the view of increaſing the price of the cow, a large udder being reckoned an important circumſtance in the value of that animal. By this cruel and unwarrantable artifice, the veſſels that ſupply the udder are kept for an unuſual length of time in a ſtate of great diſtention, which terminates frequently in a violent inflammation of thoſe parts, ſucceeded by large eruptions upon the teats and udder that ſometimes leave deep and troubleſome ſores. The matter diſcharged from these ulcers will communicate a disorder, like the other, into the hands of the milkers, when the skin is broken in any part; and often produces foul and extensive ulcers, which sometimes occasion pustules on the arms and shoulders, and prove tedious and difficult of cure.

The genuine cow-pox, however, is a distinct disease from those which have been just mentioned. It generally makes its appearance in the spring, and shows itself in irregular pustules on the teats or nipples of the udder. They are at first of a palish blue, or rather a livid colour, and contain a thin, watery, and sharp fluid. The surrounding parts are inflamed and hardened. These pustules, it seems, are very apt to degenerate into deep corroding ulcers, which, as the cow-doctors term it, *eat into the flesh*, and constantly discharge a matter, which commonly increases in thickness, and hardens at last into a scab. Now and then the cow becomes evidently indisposed, loses her appetite, and gives less milk than usual; but it often happens that the disorder, though severe, is entirely local.

It appears that the cow-pox never proves fatal to cows, nor is it infectious in the usual manner of contagious distempers, but can only be communicated to them or to the human species by actually touching the matter which proceeds from the sores. Hence, the cows which are not in milk escape the disease entirely, though constantly in the same field with those that are highly infected; and it seems to be only from the circumstance of the milker handling the teats of the sound cows, after touching the diseased, that the cow-pox ever spreads among the herd.

We are informed that the cow-pox is familiar to the inhabitants of the hundred of Berkley in Gloucestershire. It has likewise been discovered in various parts of the counties of Wilts, Somerset, Buckingham, Devon, and Hants; in a few places of Suffolk and Norfolk, where it is sometimes called the *pap-pox*; and in Leicestershire and Staffordshire. Nor is it unfrequent in the very large milk-farms contiguous to the metropolis on the Middlesex side. It is here observed generally to attack first some cow newly introduced to the herd, and is supposed to originate in a sudden change from a poor to a very rich and partly unnatural diet, which it is the practice to use, in order to bring the yield of milk to its highest point.

According to Dr. Jenner, the origin of the cow-pox is ascribed to a derivation from the horse. The horse is well known to be subject to an inflammation and swelling in the heel, called *the grease*, from which is discharged a very sharp matter, capable of producing irritation and ulcers in any other animal to the surface of which it is applied. It is supposed that this matter is conveyed to the cow by the men-servants of the farm, who, in several of the dairy counties, assist in milking. One of these, having dressed the horse, goes immediately to his occupation of milking; and having upon his hand some particles of the discharge from *the grease*, he, of course, applies it to the udder of the cow, where, if the animal be in a state for receiving the infection, it produces that specific change in those parts which gives rise to the disease of the cow-pox.

The origin here ascribed to this disorder is principally founded on the circumstance, that wherever the cow-pox appears, *the grease* is generally found to have preceded it: and the opinion of the propagation of the disease from the horse to the cow is likewise current in some of the dairy counties where the disease is known. But this opinion requires to be ascertained by further observations.

This conjecture, respecting the origin of the cow-pox, was no sooner started by Dr. Jenner, than attempts were made repeatedly, but without success, to introduce the disease in the nipple of the cow by direct inoculation of the recent matter of *the grease* from the horse's heel. The consequence of this experiment, when it took any effect, was a slight inflammation, and the production of a small pustule or pimple, but which disappeared in a few days, without exciting the specific disease of the pox. But the failure of these experiments by no means overthrows the opinion for the ascertainment of which they were made; since it is admitted that a certain predisposition in the constitution of the cow to receive the disease is also requisite for its production.

It is remarked, that the matter discharged from the sores in the horse's heel is likewise found to occasion, at times, very troublesome ulcers on the hands of the men that dress them, attended with a very considerable degree of indisposition; both of which appear to be full as severe as in the genuine cow-pox, and in many points to resemble this latter disorder. But the person who has been infected by the horse is not rendered thereby entirely secure from afterwards receiving the small-pox.

The pustular sores on the udder and teats of the cow, that constitute the genuine cow-pox, whatever be the way in which they are produced, are found by experience to possess the power of infecting the human species, when any part of the body, where the skin is broken, or naturally thin, comes into actual contact with the matter which they discharge. Hence it is, that, with the milkers, the hands are the parts that acquire this disorder accidentally, and it there exhibits the following appearances: Inflamed spots begin to appear on the hands, wrists, and especially the joints and tips of the fingers; and these spots at first resemble the small blisters of a burn, but quickly proceed to suppuration. The pustule is quite circular, depressed in the middle, and of a blueish colour, and is surrounded with a considerable redness. The blue colour which the pustule almost invariably assumes, when the disorder is communicated directly from the cow, is one of the most characteristic marks by which the cow-pox may be distinguished from other diseases which the milkers are likewise liable to receive from the cow. The matter of the pustule is at first thin and colourless; but, as the disorder advances, it becomes yellower and more purulent. In a few days from the first eruption, a tenderness and swelling of the glands in the arm-pit comes on, and soon after the whole constitution becomes disordered, the pulse is increased in quickness, shivering succeed, with a sense of weariness, and pains about the loins, vomiting, head-ach, and sometimes a slight degree of delirium.

These symptoms continue with more or less violence from one day to three or four, and, when they abate, they leave sores about the hands, which heal very slowly; resembling, in this respect, the ulcers on the nipple of the cow, from which they derive their origin.

It is to be observed, that the cow-pox eruption, though very severe on the hands, and occasioning much general illness, never produces a crop of pustules over distant parts of the body, arising spontaneously, as in the small-pox. It often happens, however, that pustules are formed in various parts which accidentally come in contact with the diseased hands, as on the nostrils, lips, and other parts of the face where the skin is thin; or sometimes on the forehead, when the milker leans with that part upon the udder of an infected cow. From this account it appears, that the cow-pox as it affects the milkers, or what may be termed the *casual* cow-pox in the human species, is often a severe disorder; sometimes confining the patient to his bed during the period of fever, and generally leaving troublesome sores, but it has never been known to prove fatal; nor are these sores, if properly attended to, followed with any lasting injury of the affected parts, though they sometimes leave sears for life.

In consequence of the close investigation which this disorder has lately undergone, the following facts may be considered as fully ascertained by the fairest experiments and most accurate observations:

*First.*—The cow-pox, in its natural state, or when propogated immediately from an infected cow, to the hands of the milkers, is capable of affecting the human species from one to another repeatedly to an indefinitive number of times; but after the first attack, it is generally much milder in its symptoms, and in particular it is much less liable to produce the fever and general indisposition which always attend the first infection, There are instances, however, where the ſecond and even third attack have been as ſevere in every reſpect as the firſt; but theſe are very rare.

*Secondly.*—The ſmall-pox in a conſiderable degree ſecures a perſon from the infection of the cow-pox; and in this reſpect appears to act in a manner very ſimilar to a previous attack of the latter diſeaſe; that is, to confine its operation to the forming of local puſtules, but unattended with general fever. Hence it is, that where all the ſervants of the dairy take the infection from the cows, thoſe of them who have previouſly undergone the ſmall-pox are often the only perſons among them able to go through the uſual work.

*Thirdly.*—The cow-pox, in its genuine ſtate, when it has been accompanied with general fever, and has run its regular courſe, ever after preſerves the perſon who has been infected with it from receiving the infection of the ſmall-pox. This aſſertion is, however, to be taken with exactly the ſame limitations as that of re-infection with the ſmall-pox preventing a ſecond attack of the ſame diſeaſe. No previous infection will entirely counteract the local effect on the arm, produced by the inſertion of variolous matter in common inoculation: this may in a few caſes go ſo far as to induce a degree of general fever, ſlight indeed, but perhaps equal to that of the mildeſt indiſpoſition cauſed by a firſt infection with this diſorder. By the inoculation of either diſeaſe, however, the ſmall-pox is equally and completely diſarmed of its virulence againſt any ſubſequent attack, which is the circumſtance that ſo much diſtinguiſhes and ſo ſtrongly recommends this operation.

*Fourthly.*—A compariſon of the two diſeaſes in reſpect of the mildneſs of their ſymptoms, and the hazard to life which they may occaſion, will ſhow a very great advantage in favour of the cow-pox. Compared with the natural ſmall-pox, the natural or caſual cow-pox is both milder and infinitely more ſafe; no inſtance having ever been known of a fatal event in the cow-pox, ſo far as it affects the people employed in the dairies. When both diſeaſes are introduced by artificial inoculation, they are each rendered much leſs ſevere; and here too the ſuperiority of the cow-pox as a ſafer and milder diſeaſe is extremely evident.

*Fifthly.*—The cow-pox, even in its moſt virulent ſtate, is not communicable by the air, nor by any other of the ordinary means of contagion, but can only be propogated, by the actual contact of matter of a puſtule from the cow-pox with ſome part of the body of the perſon who receives it. It is not yet aſcertained, whether in all caſes an inſertion of ſpecific infectious matter under the ſkin be neceſſary; but in its moſt active ſtate, as it is when formed in the cow's udder, the ſkin which covers the lips and noſtrils readily receives the infection without being broken. In this respect, the contagion of the cow-pox seems to equal that of the small-pox in activity; but the striking difference between the two diseases in the cow-pox not being communicated by the air, &c. is a circumstance fully and satisfactorily ascertained. In the dairy-farms, infected servants sleep with the uninfected: infants at the breast have remained with their mothers whilst only one of the two have had the disorder upon them; and in no instance has the disease of one been communicated by contagion to the other. It is this circumstance which gives the cow-pox its decided superiority; since, by adopting this disease instead of the small-pox, all the dread and all the mischief occasioned by the contagion of the latter are entirely removed.

The inoculated cow-pox appears to have almost as great a superiority in point of mildness and security over the ordinary inoculation of the small-pox, as this has over the natural small-pox; so that the same precautions which would be highly requisite in communicating the latter becomes less so where the disorder is to be introduced by inoculation; and still less where the cow-pox is substituted in the room of the other.

With regard to the method of performing inoculation in the cow-pox, Dr. Woodville, whose industry, judgment, and accuracy, appear to great advantage in his observations on this subject, advises "that the lancet should be held nearly at a right angle with the skin, in order that the infectious fluid may gravitate to the point of the instrument, which, in this direction, should be made to scratch the cuticle repeatedly, until it reach the true skin and become tinged with blood."

The act of inoculation having been performed, the first proof of its success is a small inflamed spot at the part where the puncture has been made, which is very distinguishable about the third day. This continues to increase in size, becomes hard, and a small circular tumour is formed, rising a little above the skin. About the sixth day the centre of the tumour shows a discoloured speck, owing to the formation of a small quantity of fluid; and this continues to increase, and the pustule or pimple to fill, till about the tenth day.

After the eighth day, when the pustule is fully formed, the effects on the constitution begin to show themselves; the general indisposition being commonly preceded by pain at the pustule and in the arm-pit, followed by head-ach, some shivering, loss of appetite, pain in the limbs, and a feverish increase of the pulse. These continue, with more or less violence, for one or two days, and always abate of their own accord, without leaving any unpleasant consequence behind them.

During, or a little after, the general indisposition, the pustule in the arm, which had been advancing in a regular manner, becomes surrounded with a broad circular inflamed margin, and this is a sign that the body in general is affected. After this period, the fluid in the pustule gradually dries up, the surrounding redness becomes fainter, and in a day or two vanishes imperceptibly; whilst the pustule no longer increases in extent, but on its surface a hard thick scab of a brown colour is formed, which, if not pulled off, remains for nearly a fortnight; till at length it falls off, leaving the skin beneath perfectly sound and uninjured.

It is a circumstance of great importance in favour of this method of inoculation, that though some attention in choosing the matter for inoculation, and performing this slight operation in such a manner as to insure success, be requisite, very little medical treatment is necessary in order to conduct the patient through it with perfect safety. In most cases it is attended with so little fever as scarcely to be detected by an attentive observer.

To conclude this account of the cow-pox with a repetition of the circumstances which gives it a decided superiority over the small-pox, Dr. Woodville affirms (and his authority is unquestionable) that of all the patients whom he inoculated with the variolous matter, after they had passed through the cow-pox, amounting to upwards of four hundred, not one was affected with the small-pox, though purposely and repeatedly exposed to the infection of the disease; and what is not less extraordinary, nearly a fourth part of this number was so slightly affected with the cow-pox, that it neither produced any perceptible indisposition, nor pustules.

From the beginning of the world, the cow has, in all countries, been esteemed a valuable animal. Besides cultivating the ground, which her species performs, she supplies us with an aliment of her own preparing, the most wholesome as well as nourishing in nature; but never before was it known, except, as appears, in some particular districts in England, that, even from a disease to which she is liable, she can likewise be further useful, in preserving us from one of the most fatal calamities that ever infested human kind.

## *Chicken or Swine-Pox.*

In many persons, this kind of pox make their appearance without being preceded by any illness or signs of their approach; but, in others, there is a slight degree of chillness, weariness, cough, loss of appetite, wandering pains, and feverishness for two or three days. The pustules, or pimples, in most cases, have the common rise of small-pox, but some are less; and they never are numerous, nor run together.

On the first day of their appearance, they are of a reddish colour; and on the second there is at the top of most of them a very small bladder, about the size of a millet-seed. This is sometimes full of a watery and colourless liquor, sometimes it is yellowish; and, the skin which contains it breaking by accident, or perhaps from rubbing to allay the itching, a thin scab is formed, on the first or second day, on the top of the pustule. On the fifth day of the eruption, they are almost all dried and covered with a crust.

This disease may be distinguished from the small-pox by its appearance on the second or third day, and from the bladder of watery liquor upon the top of the pox. It may likewise be distinguished by the crust which covers the pox on the fifth day, at which time the small-pox is not come to a state of maturity.

The disease, as above described, stands in no need of any remedies; but there sometimes appears a more malignant kind of it. For three or four days all the symptoms which precede the eruption run much higher. On the fourth or fifth day the eruption appears, with very little abatement of the fever. The pains likewise of the limbs and back continue; to which are joined pains of the gums. The pox are redder than the common chicken pox, spread wider, and hardly rise so high, at least not in proportion to their size, but go off in the same manner.

From the similarity of this disease to the small-pox, we may account for the opinion entertained by some, of persons having been affected with the small-pox twice, or having them after being inoculated. For some have been inoculated from the chicken instead of the small-pox. It is also worthy of observation, that those who have had the small-pox may have the chicken-pox; but those who have had the chicken-pox cannot be infected again by it, though to such as never had the distemper it is as infectious as the small-pox.

In this disease, if the feverish symptoms run high, they must be treated in the same manner as the small-pox under similar circumstances.

## *Measles.*

This disease resembles the small-pox in several particulars. They both made their appearance in Europe about the same time; both came from Arabia, or its neighbourhood; both are infectious, and seldom or never attack the same person more than once. The measles are most frequent in the spring, and generally disappear in summer.

Symptoms.—The measles, like other fevers, usually begin with a cold fit, which is soon succeeded by a hot one; and sometimes the fits succeed each other alternately, accompanied with sickness and loss of appetite, which are more or less considerable in different patients. The tongue is white, but generally moist. There is a hoarse dry cough, often with some difficulty of breathing; drowsiness, sneezing, a running at the nose, and a heaviness of the head and eyes; the latter of which are sometimes a little inflamed, discharge a sharp humour, and are so tender that they cannot bear the light without pain. A vomit or looseness often precede the eruption, which commonly appears the fourth day, first on the face, then on the breast, and successively on the lower part of the body. At the beginning, it resembles flea-bites, but soon after the specks run together in clusters. The eruption does not rise in evident pimples like the small-pox; however, in touching the spots, they are found to be raised a little above the skin.

This is the case on the face; but in other parts of the body the elevation or roughness is hardly to be perceived. On the face, the eruption maintains its redness, or has it even increased for two days; but on the third the colour is changed to a brownish red; and in a day or two more the eruption becomes dry, and, falling off in scales, at length entirely disappears.

The fever, cough, and difficulty of breathing, instead of being removed or abated by the eruption, as in the small-pox, are rather increased; but if there was any vomiting before, it generally ceases. During the whole time of the eruption, the face is a little swelled, but seldom to any considerable degree, Sometimes, after the eruption has appeared, the fever entirely ceases; but most commonly it increases, and continues till the complete disappearance of the spots; even after this period it is often found to remain.

Though the fever should cease when the eruption has appeared, it is usual for the cough to continue for some time longer; and when the fever continues the cough never abates, and is also accompanied with an increase of the difficulty of breathing. These unfavourable symptoms are sometimes occasioned by too hot a treatment of the patient; which error, likewise, frequently gives rise to purple spots,

Sometimes the measles are succeeded by a violent looseness; and when this happens the case is attended with danger. The most fatal period in this disease is about the ninth day from the beginning of the complaint, when many are carried off by an inflammation of the lungs. The most favourable symptoms are a moderate looseness, a moisture on the skin, and a plentiful discharge of urine.

It sometimes happens that the eruption suddenly falls in, and the patient is seized with a delirium, which is a very dangerous case. Another unfavourable symptom is when the measles become too soon of a pale colour; and the same may be said o great weakness, restlessness, vomiting, and difficulty of swallowing. Purple or black spots appearing among the measles afford also a sign of great danger. When the disease is succeeded by a continuance of the cough, accompanied with hoarseness, there is reason to apprehend that a consumption of the lungs may ensue.

In the measles, as well as in the small-pox, it is necessary to observe a cool *diet*, and to drink plentifully of watery liquors. Acids, however, as they tend to increase the cough, do not suit so well as in the preceding disease. The most proper drinks are barley-water, infusions of linseed or balm, with decoctions of liquorice and marsh-mallow roots.

Cure.—In curing this disease, the great object is diligently to assist the tendency and efforts of nature. If her strength be too weak to throw out the eruption, she must be aided by blisters and proper cordials, such as wine-whey, with a few drops of the spirit of hartshorn; but when the fever is too violent, it may be restrained by bleeding; and attention must always be paid to the most urgent symptoms, such as the cough, restlessness, and difficulty of breathing. For abating the fever, the saline draughts should be used, or a julep answering the same purpose. Take of the salt of wormwood one drachm, fresh lemon-juice three or four table-spoonfuls, mint-water a gill, loaf-sugar two drachms. Mix them, and give a table-spoonful every four or five hours; but if the patient exceed the age of childhood, the dose must be increased.

When the cough and restlessness are troublesome, a tea-spoonful or two of the syrup of white poppies should be given occasionally. To abate likewise the cough, the patient should frequently hold his head over the steam of warm water, and draw it into his lungs. With the same intention, the feet should be often bathed in warm water. For relieving the cough, it will be proper to give from time to time a little spermaceti and sugar-candy pounded together.

When purple or black spots appear, the patient's drink should be sharpened with acid of vitriol; and if the putrescent disposition o the blood increase, which may be known by the blackness and the number or enlargement of the spots, a bad breath, and high-coloured urine, recourse must be had to the Peruvian bark, in the same manner as has been directed in the small-pox.

A looseness succeeding the measles will often give way to bleeding; but if this is not rendered neceſſary by any accompanying fever, the complaint may be checked by taking for ſome days a gentle doſe of toaſted rhubarb in the morning, and a little ſyrup of white poppies, or a few drops of the tincture of opium (laudanum), at night.

After the meaſles and other ſymptoms of ſickneſs are gone off, the patient ought to take a few doſes of phyſic, in the ſame way as after the ſmall-pox. But ſhould a cough, with difficulty of breathing, and other ſymptoms of a conſumption, remain after this period, ſmall quantities of blood, as the ſtrength of the patient can bear, ſhould be drawn at moderate intervals, and he ſhould be put upon the uſe of aſſes' milk, with that of a free air, and riding on horſeback.

Several years ago, Dr. Home, of Edinburgh, made ſucceſsful experiments for inoculating the meaſles in the ſame manner as the ſmall-pox. In the hands of ſome others the practice has not proved equally favourable; but it is to be wiſhed that greater attention were paid to it; for there is ſufficient evidence that ſuch practice renders the diſeaſe much more mild.

## *Chilblains.*

Chilblains or kibes are ſmall ſhining ſwellings, moſt commonly on the heels, but ſometimes on other parts, and have at firſt a whitiſh appearance, inclining to a blue caſt. They itch violently, are frequently painful, and at length vaniſh, ſometimes with, and ſometimes without, breaking or ulceration. They uſually attack children in cold weather.

At the firſt approach of the diſorder, when it is in its loweſt degree, dip the part into water that is cold, and if near to freezing ſo much the better. Let it continue in this ſituation during a minute or two: or if the cold chills and benumbs the part very much, dip it in and take it out two or three times at ſhort intervals; after which it ſhould be gently dried, and the ſame proceſs continued every morning and evening at leaſt, until all uneaſineſs is removed.

When the chilblains begin to look red and ſwell, the patient ought to take a doſe of phyſic, and to have the affected parts frequently rubbed with muſtard and brandy, ſpirits of turpentine, of wine, or ſomething of a warming nature. Another very good application is vinegar and brandy mixed, with the addition of a little allum. Let linen rags be dipped in this mixture, and kept applied to the parts. Among the common people, even urine is made uſe of with ſucceſs. To rub the parts with ſnow is highly advantageous. Some apply to them warm aſhes between cloths; and when the parts are ſwelled, this frequently helps to reduce them. If there be a sore, it must be dressed with the ointment of tutty, Turner's cerate, or some other drying application.

Chilblains are generally occasioned by the feet or hands being kept long wet or cold, and afterwards suddenly heated. In order to prevent the complaint, when winter approaches, it is a good practice to put the parts usually affected in cold water, and avoid every occasion of subjecting them to too much warmth.

### *Scald-Head.*

The scald-head consists of little ulcers, at the roots of the hair, which discharge a humour that dries into a white scab, or thick scales, and has an offensive smell. It is not only a very troublesome complaint, but often highly contagious, and, when united with a scrofulous constitution, found extremely difficult to be cured.

Cure.—When it is merely a complaint of the skin, it may be successfully treated with topical applications. If taken early, before it is spread far over the head, and while the scabby patches are small and distinct, it may frequently be cured by an ointment made of equal parts of sulphur, flower of mustard, and powder of staves-acre, mixed up with lard; first cutting off the hair; and, through the whole course of the cure, taking care to remove the scabs by frequent washing with soap and water.

If the disease has considerably extended itself, the hair must be shaved off, and the head washed twice a day with a strong decoction of tobacco; repeating this process till the scabs disappear, and fresh hair grows up from the parts they had occupied. Instead of tobacco, water in which a good quantity of yellow soap is dissolved may be used for the purpose; but both this and the decoction of tobacco should be applied warm.

These washes frequently effect a cure of themselves; but, if the disorder prove obstinate, it is of great advantage, immediately after shaving the head, and using the soap and water, to rub in very forcibly the common pitch-ointment with a good quantity of the powder of white hellebore, for near an hour at a time, always using it very warm. The head is to be afterwards covered with a bladder, to preserve the ointment on the part, as well as to keep it from sticking to the cap or other covering made use of. This process having been repeated three or four times, not only the scabs but the hairs also will become loose, and must be pulled out. When new hair springs up, free from scabs, it is a proof that the complaint is subdued. The method here recommended is no doubt painful in the operation; but some degree of severity is unavoidable, and the disorder is generally removed by these means.

The following plaster has been strongly recommended, as proving ſucceſsful in the worſt caſes. Take of common ale, one pint; of the fineſt flour, three ounces; mix them well together; and, having ſet them over a briſk fire, add two ounces of yellow reſin, ſtirring them conſtantly till they are perfectly incorporated, and have a ſmooth jelly-like appearance. Before this plaſter is laid on, the head muſt be well waſhed, and a bread and milk poultice applied, if the ſcabs are very dry.

In ſome inſtances the milder mercurial ointment has great effect, but it ſhould be cautiouſly applied; and, inſtead of being forcibly rubbed in, like other topical remedies, ſhould be only ſpread lightly, and very thin on the head; the body being at the ſame time kept open by ſome gentle purgative, ſuch as ſenna, manna, cream of tartar, or the like.

Some, in the cure of this complaint, adviſe the application of a bliſter to the head.

When the diſorder reſiſts the means above mentioned, and ſeems to be confirmed in the conſtitution, the uſe of lime-water and a decoction of the woods is adviſable.

# BOOK III.

## *FEBRILE DISEASES.*

### CHAP. I.

*Of Fevers in general, and the Inflammatory Fever.*

FEVERS are both the moſt frequent and moſt fatal diſeaſes to which mankind are liable; and, being likewiſe of ſeveral diſtinct kinds, which demand each a different method of treatment, they generally require the aid of a phyſician; without whoſe aſſiſtance ſuch errors might be committed, in the earlier ſtages of the diſeaſe, as would render it afterwards incurable by the utmoſt ſkill and attention.

SYMPTOMS.—All fevers, however, are not equally dangerous: for ſome are very ſlight and inconſiderable, performing their courſe in a ſingle day, or at moſt in two or three; but they all partake of one common ſymptom, which diſtinguiſhes their character, namely, that of an increaſed frequency of the pulſe. This, however, is not always a certain ſign of fever in all ages of the human conſtitution; for in infants the pulſe will beat ſuch a number of times in a minute, as could not take place in a man without a very high degree of fever. In the ſtate of manhood, the moſt common rate of the pulſe is about ſeventy ſtrokes in a minute. In ſome conſtitutions it is naturally more, in others a few leſs; and according to the peculiarity obſervable in any individual, when it is known, we ought to judge of the exiſtence of a fever.

But a fever is diſtinguiſhable by other ſymptoms beſides the frequency of the pulſe. It is uſually preceded by a coldneſs, or ſhivering, which is followed by a heat, a ſickneſs or loathing of food, a ſenſe of wearineſs, a pain of the head, frequently likewiſe of the back and loins, accompanied with thirſt, want of ſleep, in many a deſpondency of mind, and other particular ſymptoms or ſigns.

CAUSES.—The moſt general cauſes of fevers are infection, errors in diet, a checked perſpiration, unwholeſome air, ſuppreſſion of ufual evacuations, violent emotions of the mind, with internal and external injuries.

I fhall now proceed to treat as briefly as poffible of the different kinds of fever.

## *Inflammatory Fever.*

SYMPTOMS.—The inflammatory fever is ufually accompanied with the fymptoms above mentioned, and with a white tongue.

CURE.—If the pulfe, befides being frequent, is alfo full, it will be proper to bleed, to the quantity of ten or twelve ounces; after which fome proper purge, fuch as the following, may be given. Take of fenua two drachms, tamarinds an ounce; boil them in a pint of water for five minutes, towards the end of the boiling adding of liquorice-root fliced two drachms. Then ftrain the liquor, and diffolve in it, of cream of tartar a quarter of an ounce, manna an ounce. Let four fpoonfuls of this be given immediately, and two fpoonfuls every hour after till it begins to take effect.

If the ftomach is foul, give a vomit, confifting of twenty-five grains of the powder of ipecacuanha; caufing the patient to drink with it a fufficient quantity of chamomile-tea. After which the feet and legs fhould now be bathed in warm water.

If the difeafe be not fubdued by thefe evacuations, it is probable that nature may make an effort to carry off the complaint through other channels, viz. by thofe of perfpiration and urine. To forward this purpofe, it will be proper to ufe the following faline mixture. Take of falt of wormwood, or tartar, or prepared kali, two drachms; juice of lemons, four fpoonfuls; mint-water, a gill; loaf-fugar, half an ounce. Mix them, and give three fpoonfuls every four or five hours. If the patient complain of much heat, ten grains of nitre may be added to each dofe; with ten or fifteen drops of the wine of antimony.

During this treatment the patient is to be kept quiet in bed, but not covered with more clothes than ufual, and the room muft not be kept too warm; a low diet muft be perfevered in, fuch as gruel, panada, roafted apples, and the like; and for drink, infufions of leaves of balm, mint, or fage, barley-water, or other watery liquors, muft be plentifully taken.

Should the fever ftill continue, and run high, it may be proper to repeat the bleeding: but this muft be done with great caution, left, by bringing on too great weaknefs, the patient might not be able to fubfift through the courfe of the difeafe, the continuance of which is uncertain. If the pain in the head does not abate, the feet and legs ought again to be put into warm water, and a blifter may be applied between the fhoulders or at the back of the neck.

In caſe of great reſtleſſneſs and want of ſleep, a moderate doſe of tincture of opium may be given in ſuch fevers; but this is by no means to be practiſed where there is much pain of the head. Through the courſe of the fever, the body ought to be kept open by a clyſter every other day; and if the pulſe ſinks, the patient muſt be ſupported by proper cordials. But to regulate the degree of their ſtrength, the advice of a phyſician is alſo neceſſary. The following may be uſed for this purpoſe. Take of cinnamon-water (not the ſpirituous kind) a gill, aromatic confection three drachms, compound ſpirit of lavender two tea-ſpoonfuls, loaf-ſugar two drachms. Mix them, and give two table-ſpoonfuls every four or five hours, firſt ſhaking the bottle. Should the patient long for any food or drink in particular, it will be proper to grant it in moderation, as ſuch a deſire is often uſefully dictated by nature herſelf.

## CHAP. II.

### *Putrid or Malignant Fever.*

THE attack of this diſeaſe is generally preceded by a giddineſs, which is followed by a burning heat, ſudden loſs of ſtrength, heavineſs, lowneſs of ſpirits, watching, ſickneſs, ſometimes vomiting; an oppreſſion of the breaſt, noiſe in the ears, purple ſpots, a delirium, a catching of the tendons, a blackiſh and thin crude urine. The pulſe is low, weak, and unequal, and there are pains in various parts of the body.

CAUSES.—This fever is uſually occaſioned by foul air, ariſing from a number of people being crowded in a cloſe place, or from putrid vapours. On this account, it is frequent in camps, jails, and military hoſpitals.

This fever is likewiſe often occaſioned by a hot and moiſt conſtitution of the air, and by great inundations in low and marſhy countries, when the body is relaxed, and the natural perſpiration much obſtructed. It is alſo produced by eating fleſh or fiſh that have been too long kept; and by living too much upon animal food, eſpecially ſuch as is ſalted, without a ſuitable quantity of vegetables; whence ſeamen, on long voyages, are much expoſed to its influence. Great ſcarcity of proviſions, approaching to a famine, may likewiſe give riſe to this fever, by weakening the conſtitution, and producing a putrid ſtate of the fluids; which latter circumſtance is not unfrequently the effect of eating corn that is much damaged, and drinking water which has become putrid either by ſtagnation, or by putrid ſubſtances contained in it. This kind of fever is extremely infectious, and often attended with ſuch mortality as to reſemble the true plague.

Distinctions.—The putrid fever may be diſtinguiſhed from the inflammatory, by the ſmallneſs of the pulſe, the uncommon dejection of mind, the diſſolved ſtate of the blood, and the extreme offenſive ſmell of the excrements. It may likewiſe be diſtinguiſhed from the low or nervous fever, by the heat and thirſt being greater, the urine of a deeper colour, and the loſs of ſtrength, dejection of mind, and all the other ſymptoms more violent. It ſometimes happens, however, that the inflammatory, nervous, and putrid ſymptoms are ſo mixed together, that it is difficult to determine, eſpecially at the beginning, to which of the three claſſes the fever belongs. Here the greateſt caution and ſkill is neceſſary in adopting the mode of cure.

The duration of the putrid fever is extremely uncertain; ſometimes finiſhing its courſe between the ſeventh and fourteenth day, and at other times continuing for ſeveral weeks. The moſt favourable ſymptoms are a gentle looſeneſs after the fourth or fifth day, with a warm moiſture of the ſkin. To have little delirium is alſo a good ſign; as it likewiſe is where the tongue is moiſt, and the pulſe riſes by the uſe of wine and cordials, with an abatement of the nervous ſymptoms. The appearance of ſmall miliary pimples, in ſome meaſure reſembling a millet-ſeed, between the purple ſpots, is likewiſe favourable, as alſo are hot ſcabby eruptions about the mouth and noſe. Swellings of the glands under the ears, towards the decline of the diſeaſe, are accounted good ſigns.

Among the unfavourable ſymptoms are, the eyes much inflamed and ſtaring; the ſpeech quick, and the ſound of the voice altered; a catching of the tendons; picking of the clothes; a high delirium; perpetual watchfulneſs; conſtant ſickneſs of the ſtomach, and vomitings; a ſinking of the pulſe; coldneſs of the feet and hands, and a trembling motion of the tongue. It is conſidered as among the worſt ſigns when the patient complains of blindneſs, and picks the bed-clothes; when he ſwallows with difficulty, or cannot put out his tongue when deſired to do it; when he can lie on his back only, and pulls up his knees; or when he makes frequent attempts to get out of bed without aſſigniug any reaſon. If without his knowledge he paſſes frequent ſtools of a very offenſive ſmell, it is a ſign of approaching death.

Cure.—In the management of this fever, one of the principal objects is, to endeavour as much as poſſible to correct the putrid tendency of the fluids; to ſupport the patient's ſtrength and ſpirits, and to aſſiſt nature in reſiſting the cauſe of the diſeaſe, by the frequent admiſſion of freſh air into the chamber of the ſick; and vinegar ought to be frequently ſprinkled upon the floor of the apartment, and likewiſe cloſe to the patient. It is proper to hold vinegar, camphor, or the freſh ſkins of lemons or oranges even to his noſe. Herbs that have a ſtrong and agreeable ſcent may be laid in different parts of the room, and of the houſe likewiſe, to correct the bad air, and prevent infection as much as poſſible.

In this diſeaſe the leaſt noiſe will affect the patient's head, and the ſmalleſt fatigue be apt to make him faint; on which account he muſt not only be kept cool, but quiet and eaſy. The food muſt be light, and eaſy of digeſtion, ſuch as beef-tea, roaſted apples, barley and currants, &c. and the patient ought to eat freely of ripe fruits when they can be procured; or, in want of them, muſt take plentifully of acids in his drink. Theſe, indeed, ought to be mixed with all his food, as well as drink. Orange, lemon, or vinegar-whey are all well ſuited to the nature of the diſeaſe, and may be drunk by turns, according to the patient's inclination; and they may be rendered cordial by the addition of wine in ſuch quantity as his ſtrength ſeems to require. When very low, a glaſs of wine unmixed may now and then be allowed; and he may drink negus with only half water, and ſharpened with juice of orange or lemon. The moſt proper wine is Rheniſh; but, if the body be open, red port or claret is preferable. Where chamomile-tea ſits upon the ſtomach, it is very uſeful in this diſeaſe, and may be ſharpened by adding to every cup ten or fifteen drops of the elixir of vitriol. When the body is bound, a tea-ſpoonful of cream of tartar may be diſſolved in a cup of the patient's drink occaſionally; or he may drink a decoction of tamarinds, which will not only quench his thirſt, but promote a diſcharge by ſtool. London porter has been recommended in this fever, and frequently with good ſucceſs; but the decline of that liquor in point of quality, of late years, renders it leſs to be depended upon. A little food and drink ought frequently to be given, and always ſeaſoned with acids or aromatics, than which nothing is here more beneficial. When the delirium prevails much, it is of advantage to foment the patient's hands and feet often with a ſtrong decoction of chamomile-flowers warm; which both relieves the head, and aſſiſts in correcting the putrid tendency of the humours.

Bleeding is inadmiſſible in this fever, unleſs there appears from the pulſe and the conſtitution of the patient a ſtrong tendency to inflammation; but it can only be admitted in the beginning of the diſeaſe, and will hardly ever bear to be repeated.

A vomit at the beginning of the fever has often a good effect; but if the fever has continued for ſome days, and the patient appears to be in a weak condition, this remedy is not adviſable.

Bliſters are of little uſe in the beginning of the putrid fever;

but if the patient's pulse sinks much, and delirium, with other bad symptoms, come on, they are often productive of the best effects. They ought to be applied to the head, and inside of the legs and thighs. One inconvenience however attends them, which is, that they are sometimes apt to occasion a gangrene; and on this account, before having recourse to them, it may be proper to try the effect of sinapisms or warm poultices of mustard-seed, crumbs of bread, and vinegar, applied to the feet.

In respect of medicines, such as the following is advisable. Take of tartarised antimony three grains; of loaf-sugar one drachm. Mix them well into a powder, to be divided into six doses; one of which to be given every six hours, with two table-spoonfuls of the following mixture: Take of spearmint-water, half a gill; tincture of cinnamon, two table-spoonfuls; syrup of oranges, three table-spoonfuls. Mix them together. This frequently produces a gentle perspiration, by which the patient is much relieved; but profuse sweats are never to be encouraged in the putrid fever, as they tend to exhaust the patient, already too much weakened by the disease.

When purple or black spots appear, no time must be lost in having recourse to the Peruvian bark, which tends both to correct the putrid and dissolved state of the fluids, and to strengthen the body. It may be given thus: Take of Peruvian bark one ounce; boil it in a pint of water a few minutes, then strain it, and add of tincture of snake-root one ounce; elixir of vitriol one drachm; syrup of oranges two table-spoonfuls. Four spoonfuls to be given every fourth hour. If there be great looseness, two drachms of the aromatic confection may be added to this mixture.

Through the course of the disease an opiate, consisting of ten or fifteen drops of laudanum, may be given every night with advantage, particularly when there is a profuse looseness; and if, on the contrary, the body is bound, a clyster should be thrown up every other day, or even daily; for it is here of great consequence to keep the bowels clear of any putrid matter, which never fails to increase the fever.

In case of convulsive symptoms or hiccup, ten grains of musk powdered may be given with three table-spoonfuls of spearmint or cinnamon-water, and a bit of sugar, and repeated in four hours, if necessary.

In removing the burning heat, which is so troublesome in this fever, good effects have been found from pouring cold water, fresh or salt, or mixed with vinegar, over the patient's head, and suffered to run down all over the body, or upon the body while laid on a blanket: but this must not be done when the patient is chilly, or in a general perspiration. The proper time for it is when the heat of the patient's ſkin is ſteadily above what is natural, and chiefly in the afternoon or evening, when the increaſe of the fever, or the exacerbation, as it is called, is uſually at its height. The earlier in the fever this method is employed the more ſucceſsful it proves. When the ſkin is hot and dry the patient's drink, as well as food, ſhould be given cold.

The uſe of yeaſt has lately been recommended in this fever; but its general utility is not yet ſufficiently confirmed.

For preventing infection in ſuch fevers, Dr. Beddoes gives the following preſcription: Take of ſalt a table-ſpoonful and half; of manganeſe half a table-ſpoonful: after mixing them well in a mortar, put them into a baſon, then add of water two table-ſpoonfuls; of oil of vitriol half a table-ſpoonful. Repeat the oil of vitriol when the ſmell from the mixture ceaſes, till it has been added four times, then make a freſh mixture in the baſon. No metal muſt be put into the mixture.

## CHAP. III.

### *Slow or Nervous Fever.*

IT is obſerved that ſlow nervous fevers have, during a century paſt, greatly increaſed in this country; and doubtleſs within that period a conſiderable change has taken place in the manner of living, even among people of all ranks. The active occupations, the hardy domeſtic cuſtoms, and the ſtrengthening diet of our anceſtors, have generally given place to a luxurious effeminacy unfavourable to the vigour of the conſtitution. Hence ariſes a weakneſs of the nerves, and a long train of real or imaginary complaints that were formerly unknown.

Symptoms.—The nervous fever makes its firſt appearance with ſlight chills and ſhudderings, uncertain fluſhes of heat, and a ſenſation of wearineſs over the whole body, reſembling that which is felt after a great fatigue. It is commonly attended with a dejection of mind, and more or leſs of a ſenſe of weight, pain, or giddineſs of the head. A great numbneſs, or dull pain and coldneſs, affects the hinder part of the head frequently; and likewiſe along the middle, from the forehead to the back part. A ſickneſs at the ſtomach and a loathing of food ſoon follow, without any conſiderable thirſt, but often with an inclination to vomit, which, if it happens, brings up little elſe than inſipid phlegm. Theſe ſymptoms are commonly ſucceeded by ſome degree of delirium.

In this condition the patient often continues for five or fix days, with a heavy, pale, funk countenance; feemingly not very fick, and yet far from being well: reftlefs, anxious, and commonly deprived of fleep, though fometimes very drowfy and heavy; appearing to thofe about him actually to fleep, but is himfelf fo infenfible of it, that he does not acknowledge he has flept at all.

The pulfe during all this time is quick, weak, and unequal; fometimes fluttering, and fometimes for a few moments flow, perhaps even intermitting: and then, with a fudden flufh in the face, immediately very quick; foon after which, it may again be furprifingly calm and equal.

The heats and chills are equally variable with the pulfe: fometimes a fudden glow arifes in the cheeks, while the tip of the nofe and ears are cold, and the forehead at the fame time in a cold dewy fweat. It is even common for high colour and heat to appear in the face when the extremities are quite cold. The urine in this fever is commonly pale; frequently of a fherry or natural colour, containing either no fediment, or a kind of loofe matter like bran, fcattered up and down in it. The tongue at the beginning is feldom or never dry or difcoloured, but fometimes covered with a thin whitifh flime; but at length it often appears very dry, red, and chapped, chiefly towards the crifis of the difeafe; though the patient fcarcely ever complains of thirft, but fometimes of a heat in the tongue. About the feventh or eighth day the giddinefs, pain, or heavinefs of the head becomes much greater, with a conftant noife in it, which is very difturbing to the fick, and frequently precedes a delirium. On fuddenly fitting up in bed the patient is apt to faint. Frequently profufe fweats break forth all at once, about the ninth, tenth, or twelfth day, commonly coldifh and clammy on the extremities. Often likewife very thin ftools are difcharged. Nature now finks apace: the extremities grow cold, the pulfe rather trembles than beats; the delirium now ends in a profound lethargy, and death foon fucceeds. Moft patients grow deaf and ftupid towards the end of this difeafe. It is not uncommon for them to languifh fourteen, eighteen, or twenty days in this fever, and fometimes a much longer period.

Causes.—This fever is in general the confequence of a weaknefs of the nerves, brought on by unwholefome food, damp, foul air, immoderate watchings, hard ftudy, fatigue, grief, and, in fhort, whatever greatly diminifhes the ftrength of the conftitution.

Cure.—This fever requires that the patient be fupported by a diet moderately generous. Chicken broth, beef-tea, and light jellies, as well as panada, fhould be allowed; and a little wine may be mixed with the latter, according as the fymptoms may require. For ordinary drink, wine-whey, or negus, fharpened with the juice of orange or lemon, will be proper. Muſtard whey* alſo is highly beneficial. There is ſcarcely any thing more uſeful in this diſeaſe than good wine, particularly claret, which may be either given alone, or mixed with water, as may be moſt ſuitable to the ſtate of the patient.

In the beginning of the diſeaſe, when there is a ſickneſs and load at the ſtomach, it will be proper to give a gentle emetic, if no ſymptom forbid. Fifteen or twenty grains of the powder of ipecacuanha will beſt anſwer this purpoſe. The bowels ought then to be gently cleared of their contents by ſome mild purgative. For this purpoſe give a ſcruple of the powder of rhubarb, or uſe the following infuſion of ſenna: Take of ſenna leaves, two drachms; coriander-ſeed, half a drachm, or a few grains of ginger; infuſe them for an hour in a pint of boiling water: then pour off the liquor, and diſſolve in it an ounce of manna. Two common tea-cupfuls of this given at the diſtance of an hour from each other will probably open the body in a little time after: if not, repeat the doſe. Through the whole courſe of the diſeaſe, if nature wants to be prompted to ſtool, a clyſter of milk, ſugar, and ſalt, may be given with advantage every ſecond or third day.

If the head ſhould be much affected at the beginning of the diſeaſe, it will be proper to apply a bliſter to the back of the neck. Indeed bliſters are of ſo much conſequence in this fever, that they ought never to be omitted; and when the diſcharge occaſioned by one bliſter abates, another ſhould be immediately applied to a different part of the body.

Beſides wine, which has been already recommended, cordial medicines to promote perſpiration are always of great benefit. Take of ſpearmint-water, and ſimple cinnamon-water, each half a gill; compound powder of contrayerva one drachm and a half; loaf ſugar two drachms. Mix them, and give two table-ſpoonfuls every four or five hours, after ſhaking the glaſs. If the patient ſhould be ſeized with convulſions, add to this mixture half a drachm of muſk, and a ſcruple of caſtor, both powdered, or Hoffmann's anodyne liquor one drachm, with forty drops of laudanum.

If the fever intermits, recourſe ſhould be had to the Peruvian bark, of which half a drachm, or more, may be given every two hours with a glaſs of wine, or wine and water, as beſt ſuits the ſtate of the patient.

A miliary eruption, or an eruption of ſmall ſpots, frequently breaks out about the ninth or tenth day of the diſeaſe. This is

* To make mustard-whey, take milk and water, of each a pint; bruised mustard-seed, an ounce and a half: boil them together till the curd is perfectly separated, and afterwards strain the whey.

ſometimes the conſequence of keeping the patient too hot: but whether it ariſes from this cauſe or not, care muſt be taken not to check it, in caſe it ſhould prove to be an effort of nature for throwing off the fever.

If a looſeneſs come on, as ſometimes happens, it may be reſtrained by ſmall quantities of Venice treacle, or giving the patient the white decoction* for his ordinary drink, or by compound powder of chalk with opium, two grains every ſix hours.

If the patient ſhould be ſeized with the thruſh, viz. little whitiſh ulcers affecting the inſide of the mouth and the adjoining parts, his mouth muſt be waſhed with gargles of honey of roſes, or honey and vinegar, and tincture of myrrh, or borax and honey.

In caſe of profuſe debilitating ſweats, the Peruvian bark muſt be given, with diluted vitriolic acid, eight or ten drops in each doſe.

When ſwallowing or breathing is interrupted by tough phlegm, recourſe ſhould be had to gentle vomits of ipecacuanha, or oxymel of ſquills, to bring it up.

After the fever is gone off, it is of great importance that the invalid ſhould enjoy a pure air, and take daily exerciſe on horſeback. He ought to uſe a nouriſhing diet, with a glaſs of wine, and take half a drachm of the Peruvian bark twice a day.

## CHAP. IV.

### *The Miliary Fever.*

THIS fever receives its name from the ſmall pimples or bladders which appear on the ſkin, reſembling, in ſhape and ſize, the ſeeds of millet. They are either red or white, or a mixture of both. Sometimes they cover the whole body, but are generally more numerous on the breaſt, or back, or wherever the perſpiration is moſt plentiful.

This fever, though ſometimes an original diſeaſe, is much more often only a ſymptom of ſome other, ſuch as the ſmall-pox, meaſles, nervous fever, &c. in all which caſes it is commonly the effect of a too hot treatment or medicines.

The miliary fever chiefly attacks perſons of a relaxed habit of body, who live upon a watery diet, and take little exerciſe. It is moſt frequent among lying-in women.

* Take of powdered chalk two ounces; gum arabic, half an ounce; water, three pints. Boil to two pints, and ſtrain the decoction. It may likewiſe be made without the gum.

CAUSE.—In general, this fever takes its origin from the ſame cauſes with the ſlow nervous fever, of which I have already treated in the preceding chapter. It may likewiſe be occaſioned by the ſtoppage of any cuſtomary diſcharge, ſuch as iſſues, ſetons, the bleeding piles in men, and in women the monthly evacuation.

SYMPTOMS.—The ſymptoms of this fever are ſhivering and heat ſucceſſively, lowneſs of ſpirits, oppreſſion about the cheſt, and ſighing. On the third or fourth day the eruption generally appears on the neck, breaſt, and back, preceded by a profuſe ſweat of a peculiar ſouriſh ſmell; and it is commonly attended with a tingling or pricking of the ſkin. The eruption being completed, the ſymptoms uſually abate; and the urine, which was before pale, becomes high coloured. In about ſeven days the eruptions commonly dry, and the ſkin peels off, accompanied with a diſagreeable itching. But the diſeaſe ends not always here; for often all the former ſymptoms are renewed, and the eruption returns as before. This is an unfavourable ſign, as it ſhows the blood to be much affected.

CURE.—It is obſerved that this diſeaſe ſometimes partakes of the nature of the inflammatory fever, ſometimes of the putrid, and at others of the ſlow nervous fever; and according to the degree in which it inclines to any one of theſe, the method of cure muſt be directed. If the inflammatory fever riſes high, there will be a neceſſity for letting blood; but this muſt be done with great caution, and not without conſidering the particular cauſe of the diſeaſe, and the natural conſtitution as well as the preſent ſtate of the patient. If the ſtomach appear to be loaded, a gentle vomit of ipecacuanha ſhould be given; and afterwards, if there be no purging, the infuſion of ſenna, recommended in the preceding chapter. The firſt paſſages being thus cleared, it will be proper to give the ſaline draughts, or julep. Take of ſalt of tartar, or wormwood, or kali prepared, one drachm; juice of lemons, ſix table-ſpoonfuls; ſpearmint-water, half a gill; loaf ſugar, two drachms. Mix them, and give two ſpoonfuls every four hours. If a delirium appears, the feet muſt be bathed in warm water, and a bliſter applied between the ſhoulders, or to the back of the neck.

If the diſorder has the appearance of a putrid or ſlow fever, and there be purple or black ſpots on the ſkin, it will be neceſſary to give the Peruvian bark, as in the putrid fever; and if low nervous ſymptoms be joined with the diſeaſe, recourſe muſt be had to the cordial medicines mentioned in the treatment of the ſlow nervous fever. In ſhort, the treatment muſt be ſuited to the particular nature of the caſe; taking care to regulate circumſtances by an attention to the ſtrength of the patient and the violence of the diſeaſe. If the mouth be affected with ulcers named apthæ, or the thrush, which for the most part accompany fevers of a putrid nature, they must be treated in the manner directed in the preceding chapter.

If a violent purging should come on while the patient is in a low state, the case is attended with danger; but the evacuation must not be suddenly restrained, otherwise the feverish symptoms will certainly increase. Before any attempt is made for that purpose, it will be proper to give about fifteen grains of the powder of toasted rhubarb; and, after this, should the discharge continue, such a mixture as the following should be given: Take of mint-water and cinnamon-water, each six table-spoonfuls; compound powder of chalk with opium,* three drachms; syrup of white poppies, two table-spoonfuls. Mix them, and give two table-spoonfuls after every stool.

This fever, on one hand, is so apt to be increased by hot treatment; and, on the other, the miliary eruption is so ready to strike in, and thereby prove dangerous, by any diminution of the patient's strength, that much attention is necessary to watch the state of the patient, and support the pulse in such a degree as is best suited to keep out the eruption, without exciting any profuse sweat, which ought always to be avoided. The diet and drink should therefore be moderately cordial; the chamber be kept in a temperature neither hot nor cold; the covering of the bed be regulated likewise with regard to moderation; and, to crown the whole, the patient's *mind* should be preserved as much as possible in a state of serenity and cheerfulness. This is not a disease of frequent occurrence.

## CHAP. V.

### *The Remittent Fever.*

THIS fever differs both from the continual and intermittent kinds, and partakes in some measure of the nature of each, but chiefly resembles the intermittent, to which it is more nearly allied; for after a certain number of hours, though not any fixed period, it is attended with a remission or abatement, but not a total cessation of fever.

Causes.—Remitting fevers attack chiefly persons of a relaxed habit of body, who live in moist situations, breathe impure air, and use watery unwholesome diet. They are particularly frequent

* For this powder, see *Appendix*.

in low marſhy countries abounding with wood and ſtagnating water; and nothing is more favourable to their production than heat and moiſture combined. They are moſt frequent in cloſe calm weather, and in the months of July and Auguſt.

Symptoms.—For the moſt part, this fever comes on ſuddenly, with weakneſs, lowneſs of ſpirits, fits of heat and cold by turns, and other feveriſh ſymptoms. The pulſe is ſmall and quick, the hands tremble, the countenance is pale or yellowiſh, the ſkin dry, and there is a difficulty of breathing. Beſides a pain and giddineſs of the head, the patient is ſometimes affected with a delirium at the very firſt attack. There is a pain, and ſometimes a ſwelling, about the region of the ſtomach, accompanied with a vomiting of bile, and ſometimes a diſcharge of it by ſtool. In ſome patients there is a looſeneſs, in others the oppoſite extreme. At length a moiſture appears on the face, and afterwards on the other parts of the body, when the remiſſion enſues.

Cure.—In curing this fever, the principal object is to bring it to a regular remiſſion, which end is moſt ſucceſsfully obtained by ſupporting the diſeaſe at a moderate pitch. Bleeding is not adviſable, unleſs there be evident ſigns of inflammation; but in moſt caſes, ſix or eight grains of ipecacuanha, with one or two of tartar emetic, may be given, as a vomit, with advantage. After this, if the body be bound, it may be opened with the following decoction: Take of ſenna leaves, a drachm and a half; tamarinds, an ounce. Boil them in a pint of water for five minutes. Then ſtrain, and diſſolve in the liquor one ounce of manna, and two drachms of cryſtals of tartar. Let the patient take four table-ſpoonfuls of this decoction every hour till a ſtool is procured.

Afterwards, to bring the fever ſooner to a criſis, or to regular intermiſſions, it will be proper to give the ſaline draughts, mentioned in the cure of the inflammatory fever, or to make uſe of the following mixture: Take of ſpearmint-water, half a gill; ſimple cinnamon-water, four table ſpoonfuls; camphor, one ſcruple; nitre, two ſcruples; tartariſed antimony, ten grains; loaf-ſugar, two drachms. Mix them, and give two table-ſpoonfuls every four hours.

As ſoon as a remiſſion is perceived, the Peruvian bark muſt be immediately given, in the quantity of half a drachm, two ſcruples, or upwards, and repeated every two or three hours; by which the uſual increaſe of the fever may be prevented, and the diſeaſe entirely ſubdued. The bark is, at this period, the great and indiſpenſable reſource, and it can hardly be given too freely, accompanied, as it ought to be, with wine and aromatics.

Fowler's ſolution of arſenic has been found an efficacious remedy both in this and the intermittent fever.

In the more advanced ſtages of this diſeaſe, in hot climates, the mouth, teeth, and inſide of the lips are covered with a black cruſt, and the tongue becomes ſo dry and ſtiff that the patient's voice can ſcarcely be heard. Among favourable ſymptoms are, inflammatory ſpots in the laſt ſtage of the diſeaſe, particularly on the breaſt, arms, or belly; as is likewiſe a plentiful and general perſpiration over the body; inſtead of which the patient is ſometimes relieved by voiding great quantities of urine.

The treatment of the patient, reſpecting diet, muſt be ſuited to the degree and ſymptoms of the diſeaſe. When there are any ſigns of inflammation, every thing of a heating quality, both in food and drink, muſt be avoided; but when the diſorder is accompanied with nervous or putrid ſymptoms, the patient muſt be ſupported with ſuch diet and cordial liquors as have been mentioned in treating of thoſe fevers. Wine, given with the bark, when the remiſſions are conſiderable, has often excellent effects; but we ought to beware of changing the fever from a remittent into a continual kind, by a management too heating and inflammatory.

In all the variations of the diſeaſe, the patient ſhould be kept cool and quiet, as in every other fever. Freſh air ought to be frequently admitted into the apartment by the windows and doors; and it will be rendered more wholeſome if often ſprinkled with vinegar. Both linen and bed clothes ſhould be frequently changed, and the excrements immediately removed: for too much attention cannot be given towards keeping the air of the chamber pure and untainted.

## CHAP. VI.

### *Intermittent Fever, or Ague.*

INTERMITTENT fevers derive their name from the manner in which they proceed; there being a perfect interruption of every ſymptom from the end of one fit to the beginning of another. An ague, on its firſt attack, may not always be diſtinguiſhed from a continued fever; but after one fit is over its character may be known, though the time of its return cannot be fixed poſitively till after a ſecond fit comes on. In one kind, called a quotidian, and which approaches near to a continued fever, the fit returns every day; in the tertian it returns every other day, or after the expiration of forty-eight hours; and in a quartan it returns every fourth day. Thoſe intermittents are called vernal which begin in

February, and prevail during the two or three following months; and thofe, on the other hand, autum nal, which appear in Auguft, or fomewhat later. The former are reckoned the leaft hurtful; indeed a tertian, in the fpring, is thought by many to contribute to health. Of all the kinds of intermittents, the tertian is the moft common, and eafily cured.

Symptoms.—The intermittent fever begins with yawning and ftretching, a naufea or ficknefs at the ftomach, fometimes a vomiting; with pain of the head, back, and limbs. Thefe fymptoms are either attended or fucceeded by cold fhiverings and chattering of the teeth, though the blood is at this time in a ftate of increafed rather than diminifhed heat. The pulfe is weak, and extremely quick; the breathing is difficult, and the urine pale. Such is the firft ftage of the difeafe, which fometimes continues several hours, but at others not more than half an hour, though in general it remains between one and two hours.

In the fecond ftage the hot fit begins, when the ficknefs, anxiety, and difficulty of breathing remain, but go off by degrees as the pulfe becomes fuller and ftronger. Befides the heat, there is exceffive thirft, violent head-ach, and frequently delirium; fometimes even a difpofition to lethargy, or apoplexy. The tongue is white, the urine now high-coloured; and there is often a heat at the pit of the ftomach, attended with pain, if not likewife with fwelling.

This ftage having no fixed period, the time of its continuance is uncertain; but it is generally followed by a fweat, in confequence of which all the feverifh fymptoms difappear.

Causes.—As intermittent fevers are moft frequent in low marfhy countries, they feem to be occafioned chiefly by vapours from putrid ftagnating water; but even in more high fituations, a long continued moifture of the air is apt to produce them in perfons of a relaxed habit of body. A poor watery diet difpofes people much to thefe fevers; as does likewife a dampnefs in the walls and the lower parts of houfes; and they are known to be frequently caught by imprudently lying upon the damp ground. Whatever relaxes the body, and diminifhes perfpiration, has a tendency to excite thefe fevers in particular conftitutions.

Cure.—During the firft fit of an ague, whether the cold or hot, there is no opportunity for giving medicine; but when the latter has come on, the patient ought to drink freely of water-gruel, weak chamomile-tea, and the like; but if his fpirits be low, he may be allowed fome weak wine-whey, fharpened with the juice of lemon. It is neceffary that all his drink be warm, for the purpofe of promoting fweat, which is the natural crifis of the difeafe.

Between the fits, the patient's food ought to be nourifhing and easy of digestion; such as broths made of the tender meats, especially beef-tea, light puddings, &c. For drink he may use wine and water, or small negus, to which is added a little of the juice of lemons or oranges. If he takes occasionally a cup of chamomile or wormwood-tea, it will serve both as drink and medicine. Much likewise depends upon his taking proper exercise between the fits. Riding on horseback, or in a carriage, when there is nothing to forbid it, is highly useful. Even walking in the apartment, or through the house, though without the advantage of a free open air, is preferable to a state of inactivity; to which, however, the patient, either from weakness or inclination, is often much disposed.

It is not uncommon for intermitting fevers, especially in those who use brisk exercise, to go off without medicine, or at least to be felt very slightly at the usual periods of their return. Some patients, in expectation of such an event, allow the disease to take its course for a considerable time, and often with impunity; especially if they guard well against watery diet and dampness, and the state of the weather be favourable to a recovery. Many likewise are inclined to this practice, not only from an opinion that an ague is good for securing the health, but that the cure of it, by the bark in particular, is accompanied with danger. It is undoubtedly true, that the repeated fits of an intermittent fever sometimes produce a favourable change in the constitution. But this happens chiefly to persons of a bad habit of body; and such being for the most part either naturally weak, or their strength being impaired by the long continuance of some complaint, they are less able to bear the repeated shocks of an intermittent fever, when violent. And I may safely affirm, that if there be any diseases which yield to the shivering, the hot fit, and the sweat, which comprise a fit of an ague, they may likewise be cured by means far less severe, and not injurious to the constitution.

It is seldom necessary to bleed in an intermittent fever, the pulse being in general not so full as to demand it; but to cleanse the stomach and bowels, in the beginning of the disease, is always attended with advantage: for nothing so much supports the fever as a foulness and load of those parts; and until they be relieved, it is in vain to expect either a speedy or perfect cure of the disorder. Indeed nature herself points out the propriety of having recourse to such means: for great quantities of bile are frequently discharged by vomiting; and the stomach is found to be lined with a tough phlegm, extremely injurious to digestion, and productive of various complaints. In order therefore to cleanse the stomach, it will be proper to employ the powder of ipecacuanha, twenty or thirty grains of which will be a dose for a grown up person. The best time for taking it is two or three hours before the return of the fit, that its operation may be completed when the fever next comes on; and the vomiting should be promoted by drinking plentifully of chamomile-tea.

The action of vomiting imitates in some measure the fit of an ague, by putting into motion, and agitating the whole frame; whence it not only cleanses the stomach, but excites a general exertion through the vessels of the body, and tends greatly to promote perspiration, which is the ordinary crisis of intermittent fevers.

Notwithstanding a vomit has been taken, and more especially if the patient has an utter aversion to vomiting, some purgative medicine will be proper; and it ought, like the vomit, to be given not only during the intermission, but immediately after the fit has ceased, that its operation should likewise be finished before the next return of the fit. This purpose may be sufficiently answered by a dose of rhubarb, Glauber's salts, or crystals of tartar; to the latter of which, dissolved in hot water, some manna may be added.

Both these discharges, viz. vomiting and purging, produce so good an effect, that an intermittent fever often yields to them, or even to one of the two, without the use of any other medicine; especially if a grain of opium or fifteen grains of opiate confection be taken after the operation of the emetics.

When, during the intermission of the fever, there is an even, steady, soft pulse, with a plentiful sediment in the urine, we may be well assured that the patient is in a proper condition for taking the Peruvian bark; but indeed there is no ground for hesitation after the stomach and bowels are cleansed.

The best form of giving this valuable medicine is in powder, with a glass of Port wine. On many stomachs it is found to sit most easily mixed with a cup of milk; but it may be given in any thing most agreeable to the patient's palate; and greater regard should be had to his taste in this respect, as a dose must be taken very often to prevent the return of the fever. It is generally found, that in an adult, or grown up person, from six drachms to an ounce of bark, begun to be taken immediately after the fit, will answer this purpose. Two scruples, or even a whole drachm, if the patient's stomach can bear it, may be given at a time, and the frequency of the dose be regulated by the usual return of the fits. Thus, in a quotidian, or an ague that returns every day, a dose ought to be taken every two hours; in a tertian, or that which returns the second day, every three hours; and in a quartan, every four hours. Where the patient cannot take so large a dose of the bark, the quantity may be diminished, and taken more frequently. A smaller quantity is likewise sufficient for young persons, and that in proportion to their age.

But though another fit of the ague has been prevented by the bark, the uſe of this medicine muſt not be immediately laid aſide, but a doſe of it be taken at leaſt three times a day, for two or three days; then twice a day for one week, and once a day for another; by which means we may inſure a ſecurity againſt the return of the complaint.

It is obſerved, however, that thoſe who have once had this diſeaſe are more liable to a return of it than others, eſpecially during a ſtate of the air favourable to its production. This diſpoſition is moſt frequent in cold moiſt weather, and when there is an eaſterly wind; on which account, ſuch perſons ought, at thoſe times, to take a doſe of the bark every morning. For this purpoſe, they may infuſe an ounce of it, with one drachm of gentian-root, and two drachms of the freſh outer rind of Seville oranges, in a quart of brandy, for three or four days; and afterwards filter it through paper. About half a wine-glaſsful of this tincture may be taken for a doſe. Inſtead of brandy the ſame quantity of white wine, if more agreeable to the taſte, may be uſed.

When the bark cannot be taken in ſubſtance, it may be given in decoction or infuſion. To make the former, Take of bark, two ounces; water, four pints; boil it to three pints and a half; then ſtrain the liquor while hot, and diſſolve in it two drachms of ſal ammoniac. Four ſpoonfuls of this decoction may be taken for a doſe.

For an infuſion, take of the powder of bark, an ounce; Virginian ſnake-root, two drachms; hot water, a pint: infuſe for twenty-four hours, and to the ſtrained liquor add, of ſtrong cinnamon-water four table-ſpoonfuls. Three or four table-ſpoonfuls for a doſe.

The bark, in whatever form it is taken, may be rendered more efficacious by the addition of other bitter medicines, ſuch as gentian-root, chamomile flowers, the rind of Seville oranges, quaſſia and the like; and it will alſo be more efficacious when aſſiſted by brandy, or other warm cordials.

When the ſtomach cannot bear the bark in ſuch doſes as are neceſſary, it may be given by clyſter. For this purpoſe, infuſe half an ounce of extract of bark in half a gill of warm water; to which add one table-ſpoonful of oil of olives, and ſix or eight drops of laudanum. Such a clyſter is to be repeated every fourth hour, or oftener, as there may be occaſion. The quantity of the extract and laudanum muſt be leſſened proportionably for children.

Children have alſo been cured of agues, by means of a waiſtcoat with powdered bark quilted between the folds of it, as they likewiſe have by being bathed frequently in a decoction of the bark. The ſame purpoſe is ſometimes anſwered by rubbing the ſpine, or back-bone with ſtrong ſpirits; or with a mixture of equal parts of compound ſoap liniment and laudanum. Wine-whey, to half a pint of which is joined a tea-ſpoonful of the ſpirit of hartſhorn, may be given to young children by way of drink. It may be added that ſuch patients have received great benefit from the following julep: Take of ſalt of tartar, or kali prepared, one drachm; freſh juice of lemons, three table-ſpoonfuls: in leſs than a minute after they are mixed, or as ſoon as the effervefcence ceaſes, add of mint-water, two table-ſpoonfuls; common water, and ſimple ſyrup, each one table-ſpoonful. Inſtead of the ſyrup a bit of loaf-ſugar may be uſed. To a child four or five years old, three tea-ſpoonfuls of this julep may be given every two hours.

It is not to children alone that this remedy proves uſeful: for medicines of the ſame nature may be taken with advantage by grown up perſons, eſpecially when the hot fit of the ague is accompanied with ſigns of inflammation.

Sometimes the bark has a tendency to paſs off through the bowels: when this happens, it it neceſſary to add a few drops of laudanum to each doſe; but if, on the contrary, the patient be coſtive, a few grains of rhubarb may be joined to the bark occaſionally.

It is a peculiar circumſtance in the intermittent fever, that it is often cured by medicines termed narcotic; ſuch as, for inſtance, the ſyrup of white poppies, and laudanum. Two or three tea-ſpoonfuls of the ſyrup given to a young child, in the hot fit, has been often known to ſtop the diſeaſe; and in grown up perſons laudanum is found no leſs effectual, when taken in the quantity of fifteen or twenty drops, half an hour after the hot fit has begun. This medicine relieves the head-ach and fever, and promotes a profuſe ſweat. The practice was introduced by the late Dr. Lind at Portſmouth, who gave the remedy in about two ounces of ſacred tincture, when the patient was coſtive, ordering the bark immediately after the fit.

When the diſeaſe does not yield to the bark, a few gallons of cold water, or brine, daſhed over the patient when the hot ſtage is completely formed, but before perſpiration comes on, brings the fit to a ſpeedy termination; and it is certain that during a perfect intermiſſion, the cold-bath has a powerful effect in preventing the return of the fever.

White arſenic has been recommended in this diſeaſe, as well as in the remittent fever, eſpecially Fowler's ſolution, which is ſold at Apothecaries-Hall, &c. and may be given in doſes of *ſeven to ten drops* every ſix hours in any pleaſant tea.

It would be endleſs to mention the great number of empirical remedies, which have been handed down by popular tradition, and indeed are daily multiplying, for the cure of intermitting fevers.

Even cobwebs, ſpiders, and the ſnuffings of candles, have each had their zealous admirers. It is probable that many of thoſe ſubſtances are entirely indebted for their reputation to ſome favourable circumſtance. Having been ſwallowed by accident, at a time when nature was inwardly, though ſecretly, conquering the diſeaſe, credulity has aſcribed the whole merit of the enſuing cure to the virtues of the viſible object.

But in the cure of agues in particular, there is certainly no occaſion for recourſe to whimſical remedies, much leſs to ſuch as are nauſeous even to think of. For, beſides the Peruvian bark, which is almoſt ſovereign in theſe diſeaſes, the preparations of iron are of acknowledged efficacy; and there is hardly an herb, or other ſubſtance, which yields either a roughneſs on the palate, ſuch as oak-bark, and alum, or a bitteriſh taſte, as chamomile-flowers, that is not highly ſerviceable againſt intermittent fevers. To theſe two claſſes I might add a third, namely, that of aromatic or ſpicy ſubſtances, which, joined to the two former, have conſiderable effect in the cure of the moſt obſtinate agues, eſpecially in rainy ſeaſons and damp ſituations, and in perſons advanced in years, or of a cold phlegmatic conſtitution.

It is however to be lamented, that amidſt the great abundance of remedies of unqueſtionable virtue, a perſon who has an ague ſhould ever truſt for a cure to any thing either of a doubtful or inſignificant nature: for, intermitting fevers being often accompanied with other diſorders, or with dangerous ſymptoms attendant on themſelves, every retardment or diſappointment of cure is apt to have pernicious effects, both by weakening the patient through the long continuance of the diſeaſe, and affording time to the other malady to increaſe, and perhaps become incurable. Though an ague is generally cured by ordinary means, if properly made uſe of, yet, as it ſometimes reſiſts the moſt powerful medicines, it ought never to be trifled with, when obſtinate; eſpecially if, during the intermiſſions, the patient is not entirely free from complaint. In all unfavourable caſes of this kind, it is proper to have recourſe to the aſſiſtance of a phyſician, before it be too late.

## CHAP. VII.

### *Milk-Fever.*

THIS fever is peculiar to women in child-bed. It frequently arises about the second, but more commonly on the third or fourth day after delivery; accompanied with swelling of the breasts, and pain shooting towards the arm-pits. The breasts are sometimes hard, hot, and inflamed. The disease is seldom of any great consequence, if the patient lies quiet, uses a thin diet, and takes freely of weak drinks. It generally continues a day or two, at which time it goes off in plentiful sweats and discharges of pale urine. Or, if the milk be suddenly driven back, the patient is sometimes relieved by a critical diarrhoea, or loosenefs.

CURE.—If the disorder should prove violent, as sometimes happens in young women of a full habit of body, the inflammation ought to be abated by bleeding; but this is seldom necessary. In every constitution, however, the body must be kept open by gentle cooling purges, or clysters. To answer the former purpose, take half an ounce of crystals of tartar; dissolve it in a pint of boiling water, and add to it an ounce of manna. A tea-cupful of this may be taken every two hours, till it produces a stool. As to the clyster, it may be made of milk, with some moist sugar, and salt, and a spoonful or two of sweet oil.

The breasts should be drawn by the child, in preference to any other person, or contrivance; but, if the mother does not intend to give suck, by some proper person who will do it gently, and in such a manner as only to lessen the fullness of the breasts, and so to diminish the pain. Both the swelling of the breasts and all these consequences might be prevented, were it not for the absurd custom of not allowing infants to suck for the first two or three days; a practice not only contrary to nature, but extremely hurtful both to the mother and child. The practice, however, of having the breasts drawn by another person is seldom required.

If the breasts are hard or inflamed, softening fomentations and poultices may be applied to them. The common poultice of bread and milk, with the addition of a little oil, or fresh butter, may be used on this occasion, and renewed twice a day, till the swelling be either discussed or brought to suppuration; and as a fomentation, warm milk, or a decoction of elder flowers. For discussing the swelling, the following fomentation, if used in time, is generally effectual: Take the heads of four white poppies: boil them

In a quart of common water to a pint; then ſtrain, and diſſolve in the liquor ſix drachms of crude ſal ammoniac.

In general, it is much better to let the tumor break of itſelf, than to open it either with the lancet or cauſtic. The ulcer is afterwards to be dreſſed with digeſtive ointments, in the uſual manner.

Chapped or ſore nipples are very frequent with thoſe who give ſuck; in which caſe, freſh cream ſpread upon fine linen, or a ſolution of gum arabic in water, is a very proper application.

If the nipples be ſoft and moiſt, apply the following liniment: Take of hog's lard, half an ounce; Armenian bole, ſtarch, and ſugar, all powdered, of each one drachm. Mix them into an ointment.

It is almoſt unneceſſary to obſerve, that whatever applications be made uſe of to the nipples, they ought always to be waſhed off before the child is permitted to ſuck.

During the milk-fever the patient ſhould uſe a thin diet, conſiſting of gruel, panada, and the like; and her drink be barley-water, milk and water, weak tea, or whatever of the watery kind is moſt agreeable to her taſte.

## CHAP. VIII.

### *Puerperal, or Child-bed Fever.*

THIS fever generally begins the firſt, ſecond, or third day, ſometimes later, after delivery, with a chillineſs, which is followed by violent pains of the belly (abdomen), and a ſoreneſs extending over the whole of that part, ſcarce capable of bearing the gentleſt touch. The belly is ſometimes ſoft, ſometimes greatly ſwelled. The pulſe is quick and weak, though ſometimes it will reſiſt the finger pretty ſtrongly. There is much thirſt; pain in the head, chiefly in the forehead, and parts about the eye-brows; a fluſhing in the face; anxiety; a ſhortneſs of breathing; a ſuppreſſion of the natural purgations after delivery; high-coloured urine; and a hot, dry ſkin. Sometimes vomiting and purging attend from the beginning; but in general, at firſt, the body is coſtive. When the diſeaſe proves fatal, however, a looſeneſs generally comes on, and the ſtools at laſt come away unknown to the patient.

Such, in general, is the courſe of the puerperal fever; the ſymptoms of which, however, may be often varied, according to the conſtitution of the patient, the degree of the diſeaſe, and its earlier or later invaſion. When the woman is naturally weak, or her ſtrength has been greatly reduced by immoderate evacuations after delivery; when the disease is violent, and immediately follows that period, its progress and termination are proportionably rapid and fatal. In such circumstances many have been known to expire within twenty-four hours from the first attack of the disease. This event, however, is generally suspended for some days; and the number of these is variable, though the eleventh from the beginning of the fever may be regarded as the period which is usually decisive. In whatever stage of the disease an unfavourable termination may happen, it would seem that the beginning of the patient's recovery is not marked by any critical symptoms in the fever, as depending on an alteration of the humours; but that the cure is gradually effected, either by vomiting, or a long continued discharge, by stool, of that corrupted matter, the existence of which, in the stomach, is usually apparent at the first attack of the disease. It is, therefore, a dangerous case, where the weakness of the patient is such as renders her unable to support so tedious a discharge as that by which the fever is carried off. When the natural purgation returns to its former state, when the swelling and tenderness of the belly abate, and there is a moisture on the skin, these symptoms afford reason to hope for a happy termination of the disease.

Though this fever may generally be known from the description now given of it, and chiefly by that remarkable tenderness of the belly which particularly distinguishes it; yet, as some of its symptoms may be confounded with those arising from other diseases, and which require a different method of cure, it will be proper to mention here the circumstances by which it may be known with greater certainty.

The pains of the belly, attending the child-bed fever, may be distinguished from those called *after-pains*, by their uninterrupted continuance, sometimes increased, through the course of the disease; whereas the after-pains often totally intermit. The latter likewise are accompanied with no symptoms of fever.

Many circumstances show a difference between the puerperal and miliary fevers, notwithstanding the symptoms of anxiety, and oppression at the breast, are common to both. In the puerperal fever, the chillness is more violent, of longer duration, and not interrupted as in the other. The pulse is fuller and stronger; the skin is more hot; and the tongue, whether moist or dry, though generally the latter, is not of a white but brownish appearance; and the urine is also higher coloured. Eruptions on the skin, which prove serviceable in miliary fevers, procure no abatement of the puerperal fever, and cordials generally increase it.

When the original attack of the puerperal fever happens to coincide in point of time with that of the milk-fever, the nature of it may at firſt be miſtaken; but the ſymptoms, and greater violence of the diſeaſe, muſt in a ſhort time diſſipate ſuch an error.

Causes.—Notwithſtanding the prevalence of this diſeaſe in all ages, its real nature has remained to the preſent time a ſubject of much diſpute and uncertainty. Some have conſidered it as proceeding entirely from an inflammation of the womb, or peritonæum; others have ſuppoſed it to be the conſequence of an obſtruction to the ſecretion of the milk; while others have been inclined to impute it to a ſtoppage of the purgation after delivery.

"The apparent indications and contra-indications of bleeding, and other remedies," ſays Dr. Manning, "ariſing from the complication of inflammatory and putrid ſymptoms; the equivocal appearance of vomiting and purging, as whether they be critical or ſymptomatical; and the different cauſes whence ſymptoms ſimilar to each other may ariſe in pregnant women; all theſe circumſtances concur to involve the ſubject in great obſcurity and indeciſion."

One of the moſt eſſential points to be aſcertained in the cure of the child-bed fever, reſpects the propriety of bleeding. A free uſe of the lancet has been generally regarded as the moſt ſucceſsful expedient in practice; but Dr. Denman thinks we may ſafely affirm from experience, that for one who will receive benefit by large bleeding, a much greater number will be injured, and that even almoſt irretrievably. Indeed, whoever regulates his practice by fact and obſervation, will be convinced that bleeding, eſpecially in any great quantity, is, in general, very far from being attended with ſucceſs. Bleeding is ſeldom proper, except in women of a full habit of body, and in whom the ſigns of inflammation run high; nor even in ſuch patients ought it to be repeated without great caution.

The genuine nature and effects of the looſeneſs in this diſeaſe, is another diſputed point of the higheſt importance. Phyſicians obſerving that women who die of the puerperal fever are generally moleſted with that evacuation, have been led to conſider this ſymptom as of the moſt dangerous and fatal tendency; and what we therefore ſhould endeavour by every means to reſtrain. In this opinion, however, they would ſeem to be governed by too partial an obſervation of facts. For experience certainly authoriſes the aſſertion, that more women appear to have recovered of the child-bed fever, by means of a looſeneſs, than have been deſtroyed by that cauſe. If it alſo be conſidered, that purging is uſually almoſt the only ſenſible evacuation in the more advanced ſtage of the diſeaſe; and is that which accompanies it to its lateſt period, there is the ſtrongeſt reaſon to think that it is critical rather than ſymptomatical, and ought therefore to be moderately ſupported, inſtead of being unwarily reſtrained. Nay, the advantage which is found to attend vomiting, as well as purging, in the earlier ſtage of the diſeaſe, would ſeem to prove beyond contradiction, that the matter diſcharged by thoſe evacuations is what chiefly foments the diſeaſe. Vomits and purges, therefore, are the only medicines on which any rational dependance is to be placed in this fever; at leaſt, they are certainly ſuch as are found the moſt ſucceſsful. It is an eſtabliſhed rule in practice, to preſcribe a vomit at the beginning of every fever attended with any nauſea or loathing of the ſtomach, and where there is no reaſon to apprehend an inflammation of that organ. Nor does the ſtate of child-bed women afford the ſmalleſt ground for prohibiting a recourſe to the ſame means for anſwering a ſimilar purpoſe.

Cure.—It is ſo ſeldom a phyſician is called at the very onſet of the puerperal fever, that he has few opportunities of trying the effects of remedies in that early ſtage of the diſeaſe. When ſuch occur, however, and the patient is in what is called the rigor of the fever, or the ſtate of chillneſs, we ſhould endeavour as much as poſſible to ſhorten that period, as the ſucceeding fever is generally found to bear a proportion to the violence and duration of it. For this purpoſe, warm diluting drinks, ſuch as gruel, barley-water, &c. ſhould be plentifully uſed, with a ſmall quantity of volatile ſpirits or brandy. In this ſituation, a diſh or two of warm ſack-whey is attended with advantage. But care muſt be taken not to give any thing too ſtrong, which is a caution that ought always to be remembered: for, though a freer uſe of the more cordial and ſpirituous kinds of liquors might perhaps ſoon abate rigor, there is danger to be feared from their influence on the approaching fever, eſpecially in women of a ſtrong and healthy conſtitution. In all caſes, warm applications to the extremities, ſuch as heated bricks, towels, or toaſted grains in a linen bag, may be uſed with perfect ſafety, and ſome advantage.

When the hot fit is come on, an injection of milk and water, or the like, ought to be immediately given, and frequently repeated through the courſe of the diſeaſe. Theſe prove beneficial, not only by promoting the diſcharge from the inteſtines, which ſeems in fact to be the means of curing the diſeaſe; but alſo by acting as a kindly fomentation to the womb and adjacent parts. With this intention they are particularly ſerviceable when the natural purgation is ſuppreſſed. Great care, however, is requiſite in giving them, on account of the tenderneſs and inflammatory diſpoſition, which at that time render the parts about the bottom of the belly extremely delicate with reſpect to the ſenſe of pain.

The next ſtep in the method of cure ought to be, to promote the diſcharge of the corrupted matter from the ſtomach and inteſtines. For this intention Dr. Denman prescribes the following remedy; Take of tartarised antimony, or emetic tartar, two grains; crabs eyes, prepared, one scruple. Mix them well together into a powder. Of this he gives from two to six grains, and repeats it as circumstances require. If the first dose does not produce any sensible effect, he repeats it in an increased quantity at the end of two hours, and proceeds in that manner, not expecting any benefit but from some evident discharge produced by it.

Should the disease be abated, but not removed (which sometimes happens) by the effect of the first dose, the same medicine must be repeated, but in a less quantity, till all danger be over; but if any alarming symptoms remain, the powder should be repeated in the same quantity as first given; though this is seldom necessary, if the first dose operates properly.

If the first dose produce any considerable effect by vomiting, procuring stools, or plentifully sweating, a repetition of the medicine in a less quantity will seldom fail to answer our expectations; but great judgment is required in adapting the quantity first given, to the strength of the patient, and other circumstances.

Saline draughts, made of salt of wormwood, tartar, or kali, and the juice of lemons, as have been before prescribed in other fevers, ought to be frequently given; which not only promote the discharge by the intestines, but likewise increase those by urine and perspiration. These medicines are particularly serviceable in subduing the remains of the fever, after its violence has been broken by the more efficacious remedies above mentioned; but when they are used even in the decline of the disease, gentle laxatives of rhubarb and magnesia ought to be frequently interposed; since, without stools, little service can be done in this disease.

Notwithstanding the discharge by the intestines appears to have the most beneficial effect in this disease; yet when the stomach has not been properly unloaded of offensive matter, though a great nausea and sickness had indicated the expediency of such an evacuation at the beginning of the fever, the continuance of the looseness is sometimes so long protracted as in the end to prove fatal. In this alarming state of the distemper, when the very frequent and involuntary discharges by stool, and all appearances, threaten danger, Dr. Denman says, that an injection made of linseed-tea, or chicken-water, and given every one, two, or three hours, or as often as possible without fatiguing the patient too much, with the following draught taken every six hours, has produced better effects than could be expected: Take of the powder of ipecacuanha one grain; opiate confection one scruple; mint-water, or cinnamon-water, an ounce and a half, which is about three table-spoonfuls. Mix them into a draught.

While these medicines are using, we should endeavour to mitigate the pains of the belly by softening applications. Take of chamomile-flowers two handfuls; the leaves of rue, or feverfew, one handful; three white poppy heads; fresh root of althæa, or marsh-mallows, one ounce. Let them be well beat, and boiled for five minutes, in a sufficient quantity of water. This decoction will serve as a fomentation, and the ingredients may be used as a poultice.

So great a variety of opinions has been entertained by late writers, respecting the nature and immediate cause of this disease, that it would be tedious to recite them: besides that such a narrative might justly be deemed unsuitable to the present work; the object of which is, not to examine the foundation of theoretical opinions, but to deliver, in the plainest manner, such practical observations and precepts as may be useful towards acquiring a competent degree of knowledge in the method of curing diseases.

Suffice it therefore to say, that the opinions of those writers are in general directly contrary to each other. But what is yet more remarkable, though they differ so widely with regard to speculative points, they come nearer to an agreement in the method of cure than could well be expected; and, in general, it is conformable to what has been delivered above.

From the account which has been given of this fever, it must appear clearly to be a disease of a very dangerous nature, when violent; and that to conduct a patient successfully through it, requires the utmost judgment and ability of a skilful physician. It is unnecessary to say any thing more towards guarding against too much confidence in the treatment of this fever. I shall therefore conclude with observing, that from all the most accurate accounts of this disease, and from the period at which it generally commenees, there seems reason to infer, that it owes its rise more immediately to accidents after delivery: for it is allowed, that it may follow a labour under the best and most favourable circumstances, though endeavours to dilate the os internum are supposed frequently to produce it. The more immediate causes generally assigned by authors are a stoppage of perspiration, the too free use of spices, and the neglect of procuring stools after delivery; sudden frights, too hasty a separation of the placenta, and binding the belly too tight. It is generally observed to be the most prevalent in an unhealthy season, and among women of a weakly and scorbutic constitution.

## CHAP. IX.

### *The Simple Scarlet Fever.*

THIS fever receives its name from the colour which it produces on the ſkin. It begins with a chillneſs and ſhivering like other fevers, but without much ſickneſs. Then follow heat, thirſt, and head-ach; ſometimes in a very moderate degree, at others more violent. About the fourth day the face ſwells, and the eruption makes its appearance, in a ſhape much broader, but leſs uniform than thoſe of the meaſles; from which it is diſtinguiſhed by a red-coloured effuſion, rather than diſtinct ſpots, and by not being accompanied with any cough, or watering of the eyes. In three or four days the redneſs diſappears, and the outer ſkin peels off in branny ſcales,. which in many caſes return for two or three times. It generally appears towards the end of ſummer, and is more frequent among children than grown up perſons. Sometimes ſpots break out on the body like the ſtinging of nettles, attended with much itching. But in three or four days, like the former, they entirely ceaſe, and are followed by a ſeparation from the ſkin in extremely ſmall ſcales.

CURE.—This is a diſorder of the moſt ſimple nature, requiring nothing more than abſtinence from animal food, viz. fleſh, fiſh, and fowl, and the keeping out of the cold air, with the free uſe of watery liquids, thin gruel, and moderate warmth whilſt in bed; but if the ſymptoms ſhould run high, and the pulſe be very quick, full, and ſtrong, bleeding may be neceſſary; and recourſe likewiſe be had to the ſaline draughts, which have already been repeatedly mentioned in the cure of fevers. The body, if coſtive, ſhould be kept gently open, by the uſe of cryſtals of tartar, manna, and the like. After the fever has entirely ceaſed, and the ſcarf-ſkin begins to peel off, two or three doſes of gentle phyſic ſhould be given.

There is another kind of this diſeaſe, called the malignant ſcarlet fever; but that being always accompanied with an ulcerous ſore throat, to which it may probably be owing, it ſhall be treated of afterwards, in the account of ſuch diſorders.

Before I conclude the account of fevers, it may be proper here to obſerve, with reſpect to thoſe of the continued kind, namely, the inflammatory, the putrid, and the ſlow nervous fevers, that though they are in general diſtinguiſhed from each other by their peculiar ſymptoms, there frequently ariſe fevers in which the ſymptoms of all the three kinds appear in various degrees and combinations. Theſe are termed mixed fevers, and require greater attention, as well as judgment, in conducting the cure; ſince no preciſe rules can be laid down for this purpoſe; but the phyſician muſt be governed by an accurate obſervation of the prevailing ſymptoms, and give his directions accordingly.

# BOOK IV.

## *ON INFLAMMATIONS.*

### CHAP. I.

*Of the Eryſipelas, or St. Anthony's Fire.*

THIS diſeaſe, otherwiſe called a blight, conſiſts of an inflammation of the ſkin, and ſubjacent fat, accompanied with an inflammatory fever, which ſeems to derive its origin from a ſharpneſs of the thinner part of the blood. It moſt frequently appears in autumn, or when hot weather is ſucceeded by cold and wet; and is very apt to return in thoſe who have once been afflicted with it. Any part of the body may be attacked by the eryſipelas, but it moſt commonly ſeizes the face and legs, eſpecially the former. Sometimes it is a primary diſeaſe, and at other times only a ſymptom of ſome other diſorder.

Symptoms.—The eryſipelas is generally preceded by cold and ſhivering, after which come on heat, thirſt, reſtleſſneſs, and other feveriſh ſymptoms. When the face is the part affected, it ſwells ſuddenly with great pain, and a ſhining redneſs, inclining to yellow, on which appears a number of ſmall pimples, containing a thin, colourleſs, liquor. One or both eyes are ſometimes ſo much affected as to be cloſed up. The inflammation ſometimes terminates in ſeven days; but at others it will continue for ten or twelve, and at laſt goes off by a plentiful ſweat. In the worſt caſes the brain is affected with the complaint, and a delirium comes on.

When the diſorder ſeizes the breaſt, the part ſwells, and becomes hard, with great pain, which ſometimes ends in an abſceſs or ulcer. A violent pain, is felt in the arm-pit of the ſide affected, and there alſo the ſame event frequently enſues.

Whatever part be affected, when the ſwelling falls, the heat and pain abate, the redneſs, which before prevailed, becomes yellow, and the ſkin falls off in ſcales.

Such is the progreſs of the diſorder in its milder ſtate: but when the ſwelling is large, deep, and affects a ſenſible part of the body, there is no ſmall ground for apprehenſion. If the red colour changes into a livid or black, a mortification is near at hand; and the ſame fatal event is apt to take place when the ſwelling, inſtead of being diſcuſſed, which is the only favourable termination, proceeds to ſuppurate; that is, to form a gathering in the part. When this diſorder proves mortal, the patient commonly dies on the ſeventh or eighth day.

CAUSES.—The eryſipelas may be occaſioned by a ſtoppage either of natural or artificial diſcharges, ſuch as the piles, iſſues, ſetons, or the like. It may alſo be produced by exceſſive drinking; by drinking of, or bathing in, water that is too cold; by a ſudden cooling of the body after it has been much heated; and, in a word, by whatever ſtops the perſpiration. It may alſo be occaſioned by violent paſſions or affections of the mind.

CURE.—The eryſipelas, like the gout, requires to be treated with great caution, eſpecially in reſpect of outward applications, theſe being in general dangerous. Even the mildeſt ſoftening fomentations and poultices are found to do great harm, and much more thoſe of the oppoſite quality, ſuch as the cold and aſtringent. No outward application anſwers the purpoſe ſo well as a bit of ſoft flannel, or ſmooth linen rag, upon which is ſprinkled ſome flour or powdered ſtarch.

When the diſorder is attended with a high fever, bleeding may become neceſſary; but, in the milder ſort, it will be ſufficient to uſe gentle purges, ſuch as ſenua, cryſtals of tartar, and manna, frequently mentioned in the other fevers. If the ſwelling attack the face or brain, the feet and legs ought to be frequently bathed in warm water; and, in this caſe, it is of great importance to keep the body open; which may be done by the purges juſt now mentioned, or by clyſters: but where the head is greatly affected the purges muſt be made ſtronger, and bliſters ought likewiſe to be applied to the neck, or behind the ears.

When the inflammation cannot be diſcuſſed, and there appears a tendency to produce matter, this ought to be promoted by warm fomentations made of chamomile-flowers and the roots of the marſh-mallow; and with poultices of bread and milk, with the addition of ſome ſweet oil; or with poultices of linſeed, than which nothing anſwers better for this purpoſe.

When, on the other hand, there appears a tendency to mortification, which may be known from the black or livid colour of the part, cloths dipped in warm camphorated ſpirits ſhould be immediately applied, and renewed often, at the ſame time that the part be frequently fomented with a ſtrong decoction of the Peruvian bark.

In this dangerous caſe the bark muſt likewiſe be given internally, in as large doſes as the ſtomach will bear. A drachm, if poſſible, every two hours, with ten or fifteen drops of the elixir of vitriol, will generally prove of great advantage.

The uſe of nitre has been much recommended in this diſeaſe, and doubtleſs nothing is more ſuitable in a ſtate of high inflammation; but when taken in large doſes, it is apt to produce a ſickneſs at the ſtomach: half a drachm, or even a ſcruple, is often attended with this effect; but it may be given with advantage, and without much chance of exciting a nauſea, in the quantity of ten or fifteen grains, every three or four hours, in a little of the patient's drink

If the ſwelling ſhould ſuddenly ſink, and the ſharp humour appear to ſtrike in, and to be followed by oppreſſion and anxiety, with a weak pulſe, it will be proper to give wine, which the patient ought to uſe freely. In theſe circumſtances the following draught may likewiſe be given every ſix hours: Take of peppermint-water three table ſpoonfuls; ſalt of hartſhorn five grains; aromatic confection half a drachm. Mix them, and diſſolve in the mixture a little loaf ſugar.

There is a kind of this diſeaſe called the ſcorbutic eryſipelas, which often continues a conſiderable time, but is attended with little danger. It may be cured by keeping the body open with gentle laxatives, and by promoting perſpiration. For the laſt-mentioned purpoſe it is common to uſe a decoction of the woods (decoct. ſarſæ comp.): but the cure will be ſooner completed by uſing every night the following draught. Take of gum guaiac one ſcruple; loaf ſugar two drachms; beat them together into a powder, and add to it gradually three ſpoonfuls of peppermint-water.

Sometimes the eryſipelas breaks forth about the middle of the body, ſurrounding it like a belt: it is then called the ſhingles. In this caſe there ariſe little pimples of a yellowiſh colour, but more frequently blackiſh, and both in appearance and their corroſive quality reſembling a tetter. The fever which attends this eruption is commonly ſlight; but if the pimples ſhould be driven back, the event might prove of dangerous conſequence. When ſuch an accident enſues, the patient muſt be treated in the ſame manner as has been already directed in circumſtances of a ſimilar kind.

When the diſeaſe is mild, it is not neceſſary that the patient be confined to bed, but he ought to keep within doors, and by the uſe of diluting liquors, drunk moderately warm, endeavour to promote perſpiration. The diet ſhould be of the ſlender kind, ſuch as gruel, barley-broth, and light pudding; avoiding fleſh, fiſh, and fowls, as well as ſpices, and every thing of a heating nature. The drink ſhould be barley-water, balm or mint-tea, and ſuch of that kind as are found to be moſt agreeable. If the pulſe be low, however, and the patient drooping, he muſt be ſupported with things of a more cordial nature; ſuch, for example, as negus, or weak wine-whey; but this muſt be done without over-heating him, as a moderate temperature, both in diet and air, is adviſable through the whole of this complaint.

Thoſe who are ſubject to frequent returns of the eryſipelas ought to be ſparing in the uſe of fat meats and ſtrong drink, and confine themſelves chiefly to a vegetable diet. They ſhould guard againſt coſtiveneſs, and avoid the extremes of heat and cold. Moderate daily exerciſe is equally advantageous to health and the prevention of the complaint; and to wear a flannel waiſtcoat next to the ſkin has by many been found highly ſerviceable.

## CHAP. II.

### *Inflammation of the Brain (Phrenitis).*

AN inflammation of the brain is, for the moſt part, a conſequence of fevers, but ſometimes, an original diſeaſe; and it is then extremely dangerous. The ſeat of it is either in the brain itſelf, or in the membranes which ſurround it.

SYMPTOMS.—In this diſorder the temporal arteries, which are thoſe on the temples, throb much, and the veins are diſtended; the eyes are very irritable, and cannot bear the light; the tongue is dry, rough, yellow, or black; there is a chattering of the teeth; a coldneſs of the external parts; a trembling of the hands, with which the patient endeavours to gather the nap of the bed-clothes: he appears to be outrageous, and often attempts to get out of bed.

CAUSES.—This diſeaſe is often occaſioned by the ſtoppage of ſome cuſtomary evacuation, either natural or artificial; ſuch as the bleeding piles in men, and the monthly diſcharge in women; the drying up of iſſues, ſetons, or any old ſores. Hard drinking, long watching, intenſe application of the mind, and violent paſſions, may alſo produce it; and it is ſometimes occaſioned by ſleeping or working out of doors with the head uncovered, and expoſed to the beams of the ſun, when the weather is hot.

CURE.—Large and repeated bleeding is neceſſary in this diſorder, and ought to be performed in the jugular vein; after which, leeches ſhould be applied to both temples. While theſe evacuations leſſen the quantity of blood in the head, endeavours ſhould alſo be made to ſolicit its motion towards the lower extremities. For this purpoſe the feet ought to be bathed in warm water, and poultices of bread and milk, or ſinapiſms, be kept conſtantly applied to them. If the patient has been formerly ſubject to the piles, and indeed whether he has or not, eminent practitioners adviſe us to apply leeches to that part. Sitting over the ſteams of hot water will alſo be uſeful; and if there be reaſon to think that the diſeaſe proceeds from the ſtoppage of any particular diſcharge, it ought to be reſtored as ſoon as poſſible, or ſome other be ſubſtituted in its place.

In the mean time the body muſt be kept open by ſtimulating clyſters, or purgatives. The head ſhould be ſhaved, and frequently waſhed with vinegar, or æther, or ſnow, &c. and, if the diſorder ſhould continue, a bliſter be applied to it.

During the courſe of the diſorder the patient ought to be kept quiet, but not debarred from the company of any perſon whom he may be inclined to ſee; and, indeed, his humour ſhould be gratified in every thing, as far as his ſafety will allow. His chamber ought to be kept in a moderate degree of temperature, and juſt ſo much darkened as not to render it melancholy; which might have a bad effect upon his mind. He ought to lie with his head conſiderably raiſed. The aliment ſhould conſiſt of water-gruel, panada, and ſuch things as are uſual in inflammatory fevers; and the drink be barley-water, or decoction of barley and tamarinds; lemonade; in either of which, or in whatever elſe of the kind he may be inclined to drink, ten or fifteen grains of nitre ſhould be given every two hours.

Every kind of phrenitis, whether a primary diſeaſe or not, is attended with great danger; and unleſs removed before the ſeventh day, it commonly proves fatal. The bad ſigns are, obſtinate watchfulneſs, with a continual and furious delirium; a diſpoſition to become ſtupid, or to faint; trembling, chattering with the teeth, hiccup, convulſions, trembling of the tongue, a ſhrill voice; thin watery urine, white ſtools, or both theſe diſcharges running off involuntarily. The laſt of all the bad ſymptoms, and which prognoſticate a ſpeedy diſſolution, is a ſudden ceſſation of pain, with apparent tranquillity. The following ſigns, on the contrary, are favourable; namely, a diſcharge of blood from the noſe, or the hæmorrhoids; a looſeneſs; ſweats, by which the complaint is alleviated; and a ſwelling of the glands behind the ears. Where the brain has ſuffered much injury by a long diſtention of the veſſels, it ſometimes happens that the patient's ſenſes never perfectly return, but there remains a degree of imbecility, or weakneſs of mind, during life.

## CHAP. III.

### *Inflammation of the Eyes (Ophthalmia).*

THE eye being a complex organ, confifting of various parts, the inflammation may here be very differently fituated; and the fymptoms will be more or lefs violent, as well as the confequences important, in proportion to the delicacy of the texture and function of the part particularly affected. In general, however, the inflammation of the eye may be diftinguifhed into two kinds: one of which is feated in the membranes or coats of the ball of the eye, and the other in the edges of the eye-lids. But though either of thefe may at firft exift feparately, yet, as one may excite the other, they are frequently connected together in the progrefs of the complaint.

The inflammation of the membranes affects commonly the white of the eye; in which it excites a rednefs, attended with pain, and generally an effufion of tears. When the affection of this membrane is confiderable, it may be communicated to the other membranes of the eye, and even to the very bottom of its orbit; in which cafe, the retina, fituated in that part, acquires fo great fenfibility, that the fmalleft impreffion of light is apt to excite great pain.

Cure.—If the inflammation be violent, bleeding is neceffary, and fhould be performed, as in the preceding article, from the jugular vein; applying afterwards feveral leeches round the eye. Blifters alfo fhould be applied to the temples, or behind the ears, and kept open for fome time; the feet ought to be bathed in warm water; and fome gentle purgative be given, and repeated every fecond or third day. For this purpofe may be ufed cream of tartar, Glauber's falts, or fenna, or even lenitive electuary. If the heat and pain of the eye be very great, a foftening poultice of bread and milk, with fome fweet oil or frefh butter, ought to be applied at night, and warm milk be ufed as a fomentation next morning. A decoction of white poppy heads may be ufed for the fame purpofe.

When the diforder is accompanied with watchfulnefs, twenty or twenty-five drops of laudanum may be given occafionally at night.

In an ophthalmia of long ftanding, a feton in the neck, or rather between the fhoulders, is attended with great advantage; and in perfons difpofed to the difeafe, the conftant ufe of it is equally beneficial as a preventive.

If the disorder arise from mere weakness of the vessels, it will be of advantage to bathe the eyes night and morning either with cold water alone, or with the addition of a little vinegar, or a sixth part of brandy. This application gradually strengthens the eye, and restores the elasticity of the vessels.

In the case last mentioned, or where the disorder proceeds from a scrofulous habit of body, and therefore proves obstinate, a dose of the Peruvian bark, in the quantity of half a drachm, should be taken twice a day, and continued for some time.

In an inflammation of the eyes, a looseness coming on spontaneously is a good sign, and frequently carries off the complaint. It is also considered as a favourable sign, when the inflammation passes from one eye to the other, in the way of infection.

In obstinate cases of ophthalmia, great benefit has been received from the use of errhine medicines, or those which excite sneezing. For this purpose the powder of asarabacca, snuffed up the nose at bed-time, has produced good effects; and even common snuff, in persons not accustomed to it, has been successfully used for the same intention.

In obstinate inflammations of the edges of the eye-lids, red nitrated quicksilver, finely levigated, and made into an ointment, with the addition of a little opium, is a very efficacious remedy. It should be carefully applied to the parts affected at bed-time, with a camel-hair pencil, keeping the eyes fast shut after it.

Inflammations are sometimes followed by specks in the eye; for removing which, it is of service to blow into the eye, by means of a small tube, some of the following substances in powder: viz. calamine-stone, tutty, white vitriol, sugar, or the like. For the same purpose, solutions of vitriolated zinc, or acetated ceruse, may be dropped into the eye.

For the cure of watery eyes, it is proper to wash them with brandy and water, as above directed, and to keep the body open by gentle laxatives; at the same time drinking a pint of the decoction of the woods (decoct. sarsæ comp.) A seton between the shoulders, or an issue in the arm, is, in such a case, also highly serviceable.

During a severe inflammation of the eyes, every thing of a heating nature must be avoided, and the patient ought to live chiefly on mild vegetables, weak broths, and gruel; using for drink barley-water, balm-tea, and the like. His chamber ought to be darkened, and he should avoid looking at any luminous or bright object, such as a candle or fire. When the inflammation arises from any mechanical cause, it should be removed as soon as possible, and the eye preserved in a state of rest.

## CHAP. IV.

### *Inflammation of the Ear (Otitis)*

BY this diſorder is to be underſtood an inflammatory ſtate of the internal parts of the ear, the membranes of which, on account of their being well ſtored with nerves, are endowed with great ſenſibility. This inflammation, therefore, is generally attended with great pain and a feveriſhneſs, which, if the more internal parts be affected, frequently runs high, and a delirium enſues.

CAUSES.—This complaint, like other inflammations, may proceed from a ſtoppage of perſpiration, or a current of cold air pouring forcibly into the ear, through narrow crevices in doors or windows. It may likewiſe be occaſioned by acrid humours falling upon the membranes of the ear; or by any thing of a ſtimulating nature that inſinuates itſelf into the cavity of this organ.

CURE.—If *cold* be the cauſe of the complaint, the head muſt be kept warm. If it proceed from acrid or ſharp defluxions, a warm infuſion, or decoction, of poppy heads in water may be injected into the ear. But if the diſorder be occaſioned by any living inſect, that has crept into the ear, a proper application is the ſmoke of tobacco, after which a little warm oil may be poured into the part; and, if the pain be very troubleſome, a few drops of the tincture of opium, or laudanum, may be added to it.

In ſlight caſes, this treatment will generally prove ſufficient; but ſhould the diſorder be ſevere, bleeding and purging may be neceſſary, accompanied with a ſlender diet, as in other inflammations; and it will be proper to apply leeches, and afterwards, if requiſite, a bliſter behind the ear; bathing the feet alſo in warm water. If the pain be violent, and the patient gets no reſt, a doſe of laudanum, ſuitable to his age may be given; reckoning twenty-five drops as a doſe for a grown up perſon.

Should the diſorder not be reſolved by the means above mentioned, but a throbbing pain ſtill continue, it is a ſign that a ſuppuration will take place; and we muſt promote it by applying externally warm poultices of bread and milk, with the addition of a little ſweet oil, or freſh butter. When the abceſs burſts, the ulcerated part muſt be kept clean by injections of warm water, in which is diſſolved a little ſoap. But a preferable injection is barley-water, to half a gill of which add an ounce and a half of honey of roſes, and a table-ſpoonful of the tincture of myrrh. This will promote the diſcharge of matter, keep the ulcerated parts clean, and forward the healing of the part. In this caſe warm balſamics are recommended to be introduced into the ear, as low as convenient: viz. pellets of cotton, or wool, dipped in eſſence of amber. For the ſame purpoſe may be uſed the tincture of myrrh, or balm of Gilead. All digeſtive or oily liniments ſhould be avoided.

## CHAP. V.

### *Quinſey, or Inflammation of the Throat (Tonſillatis.)*

THIS diſorder is divided into two ſpecies, viz. the inflammatory, and the malignant; the former of which is diſtinguiſhed by authors into ſeveral ſubdiviſions, according to the parts moſt affected. It is a complaint very frequent in this country, and is more dangerous, as it ſometimes not only obſtructs deglutition, or the power of ſwallowing, but even reſpiration, or that of breathing.

Causes.—This diſorder is moſt frequently owing to a ſtoppage of perſpiration, particularly about the neck; drinking too cold water, or any other liquid, when a perſon is overheated; the ſuppreſſion of ſome accuſtomed evacuation; or a peculiar ſtate of the air rendering the complaint epidemical. It is very apt to be occaſioned by wet feet; and a few returns of the diſorder create a diſpoſition to contract it. It occurs chiefly in ſpring and autumn, when viciſſitudes of heat and cold frequently take place; and is molt incidental to perſons of a ſanguine temperament. It terminates often by reſolution, ſometimes by ſuppuration, but very rarely by gangrene; though in ſome caſes ſloughy ſpots appear about the top of the throat.

Symptoms.—In this diſorder the tonſils and upper part of the throat are affected. For the moſt part, the inflammation begins in one tonſil, then, ſpreading acroſs the palate, ſeizes the uvula, and the other tonſil. If only one ſide of the fauces or throat be affected, though conſiderable pain attends the action of ſwallowing, ſtill that action may be tolerably well performed; but when both ſides are affected, not only ſwallowing becomes extremely difficult, but the pain is ſometimes ſo violent, as, in delicate habits, even to occaſion convulſions.

It may appear ſurpriſing that more pain ſhould be felt in ſwallowing liquids than ſolids: but ſuch is the fact; and the reaſon of it is, that a greater portion of muſcular fibres is employed in ſwallowing the former than the latter.

While the inflammation is confined to the parts above described, there is not much danger, especially if the neck appears puffed up, this being considered as a favourable sign. But if the inflammation extends itself to the muscles about the top of the wind-pipe, there is a possibility of the patient's being suffocated. There is also danger of the brain or lungs being affected by a translation of the inflammation to those parts.

The disorder is manifest from the redness, tumor, and heat of the tonsils, rendering deglutition painful; besides a quick, hard pulse, and other symptoms of fever.

Cure.—The same treatment is proper here as in other inflammatory disorders. The food must be of the lightest, and the drink of the weakest kind. The patient ought to be kept quiet, and to speak as little as possible. The temperature of his chamber should be such as to favour perspiration; and, when in bed, he ought to lie with his head a little raised, in the same way as in other inflammatory disorders affecting the head. It is particularly of great consequence that the neck be kept warm, by wrapping round it some folds of soft flannel; which expedient alone, if employed early, will often remove a slight affection of the throat.

Bathing the feet and legs in warm water is also of great importance in this disorder: and, in conjuction with the means before mentioned, might so check the complaint at the beginning, as to render the farther aid of medicinal application unnecessary.

As the parts affected by the quinsey *(cynanche)* are naturally furnished with a quantity of mucus, or slimy liquor, the retention of which would increase the complaint, the use of gargles, in this case, is attended with great advantage. For this purpose may be employed sage-tea, with a little vinegar and honey. The mixture may be improved by adding to it a little jelly of black currants, or, in defect of that, some jelly of red currants. If the patient be troubled with thick tough phlegm, a tea-spoonful of the spirit of sal ammoniac may be added to half a pint of the preceding mixture. With this the patient ought to gargle his mouth every three or four hours.

When the fever accompanying the inflammation runs high, bleeding is necessary, performed in the arm, or rather in the jugular vein; and after this evacuation, leeches ought to be applied to the throat. Great benefit is found from applying to the same part a thick piece of flannel, moistened with a mixture of two ounces of oil of olives and one ounce of spirits of hartshorn. This application ought to be renewed every four or five hours; and should it not prove effectual, a blister should be applied in its room.

The body, in the mean time, ought to be kept gently open, either by an infusion of ſenua, or a decoction of figs and tamarinds.

Where the means above recommended have been diligently uſed, it ſeldom happens that the diſorder proceeds to ſuppuration; but when there is evidently a tendency to this effect, it will be forwarded by breathing through a funnel the ſteams of warm water, in which is put a bit of camphor groſsly powdered. Softening poultices of bread and milk, with ſome oil, ought likewiſe to be applied outwardly.

In ſome caſes, the ſwelling becomes ſo large, before it is ripened, as entirely to obſtruct the entrance to the gullet (*æſophagus*) ſo that neither aliment nor drink can get down into the ſtomach. There are then no other means of preſerving the patient's life but by nouriſhing clyſters, which may be made of broth, thin jellies, gruel and milk, &c. In ſuch circumſtances, patients have been ſupported in that manner for ſeveral days, till, by the breaking of the abſceſs, the paſſage to the ſtomach has been opened.

When the abſceſs is attended with much ſwelling, if it break not ſpontaneouſly, it ought to be opened with a lancet.

When the diſeaſe runs rapidly to ſuch a height as to threaten ſuffocation, it is ſometimes neceſſary to have recourſe to an operation, as the only expedient for ſaving the life of the patient. The operation alluded to is bronchotomy, by which an inciſion is made into the wind-pipe, for the purpoſe of reſpiration; but there occur very few inſtances in practice where recourſe to this expedient is neceſſary.

There is ſometimes a difficulty of ſwallowing unattended with any inflammation. This generally proceeds from an obſtruction or enlargement of the glands about the throat, and requires nothing more than keeping the neck warm, and gargling the throat with ſome water, vinegar, and honey.

Perſons who are ſubject to inflammation of the throat are apt to have a return of the complaint upon any irregularity in point of living. They ought, therefore, to be temperate; or, if not, to carry off the ſuperabundance of humours by purging, and other evacuations. They ought, likewiſe, to guard well againſt cold, and avoid whatever is of a ſtimulating nature in diet. Drinking cold liquor immediately after violent exerciſe is very prejudicial: as is likewiſe a ſudden expoſure to cold air, after any great exertion of the throat by ſpeaking or ſinging. The ſame caution is adviſable after drinking warm liquors.

After an inflammation of the throat, the glands of that part ſometimes continue ſwelled, and acquire a degree of hardneſs which is difficult to be removed. No attempt ſhould ever be made to resolve these tumors by any stimulating application. The best way is to keep the throat warm, leaving the swellings to dissipate spontaneously by time, and only gargling twice a day with a decoction of figs, or barley, sharpened with a little vinegar.

### *Of the Malignant Quinsey, or Ulcerous Sore Throat, (Angina maligna, or Cynanche maligna.)*

This kind of quinsey is more dangerous than the preceding, and of a highly contagious nature. It seizes children more readily than adults, women than men, and the delicate than the robust.

Causes.—It originally derives its source from the same causes with putrid fevers, which it likewise resembles; but those which chiefly produce it in the first instance are, unwholesome air, damaged provisions, and obstructed perspiration, in persons predisposed to the disease: it is afterwards propagated by the breath from one patient to another.

Symptoms.—It begins, like most fevers, with fits of shivering and heat alternately. The pulse, though quick, is low and unequal. The patient complains of weakness and oppression at the breast; has great dejection of spirits; and, on being set upright, is apt to faint away: the tongue is moist; the eyes heavy and watery; the countenance frequently full, flushed, and bloated; though occasionally pale and sunk; the breathing is quick and laborious; the skin extremely hot, and, in many cases, there is an eruption or efflorescence resembling scarlet fever; the urine commonly pale, thin, and crude; but in some adults it is made in small quantity, and high coloured, or turbid, like whey. The throat is sore and inflamed, exhibiting a shining redness, of a deeper colour than in common inflammatory sore throats, and interspersed with pale or ash-coloured spots. There is sometimes a delirium, though the symptoms appear slight; the swallowing is difficult, and more so on swallowing the saliva only, than of any liquid or soft diet. The patient is troubled with a nausea, or sickness at the stomach, and often with a vomiting or purging; but the two latter are most common in children. An efflorescence or eruption frequently breaks out upon the neck, breast, and arms, about the second or third day; and when this appears, the evacuations just now mentioned generally cease.

The malignant sore throat may be distinguished from the inflammatory by the looseness and vomiting; the puffy and dark-coloured redness attending the swelling; and by the fœtid ulcers of the throat, covered with white or ash-coloured sloughs. It may also be distinguished by the slight delirium appearing early in the disease; and by the sudden weakness with which the patient is seized.

It is accounted favourable in this diforder when the eyes are bright; when there is no great degree of weaknefs or fainting; when the floughs are white, and the eruption on the fkin has a florid appearance.

But if the weaknefs be great; if the ulcers be afh-coloured, black, or livid; if the pulfe fhould be weak and fmall, accompanied with a loofenefs, or fhivering; if the eruptions difappear, or become livid; if the eyes look very dull; if the nofe bleeds; and if the body puts on a cadaverous appearance; under this accumulation of fymptoms nothing elfe can be expected but a fatal termination of the difeafe.

Cure.—The great weaknefs which accompanies this difeafe renders bleeding and all other evacuations improper. If, however, at the beginning of the complaint there be an inclination to vomit, it ought to be promoted by drinking an infufion of chamomile-flowers; and if this prove infufficient, a few grains of ipecacuanha may be given. Early vomiting is of great advantage, by cleanfing the ftomach and bowels of their putrefcent contents, which tend greatly to aggravate the difeafe; and, indeed, it is fo beneficial as frequently to put an entire ftop to the diforder.

To fupport the patient's ftrength, to correct the putrid tendency of the humours, and to keep the ulcers clean, are the objects which require our chief attention in the treatment of this difeafe.

When the violence of the difeafe threatens danger, the beft remedy is the Peruvian bark, of which half a drachm, or two fcruples, in powder, may be given in a glafs of red wine, every three or four hours. But if the patient's ftomach cannot bear the bark in fubftance, two ounces of it, grofsly powdered, with half an ounce of Virginian fnake-root, may be boiled in three pints of water for ten minutes; and to the liquor, when ftrained, two tea-fpoonfuls of the elixir of vitriol may be added. Three table-fpoonfuls of this may be given every three or four hours.

If the ficknefs at the ftomach, with an inclination to vomit, fhould continue to prove troublefome in the progrefs of the difeafe, the faline draughts, formerly mentioned in the cure of fevers, fhould be given every two hours, or oftener. For example: Take of falt of worm-wood, or kali, one fcruple; juice of lemons, a large table-fpoonful; mint-water, two table-fpoonfuls, and a bit of fugar: mix them, and give the draught in the ftate of effervefcence; that is, while the mixture continues to fend forth a fmoke and a hiffing noife. In this ftate of the difeafe, the patient ought likewife to ufe for common drink an infufion of fpearmint, adding to every dofe of the liquor an equal quantity of red wine.

If the patient ſhould be troubled with a violent looſeneſs, the bulk of a nutmeg of the electuary of catechu may be given every four or five hours.

During the progreſs of the diſeaſe, it is neceſſary to gargle the throat frequently. For this purpoſe an infuſion of ſage and roſe-leaves, to a gill of which is added a large ſpoonful of honey, and as much vinegar as will give it an agreeable ſharpneſs, may, in many caſes, prove ſufficient; but under unfavourable circumſtances of the complaint, boil half an ounce of the root of contrayerva in half a pint of barley-water for a few minutes, and add to the ſtrained liquor a large table-ſpoonful of fine honey, with four table-ſpoonfuls of the beſt vinegar, and two table-ſpoonfuls of tincture of myrrh. Beſides gargling with this mixture, ſome of it ought to be frequently injected with a ſyringe to clean the throat, before the patient takes any food or drink; as otherwiſe the ſloughs, and putrid diſcharge from the ulcers, may be carried down into the ſtomach, and aggravate the diſeaſe.

To correct the gangrenous diſpoſition of the parts about the throat, the patient ought frequently to receive into his mouth, through an inverted funnel, the ſteams of warm vinegar, myrrh, and honey.

The mineral acids, ſuch as elixir or ſpirit of vitriol, or of ſalt, ſhould be frequently given in the quantity of ten or fifteen drops, in a cupful of the patient's drink, or the infuſion of roſes.

When the pulſe is low, or the tumor about the throat conſiderable, bliſters ſhould be applied to the throat, behind the ears, and upon the back part of the neck.

In ſome caſes there happens a diſcharge of blood from the noſe, which not being critical, or tending to alleviate the complaint, requires to be ſtopped. For this purpoſe the ſteams of warm vinegar may be received up the noſtrils frequently and the acids above mentioned be freely uſed.

If the patient be troubled with a ſtrangury, or ſtoppage of water, the belly ought to be fomented with a decoction of chamomile-flowers and linſeed, and ſoftening clyſters be given every four or five hours.

When the diſeaſe has ceaſed, the belly ought to be kept gently open with ſenna, manna, rhubarb, or the like, for a little time, to carry off the putrid dregs, that may remain in the inteſtines; and if the patient continues weak, he ought to perſevere for ſome time in the uſe of the Peruvian bark, and elixir of vitriol; with daily exerciſe on horſeback. He ought likewiſe to take frequently a glaſs of ſome rich wine; and in caſe of a great debility of the digeſtive powers, to make uſe of a milk-diet.

## CHAP. VI.

### *Of a Catarrh, or Cold.*

THIS complaint is ſo univerſally known, that it would be ſuperfluous to deſcribe it. The chief characteriſtic ſymptom, however, is an increaſed diſcharge of mucus from the noſe, the top of the throat, and the wind-pipe. It is always occaſioned by a ſtoppage of perſpiration; and is of different degrees, according to the violence of the cauſe, or the conſtitution of the perſon. So many accidents may effect the diſcharge by perſpiration, that a partial ſuppreſſion of it muſt ſometimes unavoidably enſue, in all perſons, climates, and ſeaſons. Even thoſe who are the moſt careful to avoid catching cold, only render themſelves more ſuſceptible of the complaint upon the ſlighteſt expoſure to the means by which it is uſually excited.

If early attention be given to a cold, nothing is more eaſy than to remove it; but when long neglected, it may prove not only obſtinate, but fatal; and indeed the greater part of diſeaſes is originally owing to this cauſe.

As ſoon as a perſon is ſenſible of having taken cold, he ought to retrench his diet, at leaſt to diminiſh the uſual quantity in the article of ſolid food, and to abſtain from all ſtrong liquors. A ſlender diet only is proper; ſuch as light puddings, roaſted or boiled apples; veal or chicken broth, &c. The drink ſhould be barley-water, pectoral decoction, linſeed-tea with a little juice of lemon, or water-gruel ſweetened with honey: where honey diſagrees with the ſtomach, treacle or moiſt ſugar, with the addition of ſome jelly of currants, may be uſed in its ſtead. The beſt ſupper is a ſlice of toaſted bread, with ſome water-gruel and honey, to which may be added a glaſs of white wine.

Water-gruel being thus taken at bed-time, and the feet and legs bathed in warm water, the body will be diſpoſed to perſpire in the courſe of the night; and the more to favour perſpiration, the patient ſhould lie longer in the morning than uſual, and even drink ſome warm diluting liquor in bed.

In this manner a common cold may frequently be carried off in a day, which, if neglected, might be attended with the moſt pernicious conſequences. For during a cold there is a conſtant ſpaſm, or chillneſs on the ſurface of the body, which goes on increaſing the ſtoppage of perſpiration, till that diſcharge be reſtored; and if this be long delayed, the united quantity and acrimony of the fluids retained may be productive of fatal effects.

It is an opinion, acted upon by many, that nothing cures a cold more effectually than a debauch in wine, hot punch, or other ſtrong liquors: but it is a dangerous experiment; and though, by reſtoring perſpiration, it may prove a cure in ſome caſes, it may in others, convert a ſlight complaint into an inflammatory fever, perhaps an inflammation of the brain, or lungs, the iſſue of which is very precarious.

If notwithſtanding a ſlender regimen of diet, temporary warmth, and the uſe of diluting liquors, the complaint ſhould not ceaſe, but be attended with a quick pulſe, a pain of the head or breaſt, and a hot, dry ſkin, it will be neceſſary to bleed, and afterwards to open the body by ſome gentle purgative, ſuch as ſenna, rhubarb, &c.

If the ſtomach be loaded with phlegm, an emetic of ipecacuanha will be proper. At the ſame time, it will be adviſable to apply a bliſter between the ſhoulders; and to give, every two or three hours, two table-ſpoonfuls of the following ſaline mixture: Take of mint-water, half a gill; ſalt of wormwood, or kali, three drachms; juice of lemon, four table-ſpoonfuls; ſugar, half an ounce: mix them.

In perſons of a phthiſical or conſumptive diſpoſition, a catarrh may bring on a ſpitting of blood, or may inflame tubercles in the lungs, which, if already exiſting in that organ, may thence be excited to a ſpeedy and fatal ſuppuration. It may alſo prove of dangerous conſequence to perſons advanced in years, either by occaſioning a baſtard peripneumony, as it is called, or laying the foundation of a chronic catarrh, which will render both health and life extremely precarious ever after.

When a cold is unattended with any degree of fever, yet does not go off by keeping the houſe for a day or two, the perſon will be better for taking ſome exerciſe, well covered, in the open air; as too cloſe confinement will expoſe to the danger of a relapſe, and thereby protract the complaint.

A cold would be much leſs frequent, if people, when they found it coming on, were to keep cool, avoid wine and ſtrong liquors, and confine themſelves for a ſhort time to a vegetable diet, uſing only toaſt and water for drink. It would be a great preventive of this complaint, were people to take more pains to accommodate their dreſs to the ſeaſon. If we were warmly clothed in cold weather, our excitability would not be accumulated by the action of the cold.

## *Common Cough.*

A cough is moſt commonly the effect of obſtructed perſpiration; and though it does not immediately ſucceed that event, it ſupervenes in a ſhort time, if the complaint be either neglected, or treated improperly. Sometimes a cough will ſubſiſt during life, without much inconvenience to the perſon, except on uſing hard exerciſe, or being otherwiſe conſiderably heated; but as the lungs are an organ of ſo great importance to life, we ought as ſoon as poſſible to remove every cauſe that has a tendency to effect them.

In phlegmatic and relaxed habits, the cough is generally moiſt; but in thoſe of a ſcorbutic diſpoſition, for the moſt part dry. In both caſes, however, it is ſerviceable to keep the body in an uniform ſtate of warmth; and to avoid malt liquors, ſpices, and whatever tends to agitate the blood.

If the cough be violent, and the perſon young, and of a ſtrong conſtitution, with a hard quick pulſe, the ſafeſt courſe is to begin the cure with bleeding; but this evacuation is not to be recommended in relaxed habits, as in ſuch it would prolong the diſeaſe. When the patient ſpits freely, bleeding is likewiſe unadviſable, on account of its tendency to diminiſh that diſcharge, which, wherever a cough ſubſiſts, is of a ſalutary nature.

When the ſpittle is viſcid and tough, and there is no degree of fever, the proper remedies are thoſe of an attenuating kind, or ſuch as have the quality of rendering the humours more thin. Of this claſs of medicines, gum ammoniac and ſquills are the pectorals chiefly uſed. Take of gum ammoniac, two drachms; mint-water, half a pint: diſſolve the gum in the water; and let the patient, if a grown up perſon, take two table-ſpoonfuls of the mixture three times a day. Squills may be uſed either in the vinegar tincture, the oxymel, or the ſyrup. Two ounces of any of theſe may be mixed with an equal quantity of ſimple cinnamon-water, and taken in the quantity of a table-ſpoonful two or three times a day, if they do not diſagree with the ſtomach.

As a domeſtic remedy, of the ſame nature, a very ſerviceable one is a mixture of lemon-juice, honey, and ſugar-candy, in equal parts. A table-ſpoonful of this mixture may be taken at pleaſure.

Such are the medicines to be uſed when the matter diſcharged by coughing is of a viſcid and tough kind; but when, on the contrary, the defluxion is thin and ſharp, the proper remedies are thoſe which thicken and ſheath the humours; ſuch as oils, mucilages, and gentle opiates. For this purpoſe may be employed an infuſion of marſh-mallow roots, linſeed, or the flowers or leaves of colt's-foot; to any of which may be joined a head or two of the white poppy; and a tea-cupful of the infuſion be taken every two hours. Or, instead of these, the patient may take, twice a day, a tea-spoonful of camphorated tincture of opium in a cupful of his drink. For the same purpose, an infusion of liquorice-root may be used; or rather a decoction made of the root, by boiling it a little. The extract of the same root, under the name of Spanish-juice, held in the mouth, and gradually swallowing the solution, is likewise a suitable medicine. This will also be very proper, where the cough is occasioned by acrid humours tickling the throat and adjacent parts; or in room of it may be employed some barley-sugar, or common balsamic lozenges. As a substitute for these, the following lambative may be used: Take of oil of almonds, and syrup of white poppies, each an ounce; mix them with three drachms of sugar, and let the patient take frequently a spoonful.

If the cough be dry, a blister may be laid between the shoulders, and kept open for a few days.

In obstinate coughs, arising from a flux of humours upon the lungs, the cure should not be left entirely to the effect of medicines alone, but an effort ought to be made to discharge the humours by issues or setons, which often prove very successful. Some, for the same purpose, recommend a small plaster of Burgundy-pitch to be applied between the shoulders, and used for a long time.

A dry cough sometimes proceeds from tubercles, or small tumors in the lungs, which by irritating that organ, and obstructing the motion of the blood through it, excite the action of coughing. In this case, the attenuating medicines above mentioned, namely, gum ammoniac, and squills, are the remedies best adapted; but they ought to be used only in a small quantity, lest they should too much irritate the lungs, and occasion a suppuration of the tubercles. But indeed it is better to abstain from the use of such deobstruent medicines, without the advice of a physician: for, where the lungs are much affected, great caution is requisite in having recourse to remedies of an active kind. In those habitual coughs, however, of long standing, it is of great service to wear flannel next the skin, so as to support the perspiration uniformly, and prevent any increase of the complaint. Malt-liquors are improper in such cases; as is likewise all food of a viscid or tough nature. A free use of honey, in dry coughs proceeding from the cause last mentioned, is attended with advantage.

Sometimes coughs have their origin in the stomach, and not in the lungs, which are affected only by sympathy; in which case the cure depends chiefly upon cleansing and strengthening the primary seat of the disorder. After giving a vomit or two, therefore, a stomachic tincture, made of Peruvian bark, and bitters, either in wine or brandy, as directed in the chapter on intermittent fevers, will be adviſable. The patient ſhould alſo uſe exerciſe, particularly riding on horſeback; and, if of a coſtive habit, may occaſionally take, at bed-time, five grains of aloes made into a pill. The following mixture would ſerve both as a laxative, and a ſafe medicine for reſolving the tubercles in the lungs: Take of Caſtile ſoap, two drachms and a half; ſocotorine aloes, powdered, half a drachm; common ſyrup, as much as will make them into thirty-ſix pills. Three to be taken every night and morning.

When a cough proceeds entirely from an affection of the nerves, no benefit can be expected from any of the remedies above mentioned, and the only effectual means of removing it are by ſtrengthening the body. The beſt medicine is the Peruvian bark, with a light nouriſhing diet, tranquillity of mind, and daily exerciſe on horſeback. A fit of the complaint, however, may be much relieved by the occaſional uſe of fœtid medicines, ſuch as aſſafœtida, which may be taken in the following form, in the quantity of a table-ſpoonful: Take of aſſafœtida, one drachm; cinnamon-water, four table-ſpoonfuls. Diſſolve the gum in the water, and keep the mixture for uſe. For the ſame purpoſe, twenty drops of the ſpirit of hartſhorn may be taken in a ſpoonful of any liquid. Smelling to the ſame kind of medicines ſometimes produces good effects; as does likewiſe the immerſion of the feet and hands in warm water, or the tepid bath.

In children, a cough is ſometimes occaſioned by teething, and at others by worms; in both which caſes, it is to be cured by ſuch medicines as are adapted to thoſe complaints.

It is not uncommon for women to be troubled with a cough during the laſt months of pregnancy. The complaint is greatly relieved by ſmall bleeding, and keeping the body gently open by lenitive electuary, or ſome other laxative; avoiding at the ſame time all food of a flatulent nature.

A cough has by ſome been repreſented as the frequent forerunner of the gout; but it is more probable that, in ſuch caſes, both the cough and gout derive their origin from an accidental impediment to perſpiration.

In all habitual coughs it is of advantage to wear flannel next the ſkin: for there is an intimate connection between the lungs and the ſurface of the body; ſo that, by ſupporting the perſpiration uninterrupted, the lungs are preſerved from a fluxion which would otherwiſe fall upon them. It cannot be too often repeated, that guarding againſt wet feet, in particular, is of great conſequence wherever there is a natural diſpoſition to complaints of the breaſt. Cough alone is not a diſeaſe, but a ſymptom, often troubleſome enough, of the ſeveral diſeaſes above enumerated.

## CHAP. VII.

*Pleurisy (Pleuritis, Pneumonia.)*

THIS is an inflammation of the pleura, the membrane which lines the thorax. It is most frequent in men of a robust constitution, and prevails chiefly in the spring.

CAUSES.—Many of the general causes of fevers may give rise to the pleurisy. It may be occasioned by whatever obstructs perspiration; frequently by cold northerly or easterly winds; wet clothes; sleeping without doors on the damp ground; drinking cold liquors when a person is hot; plunging the body into cold water, or exposing it to the cold air, during a strong perspiration. It may likewise be occasioned by the stoppage of accustomed evacuations, natural or artificial; or by the sudden disappearance of any eruption on the skin. It may besides owe its rise to violent exercise, or to drinking strong liquors.

SYMPTOMS.—The pleurisy, in common with most of the acute diseases, generally begins with a sensation of cold and shivering, followed by heat, thirst, and the usual attendants of a fever. The pulse is quick, hard, and strong; and an acute pain or stitch is felt in one of the sides, most commonly the right, which increases upon inspiration. A difficulty of breathing succeeds, accompanied with a short cough, dry in the beginning of the disease, but afterwards sometimes moist. When matter is expectorated, it is usually phlegm, either streaked with blood, or yellowish.

CURE.—Nature frequently makes an effort to expel this dangerous disease by some of the outlets of the body, or by a bleeding in some particular part; but the most usual channel is by expectoration from the lungs, with which the membrane of the pleura is intimately connected. No crisis, however, can be expected while the motion of the blood is rapid and tumultuous, and every means must be used for bringing it to a state of moderation. The patient, as in every other fever, must be kept quiet, cool, and easy. His diet must be of the most slender kind, such as gruel, panada, and the like; and his drink barley-water, or a decoction of barley, figs, and raisins; to which, towards the close of the boiling, may be added some liquorice-root. All the food and drink ought to be taken a little warm, and never much at a time; but the patient should keep continually sipping them, to moisten and relax the throat and the adjacent parts. He ought also to take ten grains of nitre in some of his drink, every three hours, during the firſt three or four days of the diſeaſe. As a cooling attenuant, or thinning medicine, in this diſeaſe, ten or fifteen grains of nitre, with three or four grains of ſalt of hartſhorn, have great effect. His feet and hands ought to be bathed two or three times a day in warm water; and he may ſometimes ſit up in bed, both to relieve his head, and favour a diſcharge by expectoration.

Scarce any diſeaſe requires more plentiful bleeding than a pleuriſy; and the blood ſhould be taken from a large orifice. From a man of a good conſtitution, twelve or fourteen ounces, or upwards, may be taken at once; but a ſmaller quantity from a perſon of a more delicate habit. If, after the firſt bleeding, the ſymptoms ſhould ſtill continue violent, that is, if the ſtitch be very painful, and the pulſe hard, full, and ſtrong, it will be neceſſary to repeat the operation at the diſtance of ſome hours; and even a third, and a fourth time, ſhould there be no mitigation of thoſe ſymptoms, and the blood that has been drawn ſhows a ſtrong buffy coat.

Beſides bleeding from the arm, topical bleeding is of great advantage. This may be performed with leeches applied immediately over the part affected with the pain, or rather by means of cupping-glaſſes with ſcarification.

Emollient or ſoftening fomentations, made of chamomile-flowers, and common mallow roots boiled in water, may be applied to the part; and flannel cloths dipped in the decoction, and afterwards wrung out, be laid over it as warm as the patient can bear. As ſoon as the cloths cool, they ought to be changed, and great care taken to prevent the patient from catching cold. The part may alſo be anointed with a liniment compoſed of two parts of oil of olives, and one of ſpirit of hartſhorn.

If after theſe applications, and repeated bleedings, the ſtitch ſhould ſtill continue, a bliſter ought to be laid upon the part affected, and ſuffered to remain open for two days. This not only excites a beneficial diſcharge from the ſide, but has the effect of removing the ſpaſm, or conſtriction, which occaſions the inflammation of the part. To prevent a ſtrangury, which is often cauſed by bliſters, the patient may drink of the Arabic emulſion* or camphorated mixture at pleaſure.

If during the illneſs the patient be bound in the belly, a clyſter of milk and water, or of a decoction of linſeed, may be given every day, both to empty the bowels, and by its relaxing quality to draw the blood downwards from the breaſt.

* See *Appendix.*

In the mean time expectoration is to be promoted as much as poſſible. For this purpoſe mucilaginous and oily medicines are proper. Take of ſpermaceti, two drachms; ammoniac milk, half a pint; ſugar-candy, half an ounce; with as much of the yolk of an egg as is ſufficient to mix them together. Two table-ſpoonfuls of this mixture to be given every five or ſix hours.

Expectoration may likewiſe be promoted, by receiving into the lungs the ſteams of warm water, to which a portion of vinegar is added.

If expectoration proceeds well, and is ſufficiently copious for a few days, the patient is perceptibly much relieved; but if it ſhould ſtop, and not be ſucceeded by ſome other evacuation, the caſe is dangerous. In ſuch circumſtances, if the pulſe will bear it, ſome more blood ought to be taken away, and bliſters applied.

If the pulſe flags, and expectoration proceeds very ſlowly, beſides the remedies above mentioned, bliſters ought to be applied to different parts of the thorax, or cheſt.

Different opinions are entertained reſpecting the uſe of opiates in inflammatory diſorders of the breaſt. It appears, however, that in the beginning of the diſeaſe, and before bleeding and bliſtering have produced ſome abatement of the pain, and of the difficulty of breathing, opiates have a tendency to increaſe thoſe ſymptoms. But in a more advanced ſtate of the diſeaſe, when the difficulty of breathing has abated, but the cough is troubleſome, and prevents the patient from reſting, opiates may be employed both with ſafety and advantage. In ſuch circumſtances, therefore, a tea-ſpoonful of ammoniated tincture of opium, or paregoric elixir, may be given three or four times a day in a little of the patient's drink.

After bleeding and other evacuations have been premiſed, a decoction of ſeneka root* has been found of great advantage in the pleuriſy. It may be taken in the quantity of two, three, or four table-ſpoonfuls, as the patient's ſtomach will bear it, three or four times a day. If it ſhould occaſion vomiting, a third part of ſimple cinnamon-water may be added to every doſe.

After bleeding, and the bowels being cleanſed, the following remedy has alſo been uſed with great ſucceſs: Take of calomel, three grains; opium, half a grain; make them into a bolus with any conſerve. The quantity of the ingredients may be varied according to circumſtances; the doſe taken two or three times a day, and plenty of barley-water, or other diluting drinks, be uſed.

Sometimes nature endeavours to carry off the diſeaſe by tranſlating the inflammation to a different part of the body, as the ſhoulder, back, &c. On diſcovering ſuch an appearance, every aid ſhould be given, by ſoftening fomentations, and ſtimulating plaſ-

* See *Appendix*.

ters, ſuch as the compound plaſter of Burgundy-pitch, to ſolicit the tranſlation to the part.

After the loſs of much blood in this diſeaſe, care muſt be taken that the body be repleniſhed with healthy juices; for which purpoſe the patient ought to uſe a light diet of eaſy digeſtion. When the pain and fever are gone, he ſhould likewiſe take a few doſes of ſome gentle phyſic.

### *Paraphrenitis (Diaphragmatis.)*

This is an inflammation of the diaphragm, and is ſo cloſely connected with the pleuriſy, as well in its nature as in the manner of treatment, that it ſcarcely can be conſidered as a ſeparate diſeaſe. It is accompanied with a high fever, and a violent pain in the part affected, which is increaſed by every exertion in which the diaphragm is concerned; ſuch as coughing, ſneezing, going to ſtool, drawing in the breath, &c. The diſeaſe is ſometimes attended by a kind of involuntary grin. The treatment, is in every reſpect, the ſame as in a pleuriſy.

## CHAP. VIII.

### *Peripneumony, or Inflammation of the Subſtance of the Lungs.*

THIS diſeaſe is accompanied with great oppreſſion at the breaſt, and difficulty of breathing, with a fever and cough. The breath is hot, the face red, and the pulſe ſometimes imperceptible; but after bleeding, it becomes ſtronger, though unequal. It differs from a pleuriſy in the cough being more moiſt, the pain leſs acute, and the pulſe not ſo ſtrong.

Cure.—The treatment of the peripneumony, both in diet and medicines, is in general the ſame as in the pleuriſy. When the oppreſſion at the breaſt is very urgent, bleeding is neceſſary at the beginning of the diſeaſe; but is afterwards to be repeated with caution. The body ſhould alſo be opened by emollient or ſoftening clyſters. But if the matter ſpit up by the patient be of a thick conſiſtence, and he expectorates freely, there will be no occaſion for recourſe to bleeding; and it may be ſufficient to aſſiſt expectoration by remedies for that purpoſe. Take of nitre, and ſpermaceti, each one drachm; ſalt of hartſhorn, ten grains; ſugar-candy, two drachms; common water, half a gill; mix them together with a little yolk of egg, and give a table-ſpoonful every three hours.

At the ſame time, bliſters ſhould be applied to the back and ſides, firſt to one, and afterwards the other, unleſs the pain be confined to one ſide.

Should there be a free diſcharge of florid frothy blood from the lungs, more bleeding will be neceſſary, if the patient's ſtrength admit of it; but this evacuation is by no means to be employed, when the diſcharge from the lungs is thin, black, and foetid.

When an inflammation of the lungs does not yield to bleeding, bliſtering, and other evacuations, it uſually proceeds to ſuppuration, and terminates either in a vomica or empyema, as they are called. The former is an abſceſs, or collection of matter, formed within the lungs; and the latter, when the diſcharge is into the cavity of the thorax, between the membrane which lines the cheſt and the lungs. In a vomica, the matter may be diſcharged by expectoration; but in an empyema, it can only be diſcharged by an inciſion made between the ribs.

The exiſtence of a vomica may be aſcertained by the cough and difficulty of breathing continuing after the pain has ceaſed; by ſlight ſhiverings ſucceeded by heat; by a quick, weak pulſe, a general waſting of the body, and the patient being able to lie only on the ſide affected. In this caſe, there is no other proſpect of a favourable iſſue of the diſeaſe, but by the matter being gradually expectorated, without endangering ſuffocation.

In the empyema, as in the former, there is a hectic fever, difficulty of breathing, a dry cough, and often a fullneſs of the ſkin and fleſh on one ſide of the cheſt.

Both theſe caſes tend ſtrongly to terminate in a conſumption.

## CHAP. IX.

### *Spitting or coughing up of Blood (Hæmoptyſis.)*

THIS complaint is frequently the fore-runner of a conſumption of the lungs, and generally comes on between the age of ſixteen and thirty-five; though it may be produced at any time of life by external violence.

CAUSES.—It is chiefly incident to thoſe who have a narrow cheſt, prominent ſhoulders, and a long neck, eſpecially if they be of a ſanguine temperament, and formerly liable to a bleeding of the noſe, or any other diſcharge of blood. It happens often to women who labour under a ſuppreſſion of the menſtrual flux, and to perſons who have ſuffered an amputation of any conſiderable limb. Among thoſe who are diſpoſed to it, the complaint is frequently brought on in the beginning of summer by external heat, which rarefying the blood, more than it relaxes the solids, previously contracted by the cold of winter, excites the discharge. Violent exercise will likewise produce it, as will also great exertions of the lungs, in speaking, singing, or crying aloud. Among other causes, a violent fit of anger has often been known to give rise to it.

SYMPTOMS.—The complaint begins with a sense of weight and anxiety in the breast; difficulty of breathing; a pain in different parts of the chest, and some sense of heat under the breast-bone; being often preceded by a saltish taste in the mouth. Immediately before the discharge appears, a degree of irritation is felt at the top of the throat; and upon the person's attempting to relieve this by hawking, a little florid and somewhat frothy blood is brought up. The irritation returning, more blood is brought up, with a noise in the wind-pipe, resembling that of air passing through a fluid. Sometimes, however, at the very first, the blood is discharged with coughing, or at least a very fine coughing accompanies the hawking above mentioned.

At first, the blood is sometimes in very small quantity, and soon disappears; but in other cases, especially when it frequently recurs, it is in greater quantity, and often continues to appear at times for several days successively. It is sometimes profuse, but seldom in such quantity as, either by its excess or by a sudden suffocation, to prove immediately mortal.

It is not always easy to discover from what particular part the blood is discharged. When it proceeds from some part of the internal surface of the mouth, it breaks forth without any hawking or coughing; and generally, upon inspection, the source of the irruption may be seen.

When blood proceeds from the top of the throat, or adjoining cavities of the nose, it may be brought out by hawking, and sometimes by coughing. In this case, its real source may appear doubtful; but, on looking attentively into the fauces, or top of the throat, the distillation of the blood from that part will easily be perceived.

When blood proceeds from the lungs, the manner in which it is discharged will commonly show whence it comes.

When vomiting accompanies a discharge of blood from the mouth, the source of the evacuation may be ascertained, by considering that blood does not so frequently proceed from the stomach as from the lungs, and that blood proceeding from the stomach commonly appears in greater quantity than from the lungs. Blood from the lungs is likewise usually of a florid colour, and mixed with a little frothy mucus or slime only; while the blood from the stomach is of a darker colour, often consisting of lumps, and mixed with the other contents of the ſtomach. The coughing or vomiting, as one or the other happens firſt to ariſe, may likewiſe ſometimes point out the ſource of the blood.

A ſpitting of blood may ſometimes be no more dangerous than a ſimilar diſcharge from the noſe: for inſtance, when it happens to females, in conſequence of a ſuppreſſion of the natural diſcharge; when, without any marks of prediſpoſition, it ariſes from external violence; or, from whatever cauſe ariſing, when it leaves behind it no cough, difficulty of breathing, or any other affection of the lungs. But even in theſe caſes danger may ariſe from too large a wound being made in the veſſels of the lungs, from any quantity of blood being left to ſtagnate in the cavities of the lungs, and particularly from any determination being made into the veſſels of the lungs, which, by renewing the diſcharge, may produce theſe effects.

CURE.—In the treatment of this complaint, the firſt object to be purſued, is to diminiſh the force with which the blood is impelled through the lungs. This end is to be anſwered by removing the fullneſs of the veſſels, when ſuch a fulneſs exiſts; by diminiſhing the general force of the circulation; and by producing a determination of the blood to the parts remote from the lungs. To accompliſh theſe purpoſes, recourſe muſt be had to blood-letting, in greater or ſmaller quantity, and more or leſs frequently repeated as the ſymptoms ſhall require. The body ſhould be at the ſame time kept open by ſome gentle laxative, ſuch as the lenitive electuary, of which a tea-ſpoonful may be taken two or three times a day, or by Epſom ſalts. Theſe evacuations having been premiſed, take of conſerve of roſes, four ounces; nitre powdered, half an ounce; ſimple ſyrup, as much as will make them into an electuary. Of this the bulk of a nutmeg may be given four, ſix, or eight times a day, according to the urgency of the caſe; or, inſtead of the electuary, ten or fifteen grains of nitre, with an equal quantity of ſpermaceti, may be taken in the ſame manner.

When this diſcharge has reſiſted other methods of cure, bliſters, particularly when applied to the breaſt, are often uſed with advantage; as has likewiſe the elixir of vitriol, taken in the quantity of ten or fifteen drops two or three times a day.

When this complaint has appeared, the patient ought to be kept quiet and eaſy; and the diet cooling and ſlender; ſuch as panada, rice-milk, weak broths, and water gruel.

Bathing the feet and legs in warm water ſhould alſo not be neglected. Where the patient is of an irritable conſtitution, or the complaint has been brought on by ſome violent paſſion of the mind, opiates have often good effect. Ten or twelve drops of the laudanum may be taken in any weak vehicle twice a day; but if not found beneficial the uſe of it ſhould not be continued long.

## CHAP. X.

### *Of a Consumption.*

THE persons most subject to a spitting of blood are likewise the most liable to a consumption of the lungs, which constitutes a great part of the bills of mortality in this country.

CAUSES.—The chief causes are, moist air; a diminution or suppression of accustomed evacuations; a sedentary life; too luxurious living; obstructions in the lungs; fumes of arsenic, or other noxious matter, getting into the lungs; violent passions of the mind; sudden cold; frequent debaucheries; late watching, and drinking of strong liquors. To these may be added various other diseases, as the scrofula, pox, small-pox, scurvy, inflammation of the lungs, spitting of blood, and fevers. It has been supposed that it may also be acquired by contagion, and in many is an hereditary disease.

SYMPTOMS.—The disorder begins with a dry cough, flying pains and stitches, an oppression at the breast, especially after motion; colliquative, or great and weakening sweats; loss of appetite, and sometimes vomiting up the food soon after taking it. The expectorated matter is purulent, sometimes bloody and offensive, with white round lumps. Toward the end of the disease a looseness frequently comes on, and the legs are apt to swell. In general the complexion is florid; there is a burning heat in the palm of the hands, and the face generally flushes after eating; the fingers become small, and club-like at the ends, the nails are bent inwards and convex, and the hairs sometimes fall off.

CURE.—As soon as any symptoms of this disorder appear, if the patient lives in a large town, where the air is confined, he ought immediately to retire to the country, and take daily moderate exercise, either on horseback, or in an open carriage; but the former is preferable. Nothing of the kind is so good as a long journey, in which the advantage of a continual change of air is joined to that of the mind's being constantly entertained with new objects: only care must be taken to avoid catching cold from wet clothes, damp beds, or other such accidents. He ought likewise not to ride sooner than two hours after dinner, and never to continue his journey to a late hour in the evening. A voyage by sea is also of great benefit if undertaken in time, and before the disorder is too far advanced.

Besides proper air and exercise, an attention to diet is necessary.

This ought to be of a nourifhing kind, and what is eafy of digeftion. Every thing of a heating nature is hurtful. The food fhould be chiefly of the vegetable clafs; and of every fort of diet, milk is the moft fuitable, particularly that of affes: but though this be a remedy of great efficacy, when employed at the beginning of a confumption, and the ufe of it continued for fome time, yet, taken in the trifling quantity that is ufual, it can hardly be productive of any benefit. It ought to be taken as an article of diet, not of medicine, and to the quantity of half a pint, with fome light bread, three times a day. If the milk fhould happen to purge, as is not uncommon, it may be mixed with fome old conferve of rofes, or a fmall tea-fpoonful of the powder of crabs'-claws.

Butter-milk, likewife, when it agrees with the ftomach, is an excellent remedy in this diforder; and I believe it would not often be found to difagree, if a perfon began to ufe it only in the quantity of a gill at a time, and increafed by degrees, either daily or every other day, to half a pint or upwards. But butter-milk, ufed for this purpofe, ought properly to be frefh every day, as otherwife it may become too acefcent, efpecially in the fummer.

Cow's milk is of all the moft eafy to be procured, and, though inferior to that of affes or mares, in point of facility of digeftion, it is neverthelefs preferable to the other common articles of diet. To render it lighter upon the ftomach, it may be mixed with half its quantity of barley-water. Some, for this purpofe, recommend the letting it ftand five or fix hours, and afterwards taking off the cream. But it may be fufficient to take off half the cream, and ftir the remainder in the milk, eating with it fome toafted bread, which is the form moft fuitable in a milk diet. The method of adding rum or brandy to milk fhould be ufed with great caution: for when added beyond a certain quantity, they not only coagulate the milk, but heat the body, and tend to augment the difeafe.

What renders milk lefs beneficial in confumptive cafes is that many of thofe for whom it is prefcribed have been accuftomed to the ufe of animal food, which never can, with fafety, be laid afide all at once. It is neceffary for fuch perfons, that they continue to make one meal in the day, according to the former manner, in refpect both of animal food and wine; but the food fhould be of the lighteft kind; and the quantity of it, as well as the liquors, be gradually diminifhed, till they be entirely left off. Then fhould commence a diet entirely of milk and vegetables: if any animal food be ufed, it ought only to be of the lighteft kind, fuch as calves' feet, which are extremely proper. Some, who had the refolution, have found great benefit from eating white fnails, either swallowed whole or boiled in milk; a sort of food that doubtless affords much nourishment, where the taste can be reconciled to it. When there is any degree of fever, currant jelly makes a suitable addition to diet; but tarts of unripe fruits, though recommended by some, seem not well accommodated to the disease; for at the same time that they afford very little nourishment, they are apt to bind the body too much, and tend to injure the lungs, both by supporting a constant fullness of the abdomen, and by the great exertion which they render necessary for expelling the fæces.

If variety of dishes can compensate an abstinence from animal food, the mode of diet here recommended admits of considerable latitude. Milk alone may be boiled with different substances, such as rice, barley and sago; all which, with the addition of a little sugar, are very grateful to the palate; exclusive of light puddings, which form also an agreeable repast.

It ought however to be observed, that acid fruits, especially those of the austere kind, such as the ingredients of tarts, do not make a proper mixture in the stomach with milk, and ought rather to be taken at the distance of a few hours from that part of diet.

If, notwithstanding this plentiful resource, the patient's strength and spirits should decline, it will be necessary to give him strong broths, jellies, and the like; but neither food nor drink ought ever to be taken in large quantity at a time, as it might oppress the lungs, and produce bad effects.

At the same time that the diet is properly accommodated to the disease, every endeavour should be exerted to render the patient as cheerful as possible; for as a consumption is often occasioned by grief or despondency, so it is always aggravated were either of these passions prevails. Amusements, therefore, cheerful company, and whatever suspends melancholy reflections, or exhilarates the mind, are in this case highly beneficial; and if prudently mixed with the consolations of religion, they will prove still more favourable for preserving serenity of mind.

Repeated bleedings, in small quantities, are considered as highly advantageous in consumptive cases; and when the constitution apparently abounds with blood, they certainly are so, especially when the blood drawn off is extremely sizy; when there is much pain in the breast; and when bleeding is followed by an abatement of every symptom. It ought, however, to be observed, that the inflammatory appearance of the blood is not alone a sufficient reason for bleeding; but, in determining the propriety of this evacuation, the other circumstances of the patient should be considered; such as the age, strength, habit, and the state of the disease.

Dr. Simmons strongly recommends a frequent repetition of

vomits. Many physicians have supposed, that where there is any increased determination to the lungs, vomits do mischief: but Dr. Simmons is persuaded, that, instead of augmenting, they diminish this determination, and that much good may be expected from a prudent use of this remedy, than which none has a more general or powerful effect on the system. If any remedy be capable of dispersing a tubercle, he believes it to be vomits. Dr. Simmons means not, however, that vomits will be useful in every period of the disease, or in every patient. In general, it will be found that the earlier in the disease emetics are had recourse to, the more likely they will be to do good, and the less likely to do harm. The cases in which emetics may be reckoned improper are commonly those in which the disease is rapid in its progress; or in that stage of it when there is great debility, with profuse colliquative sweats.

As an emetic in this disease, Dr. Simmons has often employed vitriolated copper. Its operation, he observes, is confined to the stomach, it acts almost instantaneously, and its astringency seems to obviate the relaxation that is commonly supposed to attend the frequent use of emetics. In two cases he experienced its good effects, after vomits of ipecacuanha had been given without success. He advises it to be given in the morning, and in the following manner: Let the patient first swallow about half a pint of water, and immediately afterwards the vitriol dissolved in a cupful of water. The dose of it must be adapted to the age, and other circumstances of the patient, and may be varied from two grains to ten, fifteen, or twenty. As some persons are much more easily puked than others, it will be prudent to begin with a small dose: not that any dangerous effects will be produced by a large one, for the whole of the medicine is instantly rejected; but if the nausea or sickness be violent, and of long continuance, the patient may perhaps be discouraged from repeating it. In general, the moment the emetic has reached the stomach it is thrown up again. The patient must then swallow another half pint of water, which is likewise speedily rejected; and this is commonly sufficient to remove the nausea.

Another remedy which Dr. Simmons strongly recommends in consumptive cases, both from his own observation and on the authority also of many other eminent practitioners, is myrrh. Take of myrrh, powdered, from ten to thirty grains; let it be made into a bolus, with honey, and taken two or three times a day. If there be much tendency to inflammation, it may be combined with a portion of nitre, or cream of tartar, which has often been serviceable in cases where a consumption was beginning to make its appearance.

Besides the use of internal remedies in affections of the lungs, physicians have often prescribed the steams of resinous and balsamic substances to be conveyed into the lungs. But the simple vapour of warm water seems preferable. This, in several instances, has been found to have good effects; but when the complaint has made any considerable progress, its utility is less obvious; and when the patients have been much weakened, it has brought on profuse sweats, especially when used in hed. Considerable expectations have lately been raised from the breathing of artificial air, and living with cows, but these expectations do not appear to have been realized. Drs. Fowler, Drake, Moffman, and others, believe that fox-glove may be relied on as a specific in consumption. See Medical and Physical Journal: But this medicine can only be administered by a skilful practitioner.

Another remedy recommended by some as a specific in consumptions is an earth-bath. For this purpose a hole is made in the ground, deep enough to admit the patient up to the chin. The hole is then carefully filled up with fresh mould, so that the earth may every where come in contact with the patient's body; and in this situation he is suffered to remain a considerable time, more or less, according to the judgment of the person who directs the operation. When the patient is taken out, he is wrapped in a linen cloth, placed upon a mattrass, and afterwards his whole body is rubbed with an ointment, composed of the leaves of nightshade and hog's-lard. Some instances are related of this process having been employed abroad with success; but we have not heard of any consumptive cases in which good effects were evidently obtained from it in this country.

In respect of drains, such as blisters, issues, and setons, so frequently recommended in consumptive cases, there is less danger of abuse from them than from bleeding; for the discharge they excite does not weaken the patient much, and they have so often been found to afford relief, that they are always worthy of a trial. But that these remedies may be of advantage, they ought to be applied at an early period of the disease. The discharge produced by a seton is by no means inconsiderable: and as in consumptive cases there is generally some inflammatory stitch, some part of the breast that is more painful, or more affected by a deep inspiration than the rest, a seton in the side, as near as can be to the seat of the inflammation, is highly advisable.

The Peruvian bark is perhaps the medicine most commonly employed of any, and often confided in as an ultimate resource in consumptive cases; but the general use of it is far from being ratified by experience. Where there is any tendency to inflammation it is evidently hurtful. There are, however, two cases in which it is found to be of advantage. One of these is, the suckling of children longer than is consistent with the mother's ability. This case frequently occurs among the middling and lower classes of females, of constitutions naturally delicate and tender. In such a state of weakness, some slight cold brings on a cough, which increases gradually, till at length it produces a true consumption of the lungs. Here the bark given early, in moderate doses, and merely as a strengthening remedy, is often of excellent use. In such cases, myrrh combined with steel is a valuable remedy; viz. Take myrrh, powdered, a drachm and a half; prepared kali, a drachm; rub them together, with a few drops of peppermint-water, till they form a soap-like lather; then add salt of steel half a drachm, and mix them well by rubbing; to the whole add of colt's-foot tea half a pint. Dose, four large spoonfuls every six hours.

Wherever there is any weakening discharge, and the lungs not inflamed, the bark is likewise of great advantage; and even if they be so affected, but not beyond a certain degree, it is of great effect in preventing the progress of the consumption. Take of Peruvian bark, in powder, an ounce; old conserve of roses, four ounces; syrup of oranges, or lemons, as much as is sufficient to make them into the consistence of honey. The bulk of a large nutmeg may be taken two or three times a day. The administration of this medicine, however, requires a judicious observer; and it ought neither to be given in the inflammatory stage of the disease, nor be continued in any subsequent period, if the breath becomes more tight and oppressed, the cough dry, the pulse more quick and hard, and especially if slight transitory pains or stitches about the thorax or breast are more frequently complained of. If, on the other hand, no pain, tightness, or oppression, is perceived, and there appears an evident abatement of the symptoms, a perseverance in the use of the bark will be advisable.

Various opinions are entertained concerning the efficacy of Bristol water in this disease. Dr. Fothergill informs us, that he has seen many persons recover from diseases of the lungs after drinking these waters, whose cure seemed to be doubtful from any other process; and he thinks this circumstance, added to the general reputation of Bristol water in consumptive cases, affords sufficient inducement to recommend the trial of them in the early stages of such complaints. It is, however, before the approach of a confirmed consumption that patients ought to repair to Bristol, otherwise a journey thither will not only be without benefit, but may even prove detrimental.

When there are evident signs of an imposthume in the breast, and the matter can neither be spit up nor carried off by absorption, it will be necessary that the patient use every means to break it inwardly, by inhaling or drawing in the ſteams of warm water, or vinegar, with his breath, coughing, ſneezing, bawling aloud, &c. If it burſt within the lungs, the matter may be diſcharged by the mouth; but ſometimes it flows in ſuch quantity as to ſuffocate the patient, eſpecially if his ſtrength be greatly reduced. On ſuch an occaſion, however, without ſuffocation, he is apt to faint; in which caſe volatile ſalts or ſpirits ſhould immediately be held to his noſe.

If the matter diſcharged be of a good conſiſtence, and the cough and breathing become eaſier, there is ſome proſpect of a cure; and recourſe ſhould be had to the Peruvian bark, to promote that effect; perſevering, at the ſame time, in the diet formerly preſcribed.

If the tumor, inſtead of pouring its contents into the interior parts of the lungs, ſhould diſcharge itſelf into the cavity of the breaſt, between the pleura and the lungs, it can only be drained off by making an inciſion between the ribs: but this is an operation which can only be performed by a ſurgeon. It is, however, not ſo formidable as people are apt to imagine, and many have recovered by means of it.

The conſumption of the lungs being generally attended with a hectic fever, it will be proper here to ſubjoin an account of that diſorder.

## *Hectic Fever.*

We are indebted to Dr. Heberden for the moſt explicit and ſatisfactory account of this diſeaſe. According to him, the appearance of the hectic fever is not unlike that of the genuine intermittent, from which, however, the diſeaſe is very different in its nature, and is alſo more dangerous. In the true intermittent, the three ſtages of cold, heat, and ſweat, are far more diſtinctly marked, the whole fit is much longer, the period which it obſerves is more conſtant and regular, and the intermiſſions are more perfect, than in the hectic fever. For in the latter, even in the moſt perfect remiſſion, there is uſually a feveriſh quickneſs perceptible in the pulſe, which ſeldom fails to exceed the utmoſt limits of a healthy one by at leaſt ten ſtrokes in a minute, being commonly 108.

The chillneſs of the hectic fever is ſometimes ſucceeded by heat, and ſometimes immediately by a ſweat without any intermediate ſtate of heat. The heat will ſometimes come on without any remarkable chillneſs preceding; and the chillneſs has been obſerved to go off without being followed either by heat or ſweat. The duration of theſe ſtages is ſeldom the ſame for three fits together; and as it is not uncommon for one of them to be wanting, the length of the whole fit muſt vary much more than in the true intermittent, but in general it is much ſhorter.

A patient under the hectic fever is little or nothing relieved by the coming on of the ſweat; but is often as anxious and reſtleſs as during the chillneſs or heat. When the ſweat is over, the fever will ſometimes continue; and in the middle of the fever the chillneſs will return, which is a moſt certain mark of this diſeaſe.

A hectic fever will return with great exactneſs, like an intermittent, for two, or perhaps three fits; but Dr. Heberden does not remember ever to have known it keep the ſame period for four fits ſucceſſively. The paroxyſm or fit will now and then keep off for ten or twelve days; and at other times, eſpecially when the patient is very ill, it will return ſo frequently in the ſame day, that the chillneſs of a new fit will follow immediately the ſweat of the former. It is not unuſual to have many threatenings of a ſhivering in the ſame day; and ſome degree of drowſineſs is apt to attend the ceſſation of a fit.

Hectic patients often complain of pains like thoſe of the rheumatiſm, which either affect by turns almoſt every part of the body, or elſe return conſtantly to the ſame part; which is often at a great diſtance from the ſeat of the principal diſorder, and, as far as is known, without any peculiar connection with it. Theſe pains are ſo violent in ſome patients as to require a large quantity of opium. They are moſt common where the hectic ariſes from ſome ulcer open to the external air, as in cancers of the face, breaſt, &c. Joined with this fever, and ariſing probably from one common cauſe, one may ſometimes ſee ſwellings of the limbs, neck, or trunk of the body, riſe up almoſt in an inſtant, as if the part was all at once grown fatter. Theſe ſwellings are not painful, hard, or diſcoloured, and they continue for ſeveral hours.

Dr. Heberden has ſeen this fever attack thoſe who ſeemed in tolerable health, in a ſudden and violent manner, like a common inflammatory one; and like that, alſo, in a very ſhort time bring them into imminent danger of their lives; after which it has begun to abate, and to afford hopes of a perfect recovery. But though the danger might be over for the preſent, and but little of a fever remain, yet that little has ſoon demonſtrated that it was kept up by ſome great miſchief within; and, proving unconquerable by any remedies, has gradually undermined the health of the patient, and never ceaſed except with his life. This manner of its beginning, however, is extraordinary. It much oftener diſſembles its ſtrength at firſt; and creeps on ſo ſlowly, that the ſubjects of it, though they be not perfectly well, yet for ſome months hardly think themſelves ill; complaining only of being ſooner tired with exerciſe than uſual, of want of appetite, and of falling away. But moderate as the ſymptoms may ſeem, if the pulſe be quicker than ordinary, ſo as to beat ninety times, or perhaps a hundred and twenty times in a minute, there is the greateſt reaſon to be apprehenſive of the event. In no diſorder, perhaps, is the pulſe of more uſe to guide our judgment than in the hectic fever; yet even here we muſt be upon our guard, and not truſt entirely to this criterion; for one in about twenty patients, with all the worſt ſigns of decay from ſome incurable cauſe, which irreſiſtably goes on to deſtroy life, will ſhow not the ſmalleſt degree of quickneſs, nor any other irregularity of the pulſe, to the day of his death.

The Causes of hectic are various, as ulcerations of the lungs, of the liver, lumbar abſceſs, white ſwelling, ſcrofula, worms, giving ſuck too long, &c. Morton ſuppoſed the immediate cauſe to be purulent matter taken into the circulation; but this notion is now abandoned.

This fever will ſupervene whenever there is a great collection of matter formed in any part of the body; but it more particularly attends the inflamation of a ſcirrhous gland, and even upon one that is ſlight and only juſt beginning—the fever growing worſe in proportion as the gland becomes more inflamed or ulcered. And ſuch is the lingering nature of thoſe glandular diſorders, that the firſt of theſe ſtages will continue for many months, and the ſecond for ſome years.

If this ſcirrhous inflammation be external, or in ſome of the abdominal viſcera or bowels, where the diſturbance of their functions plainly points out the ſeat of the diſorder, no doubt can be entertained concerning the cauſe of the fever. But if the part affected be not obvious to the ſenſes, and its preciſe functions be not known, the hectic, which is there only part of the train of another diſeaſe, may be miſtaken for the primary or only one.

Lying-in women, on account of the violence ſuſtained in delivery generally die when affected with this fever. Women of the age of near fifty and upwards, are particularly liable to it; for upon the ceſſation of their natural diſcharge, the glands of the breaſts, ovaries, or womb, too commonly begin to grow ſcirrhous, and proceed to be cancerous. Not only theſe, but the glandular parts of the abdominal viſcera, or bowels of the belly, are diſpoſed to be affected at this period, and to become the ſeats of incurable diſorders.

The injuries done to the ſtomach and liver by hard drinking are attended with ſimilar ſymptoms, and terminate in the ſame manner.

It is obſerved that the ſlighteſt wound by a fine pointed inſtrument will, upon ſome occaſions, bring on the greateſt diſturbanecs, and the moſt alarming ſymptoms, nay, even death itſelf; for not only the wounded part will ſwell and be painſul, but by turns almoſt every part of the body; and very diſtant parts have been known to come even to ſuppuration. Theſe ſymptoms are conſtantly accompanied with this irregular intermittent, which laſts as long as any of them remains.

This ſpecies of fever is never leſs dangerous than when it belongs to a kindly ſuppuration, into which all the diſeaſed parts are melted down, and for which there is a proper outlet.

The inflammation of internal ſcirrhous glands, or of thoſe in the breaſts, ſometimes goes off; and the fever, which depended upon it, ceaſes; but it much oftener happens that it proceeds to cancerous and gangrenous ulcers, and terminates only in death. Death is alſo, almoſt univerſally, the conſequence of a hectic fever from tubercles of the lungs, which have, in general at leaſt, been conſidered as glandular bodies in a ſcirrhous ſtate.

Cure.—It is not to be expected that the ſame remedies will in every caſe be adapted to a fever which, ariſing from very different cauſes, is attended with ſuch a variety of ſymptoms. A mixture of aſſafœtida and opium has in ſome perſons ſeemed ſingularly ſerviceable in this fever, when brought on by a ſmall wound; but in moſt other caſes, the principal if not the ſole attention of the phyſician muſt be employed in relieving the ſymptoms, by tempering the heat, by preventing both coſtiveneſs and purging, by procuring ſleep, and by checking the ſweats. If, at the ſame time, he put the body into as good general health as may be, by air, exerciſe, and a proper courſe of mild diet, he can perhaps do nothing better than to leave all the reſt to nature. In ſome few fortunate patients, nature appears to have ſuch reſources as may afford reaſon for entertaining hopes of cure, even in very bad caſes; for ſome have recovered from this fever attended with every ſymptom of ſome bowel in the abdomen being incurably diſeaſed, after all probable methods of relief from art had been tried in vain, and after the fleſh and ſtrength were ſo exhauſted as to leave ſcarce any hopes from nature. In theſe deplorable circumſtances, there has ariſen a ſwelling not far from the probable ſeat of the diſorder, and yet without any diſcoverable communication with it. This ſwelling has advanced to an abſceſs; in conſequence of which, the pulſe has ſoon returned to its natural ſtate, as have alſo the appetite, fleſh, and ſtrength. What nature has performed in theſe rare caſes, Dr. Heberden tells us, he has often endeavoured to imitate, by making iſſues and applying bliſters near the ſeat of the diſeaſe; but he cannot ſay with the ſame ſucceſs.

It seems at present to be the opinion of many practitioners, that the gangrenes will be stopped, and suppuration become more kindly, by the use of the Peruvian bark; and therefore this remedy is always either advised or permitted in the irregular fever joined with suppurations. But Dr. Heberden has never seen any good effect from the bark in this fever unattended with an apparent ulcer; and even in gangrenes it so often fails, that in successful cases, where it has been administered, there must be room for suspicion that the success was owing to another cause. Dr. Heberden acknowledges at the same time, that he never saw any harm from the bark, in these, or indeed in any other cases, except a slight temporary purging or sickness, where it has happened to disagree with the stomach, or where the latter has been loaded by taking the medicine too fast, especially in dry boluses wrapped in wafer-paper.

In hectie illnesses, where all other means have proved ineffectual, a journey to Bath is usually proposed by the friends, and wished for by the sick; but besides the fatigue and many inconveniences of a journey to a dying person, the Bath-waters are peculiarly hurtful in this fever, which they never fail to increase, and thereby aggravate the sufferings and hasten the death of the patient. The fox-glove has been found successful in hectic arising from consumption.

## *Atrophy (Tabes) or Nervous Consumption.*

This disease consists in a wasting of the body, without any remarkable fever, cough, or difficulty of breathing; but attended with want of appetite and bad digestion.

Causes.—Sometimes this disease approaches without any evident cause, but is occasioned by one or other of the following; viz. too copious evacuations, especially of the semen, in which case it is named *tabes dorsalis;* deficiency of nourishment; abuse of spiritous liquors; passions of the mind; indigestion; scrofulous obstructions of internal glands.

Symptoms.—In the beginning of this disease the face is pale, and there is a loathing of all solid food; the patient also feels a languor, which chiefly prevails while in bed. The urine is often small in quantity, and high-coloured, but sometimes pale and copious.

This complaint, from whatever cause it arises, is very difficult of cure; and when it does not carry off the patient by excessive weakness, often terminates in a fatal dropsy.

CURE.—The treatment of this diſeaſe muſt be varied, according to the particular cauſe which gives riſe to the complaint. When the appetite and digeſtion are bad, an emetic of ipecacuanha ſhould be given to cleanſe the ſtomach; and a doſe or two of rhubarb, to produce the ſame effect in the bowels. Afterwards the patient ought to take ſtomachic medicines and the Peruvian bark. They may be combined in the following manner. Take of gentian-root, two drachms; outer rind of Seville oranges, half an ounce; Peruvian bark one ounce; infuſe them for two or three days in a quart of white wine, and filter through paper. Three table-ſpoonfuls of this to be taken twice a day, with ten drops of the tincture of muriated iron; or inſtead of the latter, may be given ſome ruſt of iron, made into a bolus with crumb of bread, and a tea-ſpoonful of water. The patient may begin with five grains of the ruſt, and increaſe the doſe daily by the addition of two or three grains, to as great a quantity as the ſtomach can bear, or the mixture of ſteel and myrrh. *See Appendix.*

The ſame medicine will be proper where the diſorder proceeds from ſcrofulous obſtructions of the glands. In this caſe the uſe of goats whey is of great advantage. If worms be the cauſe, it muſt be treated according to the manner mentioned under that article in the diſeaſes of children. If owing to a venereal taint, the method of cure muſt be by mercurials, and ſarſaparilla, as directed for that diſorder. If the complaint ariſe from weakneſs of the nerves, as in the hyſterical and hypochondriacal affection, preparations of iron, or the ruſt above mentioned, will be proper; with two of the following pills twice a day. Take of aſſafœtida, and caſtor, each a drachm; common ſyrup as much as is ſufficient to make them into twenty-four pills. If the perſon be of a ſcorbutic habit, the ſcorbutic juices, ſuch as garden ſcurvy-graſs, brook-lime, and water-creſſes, ſhould be uſed with vegetable acids; and the Peruvian bark, with goats whey, in this caſe, is likewiſe highly adviſable. If great evacuations have given riſe to the complaint, the principal remedy is alſo the Peruvian bark.

In all theſe caſes, a conſtant uſe of ſome gentle laxative, ſuch as lenitive electuary, is generally requiſite; the diet ought to be light and nouriſhing; and the patient ſhould every day take moderate exerciſe on horſeback, and uſe the cold bath occaſionally.

## CHAP. XI.

### *Inflammation of the Stomach (Gastritis) Heart, and Midriff.*

AN inflammation of the ſtomach may ariſe from drinking too largely of cold liquor when a perſon is very hot; from acrid ſubſtances taken into it; from a ſurfeit; a ſtoppage of perſpiration; repulſion of the gout; violent paſſion, &c.

SYMPTOMS.—This diſorder is accompanied with great heat, pulſation, and acute pain in the region of the ſtomach, which is increaſed by ſwallowing any thing that adds to the irritation of the part. There is a conſtant tenſion at the pit of the ſtomach, with anxiety, and continual retching; often likewiſe with a hiccup. The pulſe is ſmall, weak, and frequently intermitting.

CURE.—An inflammation of the ſtomach requires the moſt ſpeedy exertion of every poſſible means to extinguiſh it. The remedy moſt to be depended upon is plentiful bleeding, which, if the diſorder prove obſtinate, it is neceſſary to repeat ſeveral times, notwithſtanding the low ſtate of the pulſe; for this generally riſes upon bleeding. A large bliſter ſhould then be applied to the region of the ſtomach; and warm fomentations, with chamomile-flowers and linſeed boiled in water, be frequently applied to the whole belly; afterwards covering it with flannel cloths, dipped in the fomentation, and wrung out, to be renewed as ſoon as they cool. Clyſters made of the ſame materials, with the addition of two drachms of nitre to each, ought alſo to be often thrown up.

The feet and legs ſhould be likewiſe frequently bathed in tepid or luke-warm water; and if the warm bath can be procured, the uſe of it would be adviſable.

The great irritability of the ſtomach in this diſeaſe precludes the poſſibility of relief by the common channel of medicinal application. Diluting drinks, however, may be tried; as may likewiſe ſmall doſes of nitre, with ſpermaceti or ſome mucilage of gum-arabic, to which may be added now and then three or four drops of the tincture of opium.

At the ſame time, opiates given in clyſters may frequently be employed with advantage. For this purpoſe, take of barley-water half a pint; to which add a tea-ſpoonful or upwards of the tincture of opium. It is likewiſe only by clyſters that the patient can be ſupported under the diſeaſe. Warm milk, given in the quantity of a gill more than the preceding clyſter, may anſwer both as a fomentation and light nouriſhment.

If the diforder fhould not be removed by the means above mentioned, it muft unavoidably proceed either to fuppuration or gangrene; the former of which can fcarcely afford any hope of cure, and the latter is univerfally fatal.

### *Inflammation of the Heart.**

The inflammation of the heart, and of the membrane that furrounds it, is attended with all the fymptoms which accompany that of the lungs, but in a higher degree. There is a deep feated pain, weight, and anxiety, with very quick and frequent refpiration; great thirft, a heat in the cheft, and a palpitation of the heart. The pulfe is hard and unequal, and the patient frequently faints.

The fymptoms attending an inflammation of the diaphragm or midriff are, an acute pain between the fhort ribs and the back, great reftleffnefs and anxiety. The hypochondrium, or part below the fhort ribs, is drawn in towards the back; and the lower belly has little or no motion during the act of refpiration. The breathing is quick and fhort, accompanied with convulfive catchings, a dry cough, and hiccup.

CURE.—The general method of cure here is the fame as in other inflammatory difeafes. Bleeding is neceffary in as great a degree as the patient can poffibly bear. Strong blifters muft likewife be laid over the parts; and the fame cooling treatment be employed as in the pleurify and inflammation of the lungs.

## CHAP. XII.

### *Inflammation of the Inteftines (Enteritis.)*

THIS inflammation is an extremely acute and dangerous difeafe, feizing any part of the inteftinal canal, but chiefly the lowermoft of the fmall guts. It is generally brought on by external cold, fever, coftivenefs, worms, acrid or auftere fubftances in the bowels; eating unripe fruits, or hard indigeftible aliments; drinking ftale and windy malt liquors, four wines, cyder, &c. It may alfo be occafioned by tumors in the inteftines or neighbouring parts; an introfufception or running in of one part of a bowel into the other, and there confined by fome ftricture or adhefion: very high feafoned and ftimulating food frequently gives rife to it; and it is

* See *Peripneumony*, p. 180 and 183

often likewise produced by wet feet, wet clothes, and whatever obstructs perspiration.

Symptoms.—It is accompanied with nearly the same symptoms as the inflammation of the stomach. The pain is extremely acute, and occupies different parts, according to the intestine affected. In general there is a distention of the belly, attended with such flatulence that the patient is continually belching up wind. The whole body, particularly about the navel, is affected with a soreness that is aggravated with the slightest touch. The vomiting is sometimes so violent that the motion of the bowels is inverted, and even the excrements discharged by the mouth. These last symptoms are commonly called iliac passion. There is often an obstruction of urine. The pulse, from being small, hard, and quick, frequently becomes at last irregular and intermittent. The tongue is dry, accompanied with great thirst; and the prostration of strength, as in inflammation of the stomach, is in proportion to the violence of the symptoms.

If this disease be left to itself, it sometimes ends fatally in ten or twelve hours; and almost always before the end of the third day; so that there is seldom any suppuration.

But if this effect should take place, the pain diminishes, and is converted rather into a sense of distention: irregular cold fits, with other signs of internal suppuration, ensue, and the other symptoms abate.

The abscess, when formed, may break either into the cavity of the abdomen, or into the intestinal canal. In the former case, it is generally fatal, by producing a hectic fever; in the other, the matter is discharged by stool, sometimes at first pure, and afterwards mixed with the fæces, and gradually diminishing, if the ulcer proceeds favourably; or a considerable quantity of matter continuing to be discharged, a hectic fever is in this case also excited, and the patient carried off.

Clammy sweats, a small intermittent pulse, and a total cessation of pain, are signs of approaching dissolution.

The treatment of the patient with respect to food and drink is the same as in the inflammation of the stomach: the former must be of the lightest kind used in fevers, and given in small quantities; and the latter be weak and diluting, as barley-water, &c. The patient ought likewise to be kept quiet, avoiding cold, and all violent passions of the mind.

Cure.—Large bleeding is no less necessary here than in the inflammation of the stomach, and should be repeated according to the urgency of the symptoms, until the pulse become soft. Cupping-glasses may also be applied to the belly with advantage, if the patient can bear them; as may likewise the following fomentation; afterwards applying the materials by way of a cataplasm or poultice. Take of chamomile-flowers, two handfuls; the heads of white poppies without the seeds, and the root of marshmallows, each an ounce. Boil them in a sufficient quantity of water for five or six minutes. The patient's feet and legs should likewise be frequently bathed in warm water; and softening clysters be given. These may consist of milk and water; or barley-water, with salt, some sweet oil or fresh butter.

If the disease should not yield to the remedies above mentioned, recourse must be had to purgative medicines, beginning with those of the gentlest kind. For this purpose may be used castor-oil, mixed with mucilage or yolk of egg with twice as much water; or Glauber's or Epsom salts, with an ounce of manna, may be dissolved in a pint of warm water; and a tea-cupful of it taken every half hour till it operates. Should this not be retained, on account of the vomiting, it will be necessary to give fifteen or twenty drops of laudanum, in a little simple cinnamon-water, or peppermint-water, and afterwards repeat the dose of the solution.

But if the vomiting still continues, give the following saline draught in the act of effervescence, or while the mixing of the ingredients yields a hissing noise. Take of the salt of wormwood, or kali, a scruple; juice of lemons, a large table spoonful; mint-water an ounce; loaf sugar, a drachm: mix them; or let the kali or lemon-juice be taken in succession. Sometimes acids alone, such as juice of lemons, or vinegar, will have the effect of staying the vomiting.

If no liquid purgative will sit upon the stomach, we must next try those of the solid kind, combined with opium, in the following manner. Take of the powder of jalap, half a drachm; calomel, five grains; opium, one grain; common syrup, a sufficient quantity, to make five pills, to be taken for a dose.

When stools cannot be produced by purgatives, the warm bath sometimes proves effectual. The patient ought to be immersed up to the breast, and continue as long as he can bear it without fainting. But it is better to repeat the immersions at the interval of some minutes than to remain in the bath too long at a time. The skins of animals just killed, applied to the belly, have often been found of great service. And when all other purgative remedies fail, the fumes of tobacco, thrown up the fundament, have produced good effects; as has also quicksilver, taken by the mouth, in the quantity of an ounce.

When the violent constipation can be removed by nothing else, it has frequently been conquered by immersing the patient's lower extremities in cold water; or while he walks on a wet pavement, to dash his legs and thighs with cold water.

Such is often the obſtinacy of this dreadful diſeaſe, and its termination ſo frequently fatal, that people cannot guard with too much caution againſt whatever may give riſe to it. Of all the cauſes above enumerated, that of long continued coſtiveneſs is one of the moſt general; which ſhould therefore always be prevented by the uſe of ſome gentle laxative. Caution is likewiſe to be ſtrongly inculcated with reſpect to ſour unripe fruits, and ſour or very ſtale liquors; and, above all, lead in any form (See *Painter's Colic*). Nor is it leſs proper to recommend a careful attention to avoid the danger of wet clothes, and eſpecially of wet feet; which of all the various ways of catching cold is the moſt pernicious to the bowels.

## CHAP. XIII.

### *Inflammation of the Liver (Hepatitis.)*

AN inflammation of the liver, though frequent in the Eaſt-Indies, does not often occur to the obſervation of practitioners in this country.

SYMPTOMS.—This diſeaſe comes on with ſome degree of fever, and a pain under the ſhort ribs of the right ſide, increaſed by preſſing upon the part, and frequently extended ſo far up as the top of the ſhoulder. It is alſo commonly attended with a cough, which is generally dry, but ſometimes moiſt; and the patient cannot lie with caſe except on the ſide affected. The ſymptoms, however, are various in this diſeaſe, according to the particular part of the liver which happens to be affected. In ſome, it is attended with hiccup and vomiting; in others, with a jaundice, or yellowneſs of the eyes, depending on the part of the liver that is the ſeat of the inflammation.

CAUSES.—This diſorder, though it may be produced by the common cauſes of inflammation, is liable to be excited by affections of the liver itſelf, and thoſe of the contiguous parts. An indurated tumor in the liver ſometimes gives riſe to it, but is more frequently the conſequence of inflammation. Too free an uſe of hot ſpicy aliment, and of ſtrong wines or ſpirituous liquors, will alſo produce the diſeaſe; as will likewiſe ſtones obſtructing the paſſage of the bile; and any thing that ſuddenly cools the liver after it has been much heated.

This inflammation, like that of other parts, may terminate by reſolution, ſuppuration, or perhaps gangrene. The firſt of theſe is often the consequence of, or is attended with evacuations of different kinds. A bleeding at the nose, and sometimes the bleeding piles, will carry off the disease. At other times, the same effect is accomplished by a bilious looseness; and many instances occur where the resolution is attended with sweating, and a discharge of urine depositing a copious sediment. Sometimes it may be terminated by an erysipelas appearing in some external part. When the disease ends in suppuration, the matter may be discharged by the biliary ducts; or, if the suppurated tumor does not adhere any where closely to the neighbouring parts, it may be discharged into the cavity of the abdomen or belly: but if during the earlier stage of the inflammation the affected part of the liver shall have formed a close adhesion to some of the adjacent parts, the discharge after suppuration may be various, according to the particular situation of the abscess. When seated on the convex part of the liver, if the adhesion be to the diaphragm or midriff, the purulent matter may penetrate into the cavity of the lungs, and may thence be discharged by coughing; but if the adhesion be to the peritonæum, or membrane lining the abdomen, the matter may work its way outwardly, or a passage be made by incision. When, on the other hand, the abscess is seated in the concave part of the liver, the matter may, in consequence of adhesion, be discharged into the stomach or intestines, and into the latter, either directly, or by the intervention of the biliary ducts.

Cure.—The treatment in respect to food and drink, must be the same as in other inflammations. The symptoms, at the beginning of this disease, being generally not alarming, it is often too late before the remedies are employed; but as soon as the existence of this disorder is ascertained, recourse should be immediately had to bleeding; which it may likewise be necessary to repeat, though the pulse should not feel hard. After bleeding, the side should be fomented as directed in the preceding inflammations; a softening clyster should be given, and the feet and legs be bathed in warm water. A blister ought then to be applied over the part; giving afterwards the following purgative. Take of the leaves of senna, two drachms; tamarinds, an ounce; water, half a pint: boil them a few minutes, and in the strained liquor dissolve half an ounce of manna. Four table-spoonfuls to be given every half hour till it begins to operate.

In this disease great benefit is sometimes found from the use of diuretic medicines, or those which increase the discharge of urine. With this intention a scruple of purified nitre, or half a drachm, if the stomach will bear it, may be taken in a cup of the patient's drink every three or four hours; or a tea-spoonful of the sweet spirit of nitre may be used for the same purpose.

When there appears any tendency to ſweat, it ought to be encouraged by drinking plentifully of warm diluting liquors, ſuch as barley-water.

Sometimes the diſeaſe is carried off by a diſcharge through the inteſtines. Should therefore ſuch a criſis ſeem to take place, by any looſe ſtools, they muſt not be checked, unleſs the evacuation be ſo conſiderable as to weaken the patient: becauſe of all the outlets from the body, this is the channel moſt convenient for affording relief to the complaint.

When the diſeaſe proceeds to ſuppuration, and matter is actually formed in the liver, we muſt watch the motion of nature, and have recourſe to ſuch remedies as tend to encourage the diſcharge by which ſhe endeavours to operate, giving in the mean time the Peruvian bark, to guard the conſtitution againſt the efforts which might ariſe from an abſorption of the purulent matter. It may be given in powder in the quantity of half a drachm, four or five times a day.

If the matter be not carried off through ſome of the outlets of the body, but the abſceſs breaks, the only favourable event is when the diſcharge is made outwardly; and this ought to be promoted as much as poſſible by fomentations and poultices. The abſceſs may then be opened by an inciſion, but ſtill the patient's life can only be preſerved conditionally; that is, if the liver adheres to the peritonæum in ſuch a manner as to prevent the matter from falling into the cavity of the abdomen.

If notwithſtanding every effort to cure the diſeaſe by reſolution, it ſhould terminate in a ſcirrhus or hard tumor, the patient may ſurvive for many years, and even live to a great age; but he muſt be attentive to his diet. He ought to uſe more of vegetable than of animal food; and avoid both high ſeaſoned meats and ſtrong liquors. He ſhould uſe gentle exerciſe; and will find benefit from a moderate uſe of vegetable acids.

Beſides the diſeaſe above deſcribed, there is alſo a chronic kind of inflammation of the liver, depending more on an accumulation and effuſion in this organ, than on an increaſed action of its ſmall veſſels. In this ſpecies of the diſorder the patient complains rather of a ſenſe of weight than of pain, and the fever is neither acute nor conſtant, but often returns in paroxyſms or fits, ſomewhat reſembling the attacks of an intermittent. This diſeaſe is very ſlow in its progreſs, frequently continuing for many months, and at laſt terminating in a very conſiderable ſuppuration. In moſt caſes this diſeaſe may be diſcovered by a careful examination of the region of the liver externally; upon which it will generally be found that this bowel has acquired a conſiderable enlargement.

In this diſorder, the beſt remedies are the neutral ſalts, given in ſmall quantities, ſo as gently to increaſe the diſcharge by urine. Half a drachm of ſal polychreſt, or a drachm of Glauber's ſalts, diſſolved in a gill of warm water, may be taken every morning. But the remedy moſt to be depended upon is a grain of calomel, morning and evening, till the mouth becomes a little ſore, and then the diuretic ſalt, in ſuitable doſes. Or tincture of ſquills.

## CHAP. XIV.

### *Inflammation of the Spleen, Kidneys, Bladder, and other Parts.*

AN inflammation of the ſpleen is a diſorder which rarely occurs; but in conſequence of ſome fevers of the remittent or intermittent kind, this bowel is frequently loaded, and remains a long time in a hardened and indolent ſtate, excited by the general cauſes of inflammatory diſeaſes, and attacking chiefly perſons of a full and ſanguine habit of body.

SYMPTOMS.—This diſeaſe comes on with a remarkable ſhivering, ſucceeded by great heat and thirſt. A dull pain is felt under the ſhort ribs of the left ſide, accompanied for the moſt part with a protuberance externally. The fever generally increaſes every fourth day; the feet and knees grow red; the noſe and ears ſometimes pale; and there is a difficulty of breathing.

The inflammation of the ſpleen is accompanied with leſs danger than that of the liver; and a vomiting of black matter, which in other acute diſeaſes is reckoned a fatal ſymptom, is ſaid to prove ſometimes critical and ſalutary in this diſeaſe. The inflammation is likewiſe ſometimes carried off by the hæmorrhoids; but it frequently terminates by a ſcirrhus.

CURE.—The treatment is the ſame in this caſe as in the inflammation of the liver. But without much previous complaint an abſceſs is ſometimes formed in this bowel, which, burſting ſuddenly, pours its contents into the belly, and in a few days terminates in death.

The ſpleen, like the liver, is alſo ſubject to a chronic inflammation, which often happens after agues, and is called the *ague-cake*; though that name is alſo frequently given to a ſcirrhous tumor of the liver ſucceeding intermittents.

*Inflammation of the Kidneys.*

Exclusive of the usual symptoms of inflammation, this disorder is attended with frequent vomiting, and often with costiveness and colic pains. The urine most commonly is of a deep red colour, and is voided frequently, and in a small quantity at a time. In more violent cases, this discharge is commonly colourless. The pain of this inflammation is not increased by the motion of the trunk of the body so much as a pain of the rheumatic kind affecting the same region. It may also frequently be distinguished by its shooting along the course of the ureter, and it is often attended with a drawing up of the testicle, and a numbness of the limb on the side affected; though indeed these symptoms most commonly attend the inflammation arising from a stone in the kidney or ureter.

Causes.—This disorder may be occasioned by any thing of an acrid nature stimulating the kidneys; heating diuretics; fulness of blood; suppressed evacuations; external contusions; calculous concretions; strains of the muscles of the back; violent or long continued riding on horseback, or shaking in a carriage.

Cure.—The remedies here are the same as in other inflammations. Bleeding must be employed, and repeated according to the exigence of the symptoms; but though necessary in robust habits, it must be cautiously used in gouty constitutions, or such as are enfeebled. Blisters here are not advisable, on account of the irritation which might be excited by the cantharides; but fomentations and the use of the warm bath are of great advantage. A gentle laxative, such as the following, should then be given. Take of senna leaves, two drachms; boiling water, half a pint. Infuse for half an hour; and in the strained liquor dissolve two drachms of tartarised kali, or three drachms of Glauber's salts, and half an ounce of manna. Four table-spoonfuls to be taken every half hour. Let the following clyster likewise be immediately injected. Take of milk and water, a gill and a half; salt and sugar, each two tea-spoonfuls; linseed oil, three table-spoonfuls. Mix them.

The following emulsion, taken warm, should be plentifully used as common drink. Take of sweet almonds, blanched, one ounce and a half; double refined sugar, half an ounce; water, two pints. Beat the almonds with the sugar; then, rubbing them well together, add the water by degrees, and strain the liquor. An infusion of linseed or marsh-mallow root, sweetened with honey, may likewise be drunk occasionally.

In case of violent pain, fifteen drops of laudanum may be given every fix or eight hours; or a tea-fpoonful of it may be mixed with a clyfter.

If the complaint fhould terminate in fuppuration, which may be known by the abatement of the pain, a remaining fenfe of weight in the loins, with frequent fhiverings fucceeded by heat, and whitifh turbid urine, give the following electuary in the quantity of a fmall nutmeg three times a day. Take of the powder of rhubarb, one drachm and a half; nitre, one drachm; double refined fugar, three drachms; Strafburgh turpentine, half an ounce; mix them into an electuary. To complete the cure, the Peruvian bark ought to be given, in moderate dofes, two or three times a day.

This complaint has frequently been miftaken for an inflammatory lumbago, or pain of the loins; but from this it may be diftinguifhed by the following circumftances, viz. from the patient's being able to raife himfelf into an erect pofture; being bent forwards without any remarkable pain, which in the lumbago is very fevere; from the pain following the courfe of the ureters; from the difficulty of making water, and the urine being more changed from the natural appearance, which is not the cafe in the lumbago.

## *Inflammation of the Bladder.*

This diforder begins with a violent pain in the regions of the bladder, deep feated and fometimes attended with an external rednefs in that part. If the neck of the bladder be affected, there is a retention of urine, with a conftant defire to difcharge it. If the bottom be the part inflamed, there is a continual dribbling, with great efforts to make water more plentifully. Thefe fymptoms are accompanied with frequent attempts to expel the fæces, to which the patient is excited by perpetual irritation. The pulfe is frequent and hard, accompanied with ficknefs, vomiting, and fometimes delirium. There is great anxiety and reftleffnefs, and the extremities become cold.

Cure.—The ufual treatment of inflammations muft in this cafe be profecuted with vigour; fuch as bleeding, fomentations, and the warm bath. Clyfters, by preffing upon the bladder, when a part near the great gut happens to be inflamed, may prove hurtful, and fhould therefore only be ufed when there are hardened fæces, and then likewife in fmaller quantities than ufual; but gentle laxatives, fuch as fenna, Glauber's falts, manna, and the like, ought never to be omitted. Ten or fifteen grains of nitre ought likewife to be frequently given in the patient's drink. This fhould confift of barley-water, or an infufion of linfeed; but if the urine be retained from a ſtricture in the neck of the bladder, the drink ſhould be taken only in ſmall quantities. In which caſe, likewiſe, it is neceſſary to evacuate the urine by means of a catheter; but this muſt be done with great caution.

If, notwithſtanding the uſe of theſe remedies, and after ſufficient evacuation, a ſpaſmodic contraction and pain ſhould continue, opiates may ſometimes be uſeful.

In caſes of mucous diſcharge from the bladder, give the following pills. Take of ſoda and Venetian ſoap, each one drachm; oil of nutmeg, ſix drops; common ſyrup, enough to make into twenty-four pills. Four to be taken twice a day, with ſome of the compound decoction of barley.

If the bladder ſuppurate, the matter muſt be diſcharged as ſoon as poſſible, and the remedies already recommended in ulcers of the kidneys are to be employed.

## *Inflammation of the Womb.*

This diſorder is accompanied with pain, heat, pulſation, and tumor of the part; a continual painful urging to go to ſtool; and a difficulty of making water.

Causes.—All the general cauſes of inflammation may give riſe to this complaint; but it is chiefly owing to the ſudden change produced in the habit after delivery, and therefore moſt frequent with women in child-bed. It is, however, not to be confounded with the diſeaſe called the puerperal or child-bed fever.

Cure.—The means to be employed for curing this inflammation is the ſame as for that in other parts; viz. by bleeding, gentle ſoftening clyſters, and fomentations; after the latter of which, a poultice of bread and milk, with oil, ſhould be applied to the pudenda. In the mean time, the patient muſt uſe a light diet, and warm diluting liquors; taking every two or three hours ten or fifteen grains of nitre, diſſolved in ſome of her drink. If the pain continues, recourſe may be had to opiates, both with ſafety and advantage.

## *Inflammation of the Meſentery.*

This, like other inflammations, is accompanied with a fever, which however is variable, being ſometimes ſlight, ſometimes remittent, and at others violent. There is a tumor and deep ſeated pain about the region of the navel: the body is bound; there is a bitter taſte in the mouth; and, in the more advanced ſtate of the diſeaſe, a thin, red, foetid, or white matter, paſſes off by the ſtool.

CURE.—In this complaint, it is found that bleeding by eight or ten leeches, applied round the navel, has greater effect than from a vein. Softening clysters, repeatedly given, are of great advantage. Fomentations must also be diligently employed; applying after them some volatile liniment, with opium, in the following manner: Take of soap liniment, or the liniment of ammonia, one ounce; tincture of opium, one drachm. Mix. Or instead of this may be used Bate's anodyne balsam. (See *Appendix*.)

### *Inflammation of the Omentum, or Cawl.*

This complaint is distinguished by an acute darting pain through the superior and middle part of the lower belly, under the muscles and membrane of the abdomen. There is a perceptible swelling and tension, increased upon pressure, and accompanied with an inflammatory fever. The bleeding with leeches, and other applications, are here to be employed in the same way as in the inflammation of the mesentery.

### *Inflammation of the Peritonæum.*

This is discoverable by a fever, and pain of the lower belly, which is increased by the body being in an erect posture. The abdomen is extremely painful on strong pressure, and is often greatly distended. The treatment of this disorder differs in nothing from that of the two last mentioned complaints.

It may be proper here to observe, that, in all internal inflammations, it is necessary in every case to attempt to procure resolution as quickly as possible; because if the disorder proceed to suppuration, and matter be formed in a place whence it is not discharged externally by nature, nor can be by art, the disease must terminate fatally.

## CHAP. XV.

### *Of painful Diseases, not attended by Fever.*

#### *Head-ach and Tooth-ach.*

IN the whole class of human diseases there is no complaint more general than that of the head-ach; nor any that is in most cases more transitory, and, in others, more obstinate. It is distinguished into different kinds, according to the degree of the malady, or the part which it occupies. These are, *cephalalgia*, when the pain is not very considerable; *cephalæa*, when it exists in a higher degree, and extends over the whole head; and *hemicrania*, in which one side only is affected. Besides these there is a fourth, called *clavus hystericus*, where the pain is fixed within a very small compass, in one side of the forehead.

The complaint is farther distinguished into internal and external; primary and symptomatic; the last of which, viz. the symptomatic, is by far the most general.

A head-ach may be occasioned by whatever distends the vessels of that part, or obstructs the circulation through them. It consequently may arise from a stoppage of perspiration; a suppression of accustomed evacuation; such as the piles; bleeding or running at the nose; sweating of the feet; and by costiveness, or other causes which, by impeding the motion of the blood in the lower extremities, produce a greater fulness in the head.

Besides the quantity of the fluids, an acrid state of them may give rise to the disorder; and hence it is frequently a consequence of the secondary venereal disease. It likewise often owes its origin to nervous irritation; and above all to indigestion, or a foulness of the stomach.

CURE.—When the complaint proceeds from a fullness of blood, which may be concluded from a sanguine habit of body, a full pulse, and perhaps a florid countenance, the remedies are bleeding, cupping on the back of the neck or between the shoulders, and gentle purgatives.

When the pain is occasioned by a retrocession of the gout, or by gouty rheumatic humours, blisters should be applied to the back and legs, and the feet bathed in warm water; which indeed is serviceable in most kinds of head-ach. To open the body, a spoonful, or two of aloetic wine should also be taken at bed-time.

A head-ach in phlegmatic constitutions will be relieved by the occasional use of the purgative just now mentioned, and by blisters, if the diſorder be ſevere or obſtinate. The uſe of the Peruvian bark, with neutral ſalts or kali, will alſo be adviſable, and may be given in the following manner: Take of the powder of Peruvian bark, one ounce, ſal ammoniac or kali, one drachm: mix them, and divide the powder into ſixteen doſes; one of which to be taken twice a day. Perſons of ſuch a habit will likewiſe find benefit from taking, twice a day, twenty drops of antimonial wine, in a diſh of valerian tea.

If a foul ſtomach be the cauſe of the complaint, an emetic ought to be taken; after which it would be proper to take ſome ſtomachic bitters, ſuch as gentian root, the root of the ſweet-ſcented flag, outer rind of Seville orange, &c. infuſed in white wine, and taken in the quantity of two or three table-ſpoonfuls twice a day.

If the head-ach proceeds from coſtiveneſs, it muſt be cured by ſome purgative; and the return of it, if habitual, obviated by the occaſional uſe of caſtor oil, lenitive electuary, or any other gentle laxative.

When the diſorder is occaſioned by a weakneſs of the nerves, after cleanſing the ſtomach by a gentle vomit, and the bowels by ſome mild laxative, bitters and the bark, with ſteel, as above recommended, ſhould be taken, and joined with chalybeate waters; or ten drops of the tincture of muriated iron may be taken twice a day, with a doſe of the bitter infuſion. In this caſe alſo, the bark and the root of wild valerian are of great advantage. They may be taken either in the form of infuſion, tincture, powder, or an electuary, as is moſt agreeable to the patient. In ſuch conſtitutions, daily riding on horſeback and the uſe of a light diet are alſo adviſable.

When a vitiated ſtate of the humours is the canſe of the head-ach, as in ſcorbutic conſtitutions, and thoſe who have been deeply infected with the venereal diſeaſe, the decoction of ſarſaparilla, with raiſins, or that of the woods, will prove of great advantage, and ought to be plentifully uſed; with which, in caſe of a venereal taint, mercurials ſhould be joined.

When the complaint ſucceeds an intermittent fever, or is obſerved to be periodical, the bark and valerian are highly ſerviceable.

In thoſe who wear wigs, letting the hair grow, and combing it frequently, has often been attended with benefit in a habitual head-ach. Waſhing the head with vinegar has alſo good effect; as has likewiſe a little æther, dropt into the palm of the hand, and applied to the forehead; or a tea-ſpoonful of æther, in valerian-tea, every three hours, for three times.. Sometimes a bit of horſe-radiſh, ſliced and laid upon the temples, will remove the complaint in a very little time. In obstinate cases, a blister to the whole head is advisable; and in gross constitutions, much benefit is experienced from the use of issues, or setons.

When the head-ach is extremely violent, so as to produce continual watching and delirium, a recourse to opiates may become necessary; but before they are employed, the bowels ought to be cleared by some gentle purgative. A bit of linen, dipped in Bate's anodyne balsam,* may then be applied to the part; and it may be advisable that the patient take twenty drops of laudanum in a cup of valerian tea, two or three times a day. But when recourse is had to this important remedy, care must be taken to obviate costiveness by means of some laxative.

Those who are subject to a head-ach ought to guard particularly against wet feet. They never should go to bed with their feet cold, and should always lie with the head high. If the pain be accompanied with heat and pulsation in the head, the diet ought to be slender, and all strong liquors avoided.

## *Of the Tooth-Ach.*

The tooth-ach may proceed from any of the causes of inflammation, or from pregnancy, but is generally occasioned by catching cold about the head, or by cold and wet feet, which repel the blood towards the head. It appears often to be owing chiefly to an acrimony in the fluids, either of a rheumatic or scorbutic kind. The foundation of it is often laid in the mismanagement of the teeth; in not keeping them clean, by daily washing the mouth; in hurting them by an immoderate use of sugar, or acids, cracking nuts, cherry-stones, &c. and in picking them with pins, or such like instruments, which injure both the teeth and gums.

PREVENTION.—It might perhaps be thought too severe to recommend the immediate extraction of a tooth upon the first attack of the complaint, though this be the only certain means of preventing its return. Such an expedient, indeed, would be more advisable where the tooth-ach was evidently owing to an external cause, which it was possible to obviate in future; for, in constitutions apparently disposed to the complaint, the extraction of the injured tooth could afford no security against the invasion of the others, but that of preserving the neighbouring teeth from the effects of contagion. When there is reason, however, to think that a tooth will prove a martyr to the disorder, it would certainly be proper to extract it, before it has become so carious as to render the operation ineffectual.

* See *Appendix.*

We are doubtless far too inattentive with respect to the preservation of the teeth, considering of what importance they are in the chewing of food, which, without their previous exertion, would render it difficult for all the concoctive powers of the stomach to digest the aliment sufficiently. We do not often enough wash them; we injure them, as has been already observed, by too free an use of sugar, or acids, which gradually corrodes their enamel; we wantonly contribute to destroy them by cracking nuts, or otherwise exposing them to violence; and instead of picking them with care, we employ a pick-tooth rather as a weapon of hostility than defence to the teeth. They ought always to be picked before a looking-glass, to avoid wounding the gums, the slightest separation of which from a tooth paves the way to its future destruction.

Cure.—In attempting to cure the tooth-ach, the first object is to divert the flux of humours from the part affected. This is best done by purgatives, and bathing the feet in warm water. Perspiration ought at the same time to be promoted, by drinking weak wine-whey, with which, if there be much heat and tumor about the part, ten or fifteen grains of nitre may be taken two or three times a day.

Some advise the application of leeches to the gums; but this is rather an indelicate, and not very safe practice. The best applications are blisters behind the ears, at least on the side affected, if only one; and they ought to be large enough to come a good way under the cheek. A poultice of linseed should likewise be applied to the cheek, and renewed when it cools, till either the complaint entirely ceases, or matter is formed in the gum, which ought then to be scarified, and washed with a little warm water and salt.

A derivation may be made from the part affected, by gently chewing in the mouth a bit of ginger, or the pellitory of Spain. If the tooth be rotten or hollow, so that the nervous chord, which is the seat of the pain, can be reached, this part may be burnt with a hot wire introduced in a pipe, and the cavity be filled up with lead, wax or mastich. Touching that part of the ear called the antihelix, which is the interior prominent part, with a hot iron, sometimes also removes the tooth-ach, but, to have the desired effect, it must be done by surprise.

If the tooth be hollow, a very good application for easing the pain is a mixture made of equal parts of the tincture of opium and myrrh; a few drops of which may be introduced into the tooth upon a little cotton, or the smoke of hen-bane seeds, &c.

Some women, during the first three or four months of pregnancy, are subject to the tooth-ach, which is generally relieved by small bleedings. Hysteric women also are liable to it; but in these it is merely a nervous affection, and to be cured by such medicines as will afterwards be mentioned in treating of that disorder.

## CHAP. XVI.

*Pain of the Stomach.*

THIS pain, commonly termed the heart-burn, is accompanied with an anxiety, a heat more or leſs violent, faintneſs, an inclination to vomit, or a plentiful diſcharge of water from the mouth. It may proceed from various cauſes, ſuch as indigeſtion; wind; ſharp humours, whether acid, bilious, or rancid; acrid and pungent food, as ſpices, &c. from worms; a ſtoppage of cuſtomary evacuations; gouty and rheumatic humours; ſurfeits; from the natural mucus or viſcid fluid of the ſtomach being abraded, particularly in the upper orifice, &c.

CURE.—When a pain of the ſtomach proceeds from a ſtoppage of cuſtomary evacuations, in a perſon of a ſanguine and full habit, recourſe ſhould be had to bleeding; and it will alſo be proper to keep the body open by mild purgatives, ſuch as rhubarb, ſenna, or cryſtals of tartar.

In any other pain of the ſtomach, bleeding is not neceſſary, but particular attention muſt be paid to the offending cauſe. If it proceeds from indigeſtion, or any acrid matter in the ſtomach, an emetic ſhould be given, and afterwards ſuch medicines as are ſuited to the ſpecific kind of acrimony. Thus, if it ariſe from acidities, Take of the powder of crabs' claws and ſugar, each two drachms; oil of cinnamon, two drops: mix them, and take a tea-ſpoonful of it two or three times a day: or, in place of it, the ſame quantity of calcined magneſia may be uſed. Lozenges of chalk may alſo anſwer the ſame purpoſe. If attended with coſtiveneſs, eight grains of rhubarb may be taken with the magneſia, or other powder, twice a day. When acidities are the cauſe, fixed and volatile alkaline ſalts, ſuch as the ſalt of wormwood, or of tartar, and the ſalt of hartſhorn, taken in a ſmall cup of water, will alſo give relief. It is impoſſible to ſay what preciſe quantity may be neceſſary to neutralize the acid, but, at a moderate calculation, a ſcruple of either of the two firſt, or ten grains of the laſt, may prove ſufficient for the purpoſe; or a pint of lime-water daily. When the nature of the acrimony is not certainly aſcertained, a little gum-arabic, diſſolved in water, will be found a more general remedy.

If a ſharpneſs and too great quantity of bile be the cauſe, an emetic is neceſſary, as in every foulneſs of the ſtomach. In this caſe, drinking a pint, or upwards, of hot water every morning;

or Bath-water is of great advantage, as a preventive remedy; keeping the body occaſionally open by ſmall doſes of rhubarb, caſtor-oil, or other mild laxative.

If too free an uſe of ſpices, or other hot ſubſtances, be the cauſe, a draught of cold water will prove ſerviceable. If it proceed from wind, the ſame remedy is often preferable to thoſe of a cordial nature. When it ariſes from worms, the means formerly mentioned under that article muſt be employed. When from gouty or rheumatic humours, the feet ſhould be bathed in warm water, and warm wine-whey be drunk to promote perſpiration. If it ariſes from a ſurfeit, a glaſs of peppermint-water may be taken.

If the pains ariſe from any excoriation or ulceration, the complaint will be conſtant, but greatly increaſed upon ſwallowing any thing hot or acrid. In this caſe, ſoft mucilaginous medicines, as gum-arabic, linſeed-tea, &c. are the beſt remedies; but nothing will prove more uſeful than a milk diet.

When women contract this complaint after the natural ſtoppage of their monthly evacuations, they will find great benefit from opening an iſſue in the arm or leg; which may likewiſe preſerve them from other ailments.

When the pain is attended with a diſcharge of clear lymph or water, ſometimes inſipid, ſometimes acrid, it is called the *water-braſh*. In this caſe, the beſt remedies are the bark and ſtomachic bitters.

Where a pain of the ſtomach is habitual, there is generally a relaxation of that organ, which ought to be ſtrengthened likewiſe by theſe remedies, and the elixir of vitriol; fifteen or twenty drops of which may be taken in a diſh of chammolile-tea, or any other vehicle, twice a day. If attended with coſtiveneſs, the occaſional uſe of aloetic-pills, or ſome other laxative, will be proper: or both ends may be anſwered by a combination of equal parts of Peruvian bark and rhubarb in wine or brandy, and taken in ſuch quantity as to keep the body gently open.

For thoſe who are ſubject to this complaint, the beſt diet is light animal food, with little bread; and the drink ſhould be toaſt and water, or occaſionally brandy and water. Daily riding on horſeback is highly ſerviceable, as is likewiſe ſailing.

### *Pain in the Stomach and Bowels from Poiſon.*

The effects of poiſon being generally ſudden and violent, it is extremely proper that every perſon ſhould be acquainted with the means of counteracting them. The knowledge neceſſary for this purpoſe is not difficult to be acquired, and may likewiſe be eaſily put in practice.

Poisons may be distinguished into three kinds, according as they belong to the mineral, vegetable, or animal kingdom. The first of these are commonly of an acrid or corrosive nature, such as arsenic, &c. The second have generally a narcotic or stupefactive quality, as aconite, hemlock, &c. And the last is the infection which poisonous animals communicate by the bite or sting, which are only applied externally.

Upon swallowing arsenic, a burning heat and violent pricking pain are felt in the stomach and bowels, accompanied with extreme thirst, and an inclination to vomit. If relief be not soon obtained, the patient is seized with great anxiety, hiccuping, faintings, and coldness of the extremities. These are followed by the discharge of black matter from the stomach, and foetid stools, which indicate a mortification of the bowels, and approaching death. A mortification of the genitals is said to be peculiar to the poison of arsenic.

For obviating the effects of this poison, the most active exertion is necessary. The person ought immediately to drink large quantities of milk and honey mixed, of warm water and oil, or, in defect of oil, melted fresh butter. Fat broths, likewise, if they can be procured in time, will answer the purpose. These, if drunk plentifully, will be apt to excite vomiting; but to produce that effect as soon as possible, it will be proper to add to them half a drachm or two scruples of ipecacuanha, or half a drachm of white vitriol, and a tea-spoonful of volatile spirits: clysters of the same kind should also be repeatedly given. In a word, the whole tract of the alimentary canal should be filled with softening emollient liquids, both to dilute and sheath the poison. When by these means a discharge has been obtained both ways, it will be proper that the person continue to take plentifully of a decoction of barley, with some gum-arabic, and spermaceti, or the drinks before mentioned; keeping the body open for several days by the castor-oil mixture, an infusion of senna, Glauber's salts, or some other purgative, until there is reason to think that the poison is entirely expelled. Even after which it will be advisable to persevere some days longer in the use of spermaceti, and the decoction of barley, and gum-arabic, to sheath and besmear any parts of the intestines which may have been abraded by the acrimony of the poison.

If the person be of a full habit of body, or the pulse be strong and full, it will be advisable, besides the above process, to take away some blood by the lancet.

The saline preparations of mercury, lead, copper, and antimony, that is, the solutions of these metals in different acids, are, in very small doses, useful and powerful medicines; but, given in too great quantity, are active and virulent poisons. When these have been taken, it has been recommended to adopt the process above described in respect to the poison of arsenic; but no medicine will have so immediate an effect as a solution of any alkali, which, uniting with the acid, decomposes the salt, and precipitates the metal in the form of a calx, nearly or wholly inactive.

When, therefore, any of these substances has been swallowed, dissolve about one ounce of salt of tartar, salt of wormwood, or common pearl-ashes, in a half gallon of warm water, and let the person drink plentifully of it, remembering that his life is at stake. After this has been done, the method before mentioned may be used with great advantage.

Among the VEGETABLE POISONS, the plants which chiefly produce unhappy effects are some kinds of mushrooms; hemlock, gathered for parsley, and eaten in sallads; the roots of the hemlock-dropwort, eaten instead of carrots; and the berries of the deadly nightshade, which children eat by mistake for wild cherries; the aconite and henbane and opium. All the poisons of this class, as has been already observed, seem to prove mortal rather from a narcotic or stupifying, than an acrimonious and stimulating quality. The chief symptoms produced by them are a staring wildness in the eyes, confusion of sight, palpitations, giddiness, loss of memory and voice, stupor or fury, convulsions, and retchings to vomit.

When any of these poisons has been unfortunately received into the stomach, the patient should immediately take a solution of vitriolated zinc, or white vitriol, in warm vinegar and water, and repeat it till it causes him to vomit plentifully, assisted by a large quantity of oil, butter, and other softening fluids, as above recommended. If he be an adult, or grown up person, he should take fifteen grains, or a scruple of the medicine, at a time.

After the operation of the vomit, and the evacuation of the intestinal canal, by emollient and oily clysters, the patient should continue to take large quantities of water, or whey, sweetened with honey or sugar, and acidulated with vinegar, which is regarded as an efficacious remedy against this sort of poisons.

The valuable drug opium, when taken in too large quantity, produces effects equally pernicious with those of the vegetable poisons above mentioned. The method of cure, in this case, is the same as already described, except that there may be a greater necessity for immediate bleeding; the effect of this poison being to produce symptoms similar to those of the sanguineous apoplexy. Blisters may be applied between the shoulders, and to the ancles, as well as vinegar to the nostrils; and dilute vitriolic acid, cream of tartar, lemon juice, or any convenient palatable acids, may be added plentifully to the patient's drink. The common saline mixture is here particularly recommended, and that to be given freely.

To afford opportunity for these remedies, much depends upon keeping the patient from sleeping until the effects of opium be over. After the poison is discharged, two or three gentle purges should be given at stated intervals.

## *Of the Bites of Poisonous Animals.*

Of the original cause of madness in animals, and the specific nature of the poison which they communicate, we as yet know nothing with certainty. Nor has experience proved more successful with respect to the uniform accomplishment of a cure in this species of infection. The credulity which always attends ignorance, and the imposture that preys upon credulity, have both contributed to retard the advancement of science wherever investigation is difficult. In the mean time, it is a matter of the greatest importance to ascertain with precision the symptoms which accompany the madness of animals, that we may be better enabled to guard against an accident productive of the most deplorable effects.

The madness of a dog may be known by his dull heavy look. He seldom or never barks, and shows an inclination to solitude. He refuses all food, hangs down his ears and tail, and often lies down, as if going to sleep. He appears angry and snarls at strangers, but fawns upon his owner.—The symptoms hitherto enumerated appear in the first stage of madness. He next begins to breathe quick, shoots out his tongue, slavers and froths at the mouth, seems as if half asleep, flies suddenly at by-standers, and runs forward in a curve line. At length he knows not his owner; his eyes become thick and dim, and water runs from them. His tongue assumes a red colour, he grows weak and faint, often falls down, then rises, and attempts to fly at something. He now becomes furious; and the nearer he is advanced to this state, the bite is more dangerous.

Innumerable remedies have been recommended for the cure of canine madness, and some of them particularly celebrated; but experience too surely evinces, that almost all of them are frivolous, and the remainder inadequate to the effect. The only certain means of cure is to cut out the bitten part immediately. Cupping-glasses should then be applied. The part should be cauterized, or washed daily with salt water: or, applying to it the stronger ointment of quicksilver, it ought to be kept open with escharotics or caustics. If the patient be of a full habit, it will be proper to bleed. Vomit, with vitriolated quicksilver, in the quantity of four grains.

Give at night half a drachm of cinnabar, with sixteen grains of musk; to which may be added, five grains of camphor, and one of opium; giving a purge the next morning. The patient should bathe in the sea, or cold bath, every morning, for a week, and at night take some of Mindererus's spirit, or other medicine, to promote perspiration. Both the bathing and sudorific should be repeated three or four times, at the next full and change of the moon. The ointment of quicksilver, applied externally, and vitriolated quicksilver, taken inwardly, so as to raise a salivation for several weeks, are said to prove of great efficacy. In Germany, the root of deadly night-shade has been given, from three to six grains at a dose, and is reported to have proved infallible in the first stages of the malady.

For curing the bite of a viper, we are informed that the viper-catchers do nothing more than rub into the wound some of the grease of this animal; though the method of sucking the wound, as practised by the ancient Psylli and Marsi, would appear to be preferable; rubbing the part, after suction, with some warm oil of olives. A poultice of bread and milk, softened with the same, should likewise be applied to the wound; and the patient ought to drink freely of vinegar-whey, or water-gruel, with vinegar in it, to promote perspiration: for vinegar is found highly beneficial in cases of poison, and ought to be plentifully used.

Another kind of poison is that which is communicated by the stings of insects; such as the bee, the wasp, the hornet, &c. but this is seldom attended with danger, when a person is not stung by a number of them at the same time, so as to excite a considerable inflammation. To remove this effect, or rather to prevent it, some apply honey, and some bruised parsley, to the part, while others, for the same purpose, recommend a mixture of vinegar and treacle; but anointing the part with warm oil of olives is commonly found successful. Should the stings, however, be very numerous, and the consequent inflammation prove alarming, not only poultices of bread and milk, with plenty of oil, ought to be applied to the part, but the patient be bled; he should also take cooling medicines, such as nitre, in the quantity of ten or fifteen grains, every three or four hours, and drink plentifully of barley-water, or other diluting liquors.

# KETTERING'S SPECIFIC FOR HYDROPHOBIA.

*The Publisher of the present edition, having the happiness of mankind warmly at heart, and wishing to give publicity to any information which may have a tendency to relieve them from the anxiety they labour under respecting this fatal disease, deems the following extract from the Journals of the Legislature of Pennsylvania, of March 6, 1802, neither inapplicable to that end, nor to the general tenor of the publication.*

## REPORT.

"The committee appointed to hear the communication of Valentine Kettering, relative to his cure of the bite of a mad animal,

"Report. That they conferred with the said Kettering on that subject, who informed them, that he uses the herb called Red Chick-weed, which, when ripe, or in full bloom, he gathers, and dries in the shade, reduces it to a powder, and gives a small table-spoonful at one time, to a grown person, in beer or water, in weight one drachm and one scruple: for a child, an equal dose, but given at three different times, or it may be eaten on bread with butter, honey, or molasses, as the person chuses. For a beast, a large spoonful; if by weight, two drachms and one scruple. When used green for a beast, cut the herb fine, and mix with bran, &c. When given to swine, mix the powdered herb with meal of any kind (dose as above) in little balls.

"He assures us that he has given it to persons many weeks after they were bitten, and never knew it fail; and never gives more than a single dose, unless to children, as above. He further says, that it is an excellent cure for cuts or wounds on the human body.

"When green, mash it; drop of the juice into the wound, and bind the herb, so mashed, on. The proper time to sow the seed is about the beginning of April, and it should be sown thin.

"He also informs us, that he is now seventy-five years old; was born in Germany, and came from thence, with his parents, to Pennsylvania, when eleven years of age; that his mother brought the seeds of the herb among her garden seeds: that he has presented to your committee, for the use of the members, a quantity of the herb and seed; and says he will give of the seed to others, who will please to call on him for that purpose.

"They also learn, from the Rev. Henry Muhlenberg, that it is an annual plant, known, in Switzerland and Germany, by the name of Gauch-heil, Rother Meyer, or Rother Hunerdarm; in England, Red Pimpernel; by botanists, as he is informed, Anagallis Phœnicea That it should be gathered in June, when in full blossom. In Germany, he understands, the usual dose was thirty grains of the powder, taken four times a day, and continued one week, in smaller doses; the wound washed with a decoction of the herb, and some of the powder strewed in it. That the plant is cultivated in many gardens, and grows near Baltimore and Havre-de-Grace, spontaneously, in great plenty."

## CHAP. XVII.

### *Of the Venereal Diſeaſe.*

THIS diſorder may very properly be ranked after the poiſons, not only as being of a virulent nature, but communicating infection by contact. It is generally diſtinguiſhed into two kinds, or at leaſt two different modifications, viz. The *primary* or *local ſymptoms*, confined to the organs of generation, and the adjacent parts, in the forms of virulent gonorrhœa, chancre, phymoſis, &c. and the *ſecondary* or *conſtitutional diſeaſe*. The firſt is often called a clap, or lues; the ſecond, ſyphilis, or the confirmed pox.

The virulent gonorrhœa conſiſts of a running or diſcharge of matter from the parts of generation in either ſex. It ſometimes commences in two or three days after the infection has been received, and at others not before a month or upwards; but it commonly makes its appearance in eight or ten days. The uſual forerunner of the complaint is an itching at the orifice of the urethra, ſometimes extending over the whole glans, which is ſucceeded by a diſcharge from the urethra, at firſt whitiſh, but afterwards changing to yellow or green. A ſlight degree of redneſs and inflammation begin to appear about the lips of the urethra; and a pain and ſmarting are frequently felt in making water.

There is commonly a fullneſs of the yard, particularly of the glans; and frequently a ſoreneſs, either in part, or through the whole of the urethra, accompanied with pain in erection. When the inflammation, or irritability, of the urethra is great, the penis is incurvated downwards in erection, attended with conſiderable pain, and ſometimes hæmorrhage. Theſe ſymptoms are ſometimes accompanied with ſwellings of the teſticles, or ſympathetic tumefactions of the neighbouring glands.

Sometimes the infection is received by the virulent matter remaining in contact with the prepuce, or glans, in which it produces a lingering ulcer, with a hardened baſe. This is termed a chancre, and frequently lays the foundation of a confirmed diſeaſe. When the matter produced by this ulcer is abſorbed, it is followed by buboes in the groin, and frequently blotches on the ſkin, at firſt attended with inflammation. This at length diſappearing, a white ſcurf ariſes, ſucceſſively peeling off and returning. It afterwards becomes copper-coloured: and in the end forms a ſcab, with an ulcer underneath. To theſe ſymptoms ſucceed ulcers in the throat, nodes on the tendons, ligaments, perioſteum, and bones, with caries, and nocturnal pains.

Cure, or treatment.—When any suspicion arises of having caught the venereal infection, the person should immediately take to a low diet, avoiding all animal food, spiceries and strong liquors, and confine himself to mild vegetables, milk broths, light puddings, &c. His drink should be of a smooth kind, the most opposite to acrimony; such as barley-water, milk and water, linseed-tea, whey, or decoctions of marsh-mallows and liquorice; of which he ought to drink plentifully. He must avoid all violent exercise, particularly riding on horseback, as well as venereal pleasures. He must at the same time beware of cold, and, during a high state of inflammation, keep his bed.

The cure of a virulent gonorrhœa is not always to be effected in any determinate time; as it depends not only upon the virulence of the infection, but the particular constitution of the patient. Under the most judicious treatment it may continue two or three weeks, and sometimes double that space. A slight infection, however, may be carried off in a week, by fomenting the parts with warm milk and water, and injecting frequently into the urethra a little sweet oil, or linseed-tea, about the warmth of new milk. After using these two or three times a day, for some days, till the virulence of the discharge is removed, then, merely to cure the remaining weakness, astringent injections may be given in the same manner, for a similar space of time. Take of white vitriol one scruple; dissolve it in five table-spoonfuls of common water, and use it as an injection, with a syringe.

At the first onset of the disorder, it may very readily be stopped by astringent injections, but this method is not to be adopted when it can be avoided. If the person be of a sanguine full habit of body, and the inflammation runs high, it will be proper to bleed, from six to twelve ounces. Cooling purges are also advisable in this stage of the complaint. Six drachms of Glauber's salts, with half an ounce of manna, dissolved in a gill and a half of warm water, may be taken every second or third day for the first fortnight; increasing or diminishing the dose, so as to procure two or three stools. By these means, not only the inflammatory symptoms but the running will be diminished; and the latter will change both its colour and consistence, becoming gradually more white and ropy as the virulence abates.

Cooling diuretics, or medicines which promote the secretion of urine, are likewise proper in this stage of the disorder, and should be joined with those of a mucilaginous nature, to abate the irritation and pain in the urethra, which is often very troublesome at this time. For this purpose, a common remedy is an ounce of cream of tartar, and the same quantity of gum-arabic, pounded together, and taken, in the quantity of a tea-spoonful in a cup of the patient's drink, four or five times a day. This mixture, besides its beneficial effects by urine, has a tendency favourable towards keeping the body gently open.

It has been already observed, that the parts ought to be frequently fomented with warm milk and water. Soft poultices, where they can be conveniently used, are also of great service; but if there lies any great objection against them, cloths rung out of warm water may be applied in their room. These applications are of great efficacy in removing violent pains which often accompany the inflammatory stage of the disorder.

For the painful erections and chordee, which frequently attend this complaint, besides the remedies already mentioned, opiates have often good effects; as have likewise, in the latter, especially at the beginning, some leeches applied to the part.

In the treatment of the gonorrhœa, some practitioners rely on mercurials given internally in small doses; while others, for the same purpose, employ injections alone. Some there likewise are who prefer diuretics to every other remedy; and there is a fourth class who are advocates for combining these different methods. It is fully ascertained by experience, that, if proper means be employed at the very beginning of the disorder, it may be subdued without quicksilver, or any preparation of that mineral; but if the virulence of the poison has made its way beyond the urethra, it is advisable, at least in point of security, to have recourse to this celebrated antidote. When, therefore, the inflammatory symptoms have subsided; that is, when the pain is become easy, the pulse rendered soft, the heat of urine abated, and the painful erections are both slighter and less frequent, the patient may enter upon the use of mercury in the form that most suits his inclination. In general, pills are the form most convenient for internal use, as they may always be in readiness when wanted. Of the common mercurial pill, he may begin with taking two at night and one in the morning. Should they affect the mouth too much by soreness and a flux of saliva, the dose must be diminished; but if they produce no effect upon that part, he may gradually increase the dose to double the number in the day. If, instead of pills, he prefers the use of calomel, he may take two or three grains of it, formed into a bolus with a little conserve of hips and roses, or some crumb of bread, moistened with a few drops of water. This may be taken at bed-time, and likewise gradually increased to five or six grains.

These medicines may either be taken every day or every other day, according to their sensible effect upon the patient; but they ought not to be taken in such a quantity as to raise a salivation, unless in a very slight degree: for, whether the mercury runs off by the mouth, or by the intestinal canal, it is not so successful in carrying off the disease as when it continues sometime in the body, and is gradually discharged.

If, during the night, the mercury should produce any purging or griping, the patient must take an infusion of senna, or some other purgative, and drink freely of water-gruel, to prevent bloody stools, which are frequently the consequence, if either the patient happens to catch cold, or the calomel has not been duly prepared. When, on account of any weakness of the bowels, such an effect is apprehended, half a drachm or two scruples of diascordium, or of the japonic confection, may be taken with the pills or bolus."

Those who cannot swallow mercury, either in a bolus or pill, may take it in a liquid form, in the following manner. Take of quicksilver one drachm, of gum-arabic, made into a mucilage with some boiling water, two drachms. Let the quicksilver be rubbed with the mucilage, in a marble mortar, until the globules of mercury entirely disappear. Afterwards add, gradually, still continuing the trituration, half an ounce of balsamic syrup, and half a pint of simple cinnamon-water. Two table-spoonfuls of this solution may be taken night and morning.

To accommodate such patients as cannot take mercury internally, either from a natural aversion to that medicine, or a tenderness of the bowels, it may be applied outwardly with equal success, and, indeed, with less danger to the constitution, which is apt to be more or less injured by a long-continued use of mercurial medicines taken inwardly. For this purpose, the common mercurial ointment, made by rubbing together equal quantities of hog's lard and quicksilver, is very well adapted. About a drachm of it may be rubbed in at night upon the inner part of the thighs. The person should stand before a fire during the operation, and should wear flannel drawers next his skin while he is using the ointment.

If, during this process, the inflammation of the genital parts, and other symptoms, should return, or the mouth should become affected, the patient ought to take a dose or two of Glauber's salts, or some other cooling purge, and the rubbing be intermitted for a few days. But, as soon as the spitting is gone off, if any of the virulence still remains, the use of the ointment must be resumed, though in smaller quantities, and at longer intervals than before; and the mercury, in whatever form employed, must not be discontinued while any particles of virulence is suspected to remain in the body.

During the stage of the complaint in which mercury is used, there is not the same necessity for a strict attention to diet as in the inflammatory state, yet the patient must still avoid intemperance of every kind. The food must be easy of digestion, and not of a heating quality. There must be a total abstinence from spirituous liquors; and if any wine is taken, it must be diluted with a sufficient quantity of water.

When the treatment now described has entirely removed the heat of urine, and the soreness of the genital parts; when the running from the urethra is considerably diminished, and not followed by any pain or swelling in the groin or testicles; when the involuntary erections have disappeared, and the matter discharged becomes pale, whitish, thick, void of ill smell, and viscid or ropy; under these circumstances we may at length proceed to treat it as a gleet, with astringent agglutinating medicines.

## *Of the Gleet.*

This is a discharge of thin matter, resembling the white of eggs, from the urethra, occasioned by relaxation. It comes on generally after a virulent gonorrhoea, and is attended with little or no pain in making water.

For the cure of this complaint the patient must have recourse to astringent remedies; such as the Peruvian bark, alum, &c. Astringent injections may likewise be employed, consisting, as before, of white vitriol, to which a few grains of alum may be added; and, when these remedies fail to produce the desired effect, the cold bath may still be used to great advantage.

The use of Pyrmont or Bristol waters, with which a little claret or port wine may sometimes be mixed, is in this case advisable; as is likewise a decoction of sarsaparilla for common drink. Blisters applied to the perinæum greatly assist other remedies when the source of the complaint is seated high up in the urethra. If these means prove ineffectual, there is reason to suspect the existence of a callosity in the urethra, for the removal of which it will be necessary to have recourse to Smyth's metallic bougies; the size of which should be as large as the parts can bear, and their use should be continued for a considerable time.

## *Swelled Testicles.*

This symptom may proceed from the venereal poison lurking in the body a considerable time, but commonly happens from infection lately contracted; and is for the most part occasioned by cold, hard drinking, strong purgatives, violent exercise, the too early use of astringent medicines, or other errors in treatment.

In the inflammatory stage of this complaint, bleeding is necessary, and must be repeated according to the urgency of the symptoms. Leeches also may be applied to the part with advantage. Fomentations and softening poultices ought to be diligently applied when the patient is in bed; and when he is up, at the fame time that care is taken to keep the tefticle warm, it muft be fufpended in a bag or trufs. The food muft be the fame as in inflammatory diforders, and the drink be diluting.

If, by this mode of treatment, the complaint fhould not be effectually removed, there will be a neceffity for renewing the mercurial procefs. The mercurial ointment muft be rubbed on the thighs, as before directed, and the patient muft be confined to bed, if neceffary, for five or fix weeks, fufpending the tefticle, all the while, with a bag or trufs, and drinking plentifully of a ftrong decoction of farfaparilla. If thefe means fhould not fucceed, there will arife a prefumption that the complaint is fupported by a fcrofulous or cancerous habit; in which cafe, recourfe muft be had to hemlock, both inwardly and outwardly employed. The part fhould be fomented, daily, with a decoction of this herb, the leaves of which, bruifed, may likewife be added to the poultice; and the patient ought to take the fame medicine, inwardly, in the form of the extract, made into pills. The manner of ufing it, is to begin with two or three grains, and to increafe the dofe gradually till fome good effect be perceived; from which period the medicine is to be continued without any further increafe.

## *Chancres.*

Chancres are fmall callous ulcers, feated chiefly about the glans, and which may appear without any previous gonorrhoea. Their progrefs is commonly as follows: firft, there arifes a red pimple, which becomes pointed at the top, and contains a whitifh matter inclining to yellow. After breaking, it degenerates into an obftinate ulcer, the edges of which gradually become hard and callous. Sometimes, at its firft appearance, it refembles a fimple excoriation of the cuticle.

A chancre fometimes appears with gonorrhœa, but is more frequently the eanfe of a confirmed lues. When it arifes foon after impure coition, its treatment differs little or nothing from that of the virulent gonorrhœa. The fame cooling diet muft be ufed, with moderate bleeding, and fome gentle dofes of phyfic; befides which, the parts muft be fomented with warm milk and water, and foftening poultices applied. In confequence of this treatment the inflammation commonly abates, and the patient is thus prepared for entering upon a courfe of mercury.

Symptomatic chancres, or thofe which arife from a confirmed lues, are commonly attended with other effects, characteriftic of their origin; fuch as ulcers in the throat, fcurfy eruptions about the roots of the hair, nocturnal pains, &c. They commonly appear upon the private parts, or the inside of the thigh, but are not always confined to these limits. They are also less painful than primary chancres, but frequently larger and more hard.

Besides the symptoms above enumerated, there are various other affections attendant on this disorder, according to the parts which are most exposed to its virulence; such as a strangury or obstruction of urine, a phymosis, paraphymosis, &c. The first of these complaints may arise either from a spasmodic constriction, or an inflammation of the urethra and parts about the neck of the bladder. In the former case, the patient at first voids his urine without any impediment; but as soon as it touches the inflamed and tender part of the urethra, a sudden constriction ensues, and the urine is evacuated by spirts, sometimes even by drops only. When the strangury proceeds from an inflammation about the neck of the bladder, there is a constant heat and uneasiness of the part, with a constant desire to make water, and a troublesome tenesmus, or an inclination to go to stool.

When the strangury arises from a spasm or constriction, the proper remedies are those which tend to sheath and dilute the salts of the urine. For this purpose may be used a decoction of marsh-mallows, linseed-tea, barley-water, and the like, with soft and cooling emulsions, which may be sweetened with the syrup of poppies. Should the complaint not yield to these means, recourse must be had to bleeding, and the use of emollient or softening fomentations.

When the disorder proceeds from an actual inflammation about the neck of the bladder, it will be requisite to bleed more freely and to repeat the operation according to the urgency of the symptoms. After bleeding, if the complaint be not removed, soft clysters must be given, to which may be added a tea-spoonful of the tincture of opium, or laudanum; applying also softening fomentations to the region of the bladder. At the same time the patient may take frequently a dish of the decoction of marsh-mallows, with ten or fifteen grains of nitre dissolved in it. If the complaint should still prove obstinate, bleeding must be repeated, and the patient put into a warm bath up to the middle. It will now be proper to lay aside the diuretics, and draw off the water by a catheter; or what will give the patient less pain, to have recourse to Smyth's hollow bougies, which tend to lubricate the passage, and greatly facilitate the discharge of urine. But as soon as they begin to stimulate, or give any uneasiness, it will be proper to withdraw them.

The phymosis is a constriction of the prepuce over the glans, so tight as to hinder it from being drawn backwards; and the paraphymosis, on the contrary, is a similar constriction behind the glans, which hinders the prepuce from being brought forwards.

in general, bleeding, and gentle purgatives, with softening fomentations and poultices, are sufficient to remove these complaints. Should these means, however, not produce the desired effect, and the parts be threatened with a mortification, it will be advisable to procure a revulsion by a vomit, consisting of a scruple or half a drachm of ipecacuanha, and one grain of tartarised antimony, or tartar emetic; working it off with an infusion of oatmeal-water, or thin gruel.

When, in spite of all endeavours to the contrary, the inflammation proceeds, and a mortification seems to be approaching, to obviate that effect, and prevent a strangulation of the parts, it will be necessary to scarify the prepuce, or divide it; which being the province of a surgeon, it is unnecessary here to be described. When a mortification has actually commenced, it will be necessary likewise to foment the parts frequently with cloths rung out of a strong decoction of chamomile flowers and the Peruvian bark, and that the patient take a drachm of the latter in powder every two or three hours.

In respect of some other symptoms, such as a priapism, and distortions of the penis, they must be treated in the same manner as the virulent gonorrhœa. When they prove very troublesome, they may commonly be relieved by a moderate dose of the tincture of opium taken at bed-time.

## *Of Buboes.*

These are hard tumors seated in the groin, and are distinguished into two kinds, viz. such as proceed from a recent infection, and such as accompany a confirmed lues. The cure of the former may be first attempted by discussion, or, that not succeeding, by suppuration. For discussing a bubo, the treatment is the same as has been recommended in the first stage of a gonorrhœa. The patient must likewise be bled, and leeches applied to the part affected; after which it will be proper to take some gentle purgative, such as a decoction of tamarinds and senna, Glauber's salts, manna, &c. Some mercurial ointment should then be rubbed upon the part. By such means, it frequently happens that the tumor is dissolved in two or three days; but if the heat, pain, and pulsation, still continue, it will be advisable to promote suppuration; which is to be effected by softening poultices, or the galbanum-plaster, applied to the part twice or thrice a day; the patient at the same time using his ordinary diet. When the tumor is ripe, which may be known from its appearance, and the fluctuation of matter, it may be opened either by a caustic or lancet, and afterwards dressed with digestive ointment. Should it not however yield to the means either of discussion or suppuration, but remain a hard scirrhous tumor, an endeavour must still be made to dissolve it by the application of hemlock, both externally and internally, as directed with regard to the testicle. The last expedient respecting a hard indolent tumor is to destroy it with caustic.

When, either by neglect, or imperfect treatment, the venereal poison has remained so long in the body as to contaminate the whole habit, there ensues that degree of the disease which has received the name of syphilis or a confirmed lues, and may be known from particular symptoms. There is reason to suspect that the poison is universally diffused, if the local symptoms, such as chancres, buboes, &c. do not give way to the usual methods of cure; or, when cured, if they break out again without any fresh infection. But if, at the same time, we find ulcers breaking out in the throat, dry scabby eruptions on the skin, or hard callous tubercles, or pustules covered with a yellow scab, and appearing chiefly on the hairy parts, we may be almost certain that the disease is confirmed.

Sometimes, however, these symptoms appear without any previous affection of the genitals, and may be the consequence of other species of acrimony; but the following may be considered as characteristic signs of the disease.

Venereal eruptions have a branny appearance, and are superficial, unattended with itching; and the scales being plucked off, the skin appears of a reddish brown, or rather copper-colour underneath. The tubercles, or pustules, seldom occupy the cheeks or the nose, and are covered at the top either with a dry branny scurf, like the eruptions just mentioned, or with a hard, dry scab of a tawny-colour. They particularly break out amongst the hair, or near it, on the forehead or temples.

Venereal ulcers of the mouth first affect the tonsils, uvula, and top of the throat; afterwards sometimes, though very rarely, the gums. They frequently extend to the nose, and are callous or hard in their edges; are circumscribed, and for the most part circular, at least they are confined to certain places; are generally hollow, and most commonly covered with a white or yellowish slough at the bottom. They are red in their circumference, and frequently corrupt the subjacent bones; being also in general combined with symptoms known to be venereal.

With regard to pains, those which are deep seated, particularly of the arms, head, and shins, always fixed in the same place, and which affect the middle and more solid part of the bones of the arms and legs, and those of the head, raging chiefly and with great violence in the *fore-part of the night*, may be regarded as sure symptoms of this disease. But other wandering pains of the membranes of the muscles, and the ligaments of the joints, though they may arise from a venereal taint, cannot be considered as certain signs, unless other symptoms of the lues appear at the same time.

Hard indolent swellings in different parts of the body, as in those which are fleshy, in the periosteum, upon the tendons, ligaments, or bones, or those protuberances at the verge of the anus, called fici; though they all are signs of a confirmed lues, yet if not preceded or accompanied by other signs of this disease, cannot be regarded as decisive in forming an opinion of its real existence, because it is possible they may depend upon some lurking scrofulous humour. When they proceed from this source, they are very seldom painful, or tend to inflame and suppurate, as those which are venereal generally do; and if they lie upon a bone, they commonly produce a caries.

Frequent abortions, or the exclusion of scabby, ulcerated, half-corrupted, and dead fœtuses, happening without any manifest cause to disturb the fœtus before its time, or to destroy it in the womb, may be regarded as a certain and infallible sign of one of the parents being tainted with the venereal disease.

Various are the remedies which have been recommended by different practitioners for the cure of this virulent disease; but experience evinces, that the only antidote to be depended upon is mercury; and that in most constitutions, the application of it externally by unction, is in general the method to be preferred. Every preparation of this mineral is not found equally successful. The solution of corrosive sublimate, once greatly extolled, has now declined in reputation. In the mean time, acids, especially the mineral, have acquired a degree of celebrity in the cure of the venereal disease; and the nitrous acid is by some regarded, as more efficacious than even mercury itself. It seems indeed, in many instances, to palliate the disease, and even to cure, at least for a time, some of the symptoms; though mercury must still be regarded as the resource which has the justest claim to be infallible. Its efficacy, however, in a confirmed lues, especially when of long standing, may be assisted by a decoction of the woods, particularly sarsaparilla; in these cases the cure can rarely be depended upon, unless the mercurial course be continued six weeks or two months.

I cannot conclude this subject without cautioning my readers against the frauds and villainy of quacks. No person that advertises by hand-bills or in news-papers can be trusted. The expence of their nostrums is from seventeen to twenty-eight times greater than that of the medicines I have recommended; and the consequences produced by their solar tinctures, balms of Gilead, and botanical or vegetable syrups are often too shocking to be mentioned.

## CHAP. XVIII.

### *Of Scirrhus and Cancer.*

A SCIRRHUS is a hard indolent tumor, generally occupying ſome gland; ſuch as the breaſts, arm-pits, groins, &c. Should it neither be diſperſed, brought to ſuppuration, nor extirpated, it may nevertheleſs remain many years without proving injurious to the conſtitution. But if it become large, unequal in its ſurface, of a livid colour, with acute darting pains, it obtains the name of an occult cancer. This likewiſe, under a temperate and cooling diet, may continue for many years without greatly moleſting the patient; but if the ſkin break, and an ulcer be formed, which generally diſcharges a thin acrimonious matter, of an extreme fœtid ſmell, it is called an open or ulcerated cancer; a diſorder moſt incident to the decline of life, and to the female ſex, more than the male.

CAUSES.—It may be occaſioned by habitual grief, melancholy, and deſpondency of mind; by a blow, bruiſe, or other internal violence; and frequently by the ſuppreſſion of ſome accuſtomed evacuation.

This diſorder, at the beginning, appears generally inconſiderable, in reſpect of its ſize, and will often remain ſtationary a long time, without any ſymptom of future uneaſineſs or danger; but if either the health be much affected by any cauſes of relaxation, or the tumor be exaſperated by preſſure or internal excitement, it extends its limits towards the neighbouring parts, by an elongation in the form of roots or limbs; from a fancied reſemblance between which and the claws of a crab, it has been denominated a cancer.—The ſkin then changing its natural colour, becomes red; and, after various tranſitions into purple, blue, and livid, aſſumes at laſt a black, of which colour it ever after remains. The patient complains of a burning heat, and lancinating pain. The tumor, meanwhile, continues increaſing, and the ſurrounding veins, diſtended with blood, become likewiſe black. At length the ſkin gives way, and a thin acrimonious fluid begins to flow from the orifice, corroding by its ſharpneſs the neighbouring parts, until it forms a large ulcer of a hedious appearance. More tumors of the ſame kind are now generated, and communicate with the neighbouring glands. The ſhooting pains, which formerly were troubleſome, now increaſe in violence; and the ſtench, which iſſues from the ulcer is intolerable, even to the patient. Such is the acrimony of the ichor diſcharged, as to excoriate, and even deſtroy the neighbouring parts. In the more advanced ſtages of the diſeaſe, by the eroſion of blood-veſſels which occurs, conſiderable quantities of blood are ſometimes alſo diſcharged.

There is perhaps no diſorder which ſo much requires a ſlender light regimen and an eaſy diſpoſition of mind, as a cancer. The diet ought to conſiſt chiefly of milk and vegetables, avoiding all high ſeaſoned or ſalted proviſions, and ſpirituous as well as fermented liquors. Even wine, though ſometimes admiſſible as a cordial, muſt be uſed with moderation. The beſt drink is a decoction of the woods, or ſarſaparilla. The patient ought to uſe daily moderate exerciſe in the open air; defending, however, the part affected from cold, by light warm covering; and guarding likewiſe againſt all preſſures. The mind, in the mean time, ſhould be conſtantly kept as eaſy and cheerful as poſſible.

Cure.—The cancer has hitherto baffled all the efforts of medicine for a certain and radical cure. When an induration of a gland is the conſequence of ſome external injury, the moſt adviſable method of cure is that of extirpation, provided the part be ſo ſituated as to admit of this reſource. But when it proceeds from a vitiated ſtate of the humours, is of long ſtanding, and the habit of body debilitated, the moſt that can be done for a confirmed, eſpecially an ulcerated cancer, is to defend it as much as poſſible from all irritation. In its incipient ſtate, if there be any inflammation, a little bleeding is proper, and the patient ſhould frequently take cooling laxatives, ſuch as Glauber's ſalts, manna, &c. Some leeches may likewiſe be applied to the neighbourhood of the part affected, and a little of the mercurial ointment rubbed gently upon it every day, keeping it afterwards covered with ſoft flannel or fur.

Both in this ſtate of the tumor, and an ulcerated cancer, fomentations with hemlock are of great advantage; as is likewiſe the extract taken internally, in the form of pills. The proper way of uſing it is to begin with two grains twice a day, and increaſe the doſe gradually, as far as the patient can bear it. In tender habits it is apt at firſt to affect the head; but this ſymptom commonly goes off by uſing it a little time; or if it continues, the uſe of the medicine may be occaſionally ſuſpended for two or three days. The freſh juice of hemlock is thought more efficacious than the extract; and ought to be begun in the quantity of four or five drops, gradually increaſing the doſe.

Salt water has been found a very efficacious alterative in many cancerous caſes, particularly in the beginning of the progreſs. A grain of corroſive ſublimate of mercury, diſſolved in ſome brandy, and taken night and morning, produces often good effects in cancers of the face and noſe. An infuſion of night-ſhade is alſo recommended in cancers of the breaſt: and, wherever ſituated, a ſolution of arſenic has proved highly ſerviceable, particularly in cancers of the occult kind. It is adviſed to be given in the following manner: Take of white arſenic four grains; diſſolve it in a pound of diſtilled water. Take of this ſolution, cow's milk, and the ſyrup of white poppies, each a table-ſpoonful. Mix and take them every morning, doubling the doſe every week.

Wort, or an infuſion of malt, has been recommended, not only as a proper drink, but an efficacious medicine in this diſeaſe. It may be drunk at pleaſure, and ſhould never be more than two days old.

It is of great conſequence in an ulcerated cancer, that the part be kept clean. The beſt application for this purpoſe is found to be the carrot poultice; which is made by grating the root of the common carrot, and moiſtening it with a ſufficient quantity of water, to make it into a proper conſiſtence. This ought to be applied to the part, and renewed twice a day. Beſides cleanſing the ſore, which it generally does, it allays the pain, and greatly diminiſhes the ſmell, ſo extremely offenſive in this complaint.

For preventing this diſagreeable ſymptom, nothing is ſo effectual as the external application of carbonic acid air and carrot poultices.

Setons, or iſſues, in the neighbourhood of a cancer, have ſometimes been found ſerviceable.

When all other medicines prove ineffectual for curing or palliating this dreadful complaint, the laſt reſource is to opium; not, however, to remove the diſorder, but to mitigate the pain, and compenſate, in ſome degree, the impoſſibility of affording more permanent relief.

To guard againſt the invaſion of this terrible diſorder, care ſhould be taken to avoid all unwholeſome food; to preſerve the health by daily exerciſe in the open air; to baniſh all ſadneſs and deſpondency, by habitual cheerfulneſs; and to beware of any accident that might hurt a glandular part, and lay a foundation for the diſeaſe.

# CHAP. XIX.

## *Diseases of the Brain and Nervous System.*

### *Of the Apoplexy.*

AN apoplexy is a sudden deprivation of sense and voluntary motion, without convulsions. The face appears red and bloated; the mouth is commonly open; the pulse, especially at first, is strong and quick; the respiration is likewise strong, and attended with snorting. It is most incident to people in the decline of life; and to those chiefly who have short necks, and use a rich and plentiful diet, without much exercise. It is frequently preceded by a pain or giddiness of the head, drowsiness, noise in the ears, loss of memory, and a difficulty of breathing.

Causes.—The immediate cause of an apoplexy is a compression of the brain, proceeding from an excess or effusion of blood, or a collection of watery humours in the ventricles. The former is called a *sanguineous*, and the latter a *serous* apoplexy. It may be occasioned by any thing that increases the motion of the blood towards the brain, or prevents its return from that part; violent passions; rich and luxurious diet; excessive use of spiceries, or high-seasoned food; hard drinking; excess of venery; suppression of urine; the stoppage of any customary evacuation; suffering the body to cool suddenly, after having been much heated; wearing any thing too tight about the neck; viewing objects for a long time obliquely; the sudden disappearance of any eruption; long exposure to excessive cold; a mercurial salivation suddenly checked by cold, &c.

Cure.—In the sanguineous apoplexy, which may be known from the plethoric constitution of the person, and the florid and turgid appearance of the face during the fit, every effort must be made to relieve the oppression of the brain. The patient should be placed on a chair, and his clothes about the neck be loosened; tightening at the same time his garters, to retard the motion of the blood from the lower extremities. The apartment ought to be kept cool. He should then be bled freely from the jugular vein, or arm; and in two or three hours the operation, if necessary, be repeated. Bleeding in the foot is also proper; as is likewise cupping the back part of the head, with deep scarification. A laxative clyster should now be given, with four table-spoonfuls of sweet oil, or some butter, and two spoonfuls of common salt. This likewise ought to be repeated every two hours, and made stronger, by the addition of some resin of jalap, or other stimulating substance, if the patient still remains in a state of insensibility. Under the same circumstances, blistering plasters should be applied to the legs and thighs, and also to the head, and between the shoulders.

As soon as the symptoms have so much abated that the patient is able to swallow, he ought to take some opening medicine, such as Glauber's salts, an infusion of senna, or the like. Or these may be combined in the following manner, and taken at intervals, in the quantity of a cupful, till an effect is produced: Take of senna three drachms; infuse for some minutes in a pint of boiling water; and in the strained liquor dissolve an ounce of Glauber's salts, and an ounce of manna.

It being common in swoonings to apply volatile salts or spirits to the nose, and, if possible, to give the patient cordials by the mouth, a caution ought to be given against all such resources in the sanguineous apoplexy. Vomits likewise must be prohibited, on account of their preventing the motion of the blood from the head.

In the serous apoplexy, which may be ascertained from the constitution of the patient, as well from the pulse being less strong, and the countenance less florid than in the preceding, bleeding is not always requisite, and sometimes not even admissible, though generally it may be performed once in a moderate degree. Leeches, however, may be applied to the temples with advantage; and, besides clysters, purgatives, and blisters, as in the former case, quick and brisk vomits, of white vitriol, or tartarised antimony, are to be given as soon as possible. If the patient be inclined to sweat, it ought to be promoted by drinking small wine-whey; as this evacuation sometimes proves critical of the disorder.

When an apoplexy is occasioned by opium, or other narcotic substances taken into the stomach, the most effectual remedy is a vomit, which ought to be administered immediately.

Those who have suffered an apoplectic fit, especially if predisposed to the complaint, should avoid the extremes of heat and cold, and guard against all violent commotions of the mind. They ought to keep their feet warm, as well as free from wet; to abstain from heavy suppers; to wear nothing too tight about the neck, and to lie with the head high. Perpetual issues, or setons, have likewise great effect in preventing a return of this disorder. To avoid both kinds of apoplexy, the body should be kept open. In the sanguineous kind, prevention is best effected by a cooling vegetable diet; but in the serous, by a diet of light animal food, with a few glasses of wine, and moderate exercise.

## CHAP. XX.

### *Epilepſy, or Falling Sickneſs.*

THE epilepſy is a deprivation of all the ſenſes, accompanied with violent convulſive motions. It is commonly preceded by a pain in the head, laſſitude, diſturbed ſleep, noiſe in the ears, a palpitation of the heart; and in ſome there is a ſenſation of cold air aſcending from the lower extremities towards the head.

When it comes on during infancy or childhood, there are ſome hopes of its going off at the age of puberty; but if it attacks after the twenty-firſt year, and ſtill more at a later period, there is reaſon to apprehend that the perſon will continue ſubject to it for life.

Causes.—This diſeaſe may be occaſioned by various accidents within the brain; blows, wounds, or bruiſes on the head; exceſſive drinking; violent paſſions; intenſe application of mind; ſuppreſſion of cuſtomary evacuations; venereal exceſſes; hyſteric affections; too great emptineſs or repletion, &c.

Symptoms.—The perſon, when ſeized with an attack of epilepſy, falls ſuddenly to the ground. In general, the limbs are violently convulſed; but ſometimes, inſtead of being agitated, they are ſtiff and immoveable. It often happens that the patient diſcharges the urine and fæces involuntarily; and during the violence of the fit, he ſometimes bites his tongue. But the ſymptoms moſt characteriſtic of the diſeaſe are, that he froths at the mouth, and his thumbs are ſhut up ſo cloſe in the palms of his hands, that it is difficult to diſengage them. When the fit is over, his ſenſes gradually return, and he complains of a wearineſs and pain of his head; but is utterly inſenſible of what happened during the paroxyſm, and commonly falls aſleep.

Cure.—The method of curing this diſeaſe muſt be various, according to the cauſe that produces it. When occaſioned by any injury of the head or brain, the previous effect muſt be removed: but if this cannot be done, or at leaſt not immediately, the treatment muſt be ſo directed as to moderate the violence of the convulſive ſymptoms. If the perſon be of a plethoric conſtitution, and there be reaſon to ſuſpect an accumulation of fluids in the head, it will be proper to bleed from the jugular vein. But, during this operation, the ſurgeon ſhould put his finger to ſome artery, and if he finds the pulſe riſe while the blood is flowing, he may perſiſt; but if otherwiſe, it will be prudent to ſtop. Bliſters, however, or poultices of muſtard, ſhould be applied to the lower extremities; and clyſters, with which two drachms, or an ounce, of milk of aſſafœtida is mixed, ſhould be injected; rubbing, likewiſe, along the ſpine or back-bone ſome of the compound camphor liniment,* or other ſtimulating and antiſpaſmodic application. If the diſorder be ſuppoſed to proceed from worms, recourſe muſt be had to the medicines adapted to that purpoſe, as directed in the diſeaſes of children. If from teething, the gums ſhould be lanced, the body ſhould be kept open by ſoftening clyſters, and the feet frequently bathed in warm water; at the ſame time that a bliſter may be applied between the ſhoulders. This method of cure is alſo to be practiſed when the epileptic fits precede the eruption of the ſmall-pox, meaſles, &c.

During the fit, care ſhould be taken to prevent the patient from bruiſing himſelf by the convulſive agitations; and particularly to prevent his hurting the tongue with his teeth, by holding a piece of ſoft wood between the teeth.

When the fits have ceaſed, the attention ſhould be directed towards obviating their future return. When the diſorder depends upon any ſenſible and determinate cauſe, ſuch as worms, the ſuppreſſion of any cuſtomary evacuation, &c. the proper remedies are evident; but, in other caſes, preſcription can only be guided by experience. Various medicines have been celebrated by different authors for the cure of this diſorder, though none of them has been found univerſally ſucceſsful, either by practitioners or patients. That many of them, however, have really proved efficacious, the reſpectable authorities on which they have been recommended leave no room for any doubt; and it is therefore adviſable to make trial of their virtues in every diſeaſe of the ſame nature. The medicines moſt extolled in this caſe, are muſk, the root of wild valerian, the flowers of zinc, and ammoniacal copper, nitrated ſilver, and the flowers of the cardamine or ladies-ſmock. The doſe of muſk may be from ſix grains to half a drachm, twice a day; valerian from a ſcruple to a drachm in powder, and in infuſion, more than double that quantity; zinc, from half a grain to eight grains and upwards; and ammoniacal copper, from a quarter of a grain to five grains; nitrated ſilver, from one eighth of a grain to one grain. In adminiſtering the three latter, it is always proper to begin with ſmall doſes, and increaſe them gradually.

Among the moſt effectual remedies for this diſorder are, likewiſe, the Peruvian bark, and the cold-bath; the powerful virtues of both which, in ſtrengthening the conſtitution, are ſufficiently well known. Whatever remedies are employed, the patient ought

* See *Appendix*.

to persevere in the use of them for a considerable time: for no disease, to which there is any pre-disposition in the habit, can very soon be eradicated.

Persons subject to the epilepsy, should endeavour to breathe a free and pure air. Their diet should be chiefly light animal food; and they ought to avoid strong liquors. Daily moderate exercise is of great service, as well as tranquillity of mind; and it must occur to their own observation, that they ought to avoid fording deep rivers, or placing themselves in any situation where a sudden attack of the disorder might prove irretrievably fatal.

## CHAP. XXI.

### *Of the Hysteric Disease.*

THIS disease affects women of a great sensibility of constitution, and who are frequently liable to obstructions of the natural discharge. It is of all disorders the most various in its appearance; and generally comes on between the age of puberty and thirty-five. It also more frequently seizes barren women, and young widows, than such as are bearing children.

SYMPTOMS.—The disorder commonly begins with a languor and debility of the whole body; yawning, stretching, and restlessness. A sense of coldness in the extremities almost always precedes, and for the most part continues during the whole of the hysteric fit. Sometimes, however, this is alternated with a sense of heat in different parts of the body. The colour of the face is variable, being sometimes flushed, and sometimes pale. There is a violent pain in the head; the eyes become dim, and pour out tears. There is a rumbling and inflation of the intestines. A sensatiou is sometimes felt like that of a globe ascending from the lower part of the belly, and which rolls along the whole alimentary canal. It ascends to the stomach, sometimes suddenly, sometimes slowly; and there produces a sense of weight and anxiety, nausea, and vomiting. At last it comes up the throat, where it produces a sense of suffocation, and difficulty of breathing or swallowing. During this time, violent pains are felt, both in the external and internal parts of the abdomen, accompanied with convulsive motions of the muscles. Sometimes the fit ceases after these symptoms have continued for a certain time; but more frequently the patient falls into a fainting fit. Sometimes she lies quite motionless, as if in a profound sleep; sometimes she beats her breasts violently with her hands. At other times, she is seized with general convulsions, and the disease assumes the appearance of an epilepsy. In some patients, a violent beating pain takes place in some part of the head, as if a nail was driving into it, and all objects seem to the person to turn round. Sharp pains, likewise, attack the loins, back, and bladder, and the patient makes an extraordinary quantity of urine as limpid as water; which is one of the most characteristic signs of the disease. The mind, as well as the body, is greatly affected. Sometimes the person is tormented with vain apprehensions; sometimes she will laugh, at other times cry immoderately.

The appearances which take place in this affection are, indeed, so various, that they cannot be enumerated; but all the symptoms of the disease seldom concur in the same person: for they vary extremely in every circumstance. When the fit remits, the pulse becomes more strong; the heat returns to the extreme parts; a rumbling noise arises in the belly; and at last, as if awaking from a profound sleep, the patient regains her voice, sense, and motion; but complains of a heavy pain of the head, and a general weakness.

CURE.—During a violent hysteric fit, if the patient be of a sanguine constitution, some bleeding may be of service; but otherwise, especially in delicate habits, this operation is not advisable. Foetid volatiles, singed feathers, and the like may be applied to the nostrils; and cold water, and foetid volatiles, administered internally, if the patient can swallow. Cold water may also be sprinkled on the face and breast. Cool fresh air should be admitted into the apartment, and the patient's feet and legs be placed in warm water. Friction of the lower extremities is also useful. Particular attention should be paid to the state of the monthly evacuation. If deficient, it ought to be promoted; and if too copious, should be restrained, as will afterwards be directed in the treatment of these complaints. If the patient be costive, it will be proper to give a laxative clyster with milk of assafoetida.

For the radical cure of the hysteric disorder, recourse must be had to those means which strengthen the nervous system, the chief of which are chalybeate medicines, or the preparations of iron, the Peruvian bark, and the cold-bath. But medicines which allay irritation are likewise advisable occasionally. Take of the tincture of assafoetida, and of castor, each two drachms; compound spirit of lavender, four drachms. Mix and preserve them for use. A tea-spoonful of this mixture may be taken, in a little water, upon the approach of any languor; and when the person feels herself under any agitation, ten or twelve drops of laudanum may be added to a dose of it. On such emergencies, likewise, as well as during a fit, the application of the anti-hysteric plaster* to the belly will be found of great advantage.

An attention to diet is highly proper for the removal of this disorder. Milk, where it agrees with the stomach, has frequently good effects; but, otherwise, the diet should consist of light animal food. In general, malt-liquors, as being flatulent, are not advisable; except good porter. The best drink is water, with the addition of red-wine, if it agrees with the patient; but if not, a small quantity of spirits. If the patient cannot comply with a total interdiction of tea, she ought to use it sparingly. Exercise, particularly riding on horseback, is of great service; as are, likewise, amusements and cheerful company.

## CHAP. XXII.

### *Of the Hypochondriac Disease.*

THIS complaint is chiefly incident to persons of a sedentary life and studious disposition; especially such as have indulged grief or anxiety, and are advanced in years. It is attended with pains, more or less violent, under the short ribs in the left side; frequently with an inflation, which sometimes becomes stationary. It is also accompanied with indigestion, watchfulness, palpitations of the heart, sometimes a looseness, but generally costiveness. Besides these symptoms, there occurs a peculiar depression of the spirits, with ridiculous fancies, and a strong apprehension of danger, which may be regarded as the characteristic sign of the disease. The patient is frequently troubled with a spasmodic constriction of the throat, sour belchings, and vomiting: when the matter thrown up is sometimes so acrid as to prove corrosive.

Causes.—This disorder may be occasioned by a high and full diet; indolence; the suppression of customary evacuations; violent passions of the mind; great, or long-continued evacuations; obstructions of some of the bowels, &c.

The immediate cause of the hypochondriac disease appears to be great weakness of the organs of digestion, often inherited, in consequence of which the aliment is not properly digested, and the constitution, for want of due nourishment, is enfeebled.

Cure.—The first step in the cure is to clear the stomach and intestinal canal, of their acrid, or viscid, contents, by means

* See *Appendix*.

of gentle vomits and purgatives; and, until the ſtrength of thoſe parts can be reſtored, the production of freſh impurities will be retarded by the uſe of abſorbent medicines, ſuch as crabs' claws, chalk, magneſia, and the like, which are well adapted to correct the prevailing acrimony, and ſluggiſh humours, in this diſeaſe. The moſt ſuitable vomit will be ipecacuanha; and the purgative, either ſome aloetic pills, taken at bed-time, or half a ſcruple of rhubarb, with a drachm of calcined magneſia, taken once or twice a day, according as it operates on the conſtitution of the patient. In the mean time, the ſymptoms will generally be abated by frequently bathing his feet in warm water at going to bed.

A vomit and purge having been premiſed, the patient ought to enter upon a courſe of ſuch medicines as are calculated to ſtrengthen the ſtomach and bowels, and thereby promote digeſtion. The great remedies for anſwering this intention are, the Peruvian bark, bitters, and the different preparations of iron, which may be taken in any form moſt agreeable to the patient. The cold-bath, as a general ſtrengthener, is inferior to no remedy yet known; but it is not ſo adviſable, at firſt, to hypochondriac patients, until their bowels have acquired a degree of firmneſs by the previous uſe of corroborants adminiſtered internally.

Moderate exerciſe is indiſpenſable in the cure of this complaint; and it cannot be taken any way with ſo much advantage as in long journies, when convenient, accompanied with ſuch circumſtances as may convert them into an agreeable amuſement. The patient ought to endeavour to guard againſt all the depreſſing paſſions, as well as againſt that ſplenetic humour peculiar to the diſeaſe, and which, if indulged, contributes not a little to increaſe it.

Proper diet conſtitutes an eſſential part in the treatment of this malady. In general, light animal food is what alone agrees with ſuch patients: for there are few, if any, vegetables which do not prove flatulent in their bowels. Acids are particularly injurious. All malt liquors, except porter, are apt to excite too high a fermentation in the ſtomach; and wines, for the moſt part, are liable to the ſame objection. If an exception can be made in favour of any, it is good old Madeira, if they can get it, which not only promotes digeſtion, and invigorates the concoctive powers, but acts, immediately, as a generous and wholeſome cordial. The uſe of ſpirituous liquors is not to be recommended as a habitual reſource, though they may be taken occaſionally, in a moderate quantity, diluted with water. Pyrmont water is, in this caſe, the moſt ſuitable drink, or the artificial imitations of it, which are much cheaper, and quite as efficacious.

## CHAP. XXIII.

*Diſorders called Nervous.*

NERVOUS diſorders are ſo various in their appearances, that a minute deſcription of them would be equally tedious and unprofitable. Though chiefly incident to women, and men of delicate conſtitutions, perſons apparently vigorous are not exempt from their influence. In fact, there is ſcarcely an individual who is not occaſionally liable to ſome ſlight and tranſient nervous affection; and it is only when they become habitual, and troubleſome or violent in degree, that they merit the name of a diſeaſe. Their ſource is generally in the ſtomach and inteſtines, where they produce acidities and diſtenſions; ſometimes a craving appetite, and frequently a rumbling noiſe in the bowels. The urine is ſometimes in ſmall quantity, and other times very copious and quite clear. The perſon is occaſionally ſubject to a palpitation of the heart, and a difficulty of breathing; has often ſlight ſpaſms, or ſtartings, and his ſleep is generally unſound and diſturbed with dreams. This affection is commonly accompanied with an irritability of mind, and ſometimes with low ſpirits.

CAUSES.—A diſpoſition to nervous complaints is often hereditary, and may be brought on by every thing that relaxes or weakens the body. The moſt common of theſe, are great, or long-continued evacuations of any kind; too watery a diet, or an immoderate uſe of tea; an indolent life; intenſe application to ſtudy; extreme grief, anxiety, or vexation.

CURE.—The cure of nervous affections depends far more upon diet and exerciſe than medicine. The latter, however, is by no means of ſmall importance. Stomachic bitters, with the Peruvian bark, and preparations of iron, have great efficacy in ſtrengthening the nervous ſyſtem, and ought never to be omitted in thoſe caſes. The cold-bath is yet more powerful for the ſame purpoſe, where no particular weakneſs of the bowels renders the uſe of it improper. Sea-bathing is preferable to that with freſh-water; and from March to November, is the fitteſt ſeaſon for uſing them. Three or four times a week is ſufficient; and the beſt periods, either an hour or two before breakfaſt, or two hours after it.

No diſeaſe requires a more ſtrict attention to diet than the nervous affection. This ought to conſiſt chiefly of light animal food; vegetables, in general, diſagreeing with ſuch conſtitutions. With moſt nervous patients, potatoes are found to agreee better than any other vegetable; but there are exceptions in different constitutions. Acids, for the most part, are hurtful, but the moderate use of spiceries beneficial to their stomach and bowels. They ought never to eat of new bread, and all their bread should be well baked. They may eat of mild apples in tarts, but the juice of this fruit in cyder is commonly hurtful.

The best drink for nervous persons is good porter or ale; but where this cannot be had, pure water with a toast in it. Except good Madeira, as has been observed in the last chapter, all wine is apt to sour on the stomach, and occasions pains in the bowels and watchfulness in the night. A little brandy may sometimes be taken with the water, but the practice should not become habitual.

Daily exercise, without fatigue, is highly conducive to the health of nervous persons. The most beneficial is riding on horseback, though sometimes a carriage, and sometimes walking may be preferable. Sailing, likewise is of considerable advantage in this complaint. But to all the conjunct influence of medicines, diet, and exercise, must be added tranquillity of mind, which is an indispensable auxiliary in the cure of nervous disorders.

## *Flatulencies, or Wind.*

This symptom, which proceeds from a relaxation of the stomach and bowels, is peculiarly incident to nervous patients, and greatly contributes to aggravate their complaints. The radical cure of flatulencies can only be effected by that of the primary disorder, but they may be moderated by a strict attention to the diet already prescribed, and by palliative remedies. Among the most efficacious for this purpose, are assafœtida, æther, and opium. Æther may be taken in the quantity of two tea-spoonfuls, or upwards, mixed with four table-spoonfuls of water. Ten grains of assafœtida, with half a grain of opium, made into two pills, may be taken for the same purpose; and it is observed, that the good effects of opium are equally conspicuous, whether the flatulence be contained in the stomach or intestines; whereas the warm medicines, commonly called carminatives, such as juniper-berries, ginger, seed of anise, &c. do not often give immediate relief, except when the wind is in the stomach. When laudanum is used for the purpose, fifteen drops of it may be taken in some peppermint-water, with double the quantity of tincture of castor, or sweet spirit of nitre.

External applications may likewise be employed with advantage against this complaint. Take of Bate's * anodyne balsam, an

* See *Appendix*.

ounce; of the expressed oil of mace, half an ounce; oil of mint, two drachms. Mix them together, and let a table-spoonful of the composition be well rubbed on the parts at bed-time. A more permanent remedy may be composed of equal parts of the anti-hysteric and stomach plaster,* spread upon a soft leather, of such size as to cover the greater part of the belly. This should be kept on for a considerable time, provided the patient be able to bear it; but if it give great uneasiness, it may be removed, and the liniment, just now mentioned, used in its room.

### *The Hiccup.*

The hiccup is a convulsive motion of the diaphragm, or midriff, and the muscles which close the passage leading into the wind-pipe. It is sometimes a primary disease, but commonly only symptomatic.

This complaint may proceed from too great a repletion of the stomach, whether by eating or drinking; from irritation, or acrimony; poisons; inflammation, or scirrhous tumor, of the stomach, or neighbouring parts. In malignant fevers, and gangrenes, it is often the harbinger of death.

Cure.—When the hiccup is owing to a surfeit, or any thing hard of digestion, it may generally be removed by a glass of pepper-mint-water, or a drachm of some spirituous liquor. When occasioned by acrimony, some troches, or lozenges of liquorice, or a drachm of gum-arabic dissolved in some water, may be taken. If the cause be poison, milk and oil, as formerly directed, must be taken in large quantities. When it proceeds from an inflammation of the stomach, which is a very dangerous case, it must be treated in the same manner with that disorder. If from a foulness of that organ, the proper remedies are a gentle vomit and purge; and if from flatulence, a bit of ginger may be chewed, or some of it powdered, may be taken in half a glassful of water One of the most dangerous causes of a hiccup is an internal gangrene or mortification; against which if any medicine can prove effectual, it must be the Peruvian bark.

In an obstinate hiccup, fifteen or twenty grains of musk, made into a draught with three table-spoonfuls of pure water, thirty drops of the compound spirit of lavender, and a small bit of sugar, may be taken two or three times a day. Of antispasmodic remedies, the last recourse is to opium, which in this case operates more safely when joined with other medicines than when taken alone. Twelve or fifteen drops of laudanum may be added to the preceding draught. Besides internal remedies, the compound plaster of

* See *Appendix.*

laudanum, or Venice treacle, applied to the region of the ſtomach, has frequently good effects.

Sternutatories, or thoſe remedies which excite ſneezing, are often beneficial in this complaint. When it proceeds from no fixed cauſe, retaining the breath for a conſiderable time; any ſudden ſurprize or fright; ſwallowing a little cold water, or a tea-ſpoonful of vinegar very ſlowly, holding the breath at the ſame time as long as poſſible, often puts a ſtop to it.

## *Cramp of the Stomach.*

This painful and dangerous complaint is chiefly incident to people advanced in years, eſpecially thoſe who are ſubject to the gout, or any nervous diſorder. When it is attended with an inclination to vomit, the diſcharge ſhould be promoted by chamomile-tea. A laxative clyſter then may be given; and afterwards a ſmaller clyſter of warm water, to which a tea-ſpoonful of laudanum is added; as an opiate given by the mouth has often the effect, at firſt, of increaſing the complaint of the ſtomach. If the pain return with violence after the mitigation produced by the anodyne clyſter, another ſhould be given with about a third part more of laudanum. The patient ought alſo, every four or five hours, to take half a ſcruple of muſk, made into a bolus with half a drachm of Venice-treacle.

During the uſe of theſe means, ſome of Bate's anodyne balſam ſhould be rubbed on the part affected, and anti-hyſteric plaſter, or a cataplaſm of Venice-treacle worn upon it for ſome time, to prevent a return of the diſorder.

When the complaint proceeds from a ſuppreſſion of the menſes, the patient's feet and legs ought to be put into warm water, and ſome blood taken away; and in general, when the cramp is violent, ſome blood ſhould be let, if the perſon can bear the evacuation. If the diſorder proceed from the gout, a glaſs of brandy, or ſpirit of peppermint with a tea-ſpoonful of the compound ſpirit of lavender, or æther, ſhould be taken; applying at the ſame time bliſtering plaſters to the ancles, and previouſly bathing the feet and legs in warm water.

## *Incubus, or Night-Mare.*

This complaint attacks a perſon during ſleep, and when he lies on his back, particularly after eating a heavy ſupper. It is felt in the form of a great weight or oppreſſion about the breaſt and ſtomach, and is generally accompanied with frightful apprehenſions. The perſon groans, and ſometimes cries out, but more frequently attempts to ſpeak in vain.

This diſorder ariſes chiefly from indigeſtion, in perſons of weak nerves, who uſe a plentiful diet, and do not take proportionable exerciſe. Flatulence in the ſtomach, as well as too heavy a ſupper, is apt to produce it. The beſt preventive is exerciſe, and a light ſupper. If any oppreſſion of the ſtomach be felt at going to bed, it may be relieved and the complaint prevented, by taking a moderate glaſs of brandy, or rather a glaſs of peppermint-water.

Somnambuliſm, or the cuſtom of walking during ſleep, is juſtly conſidered as a different modification of this diſeaſe, and requires the ſame method of prevention.

## *Swoonings, or Fainting Fits.*

Theſe complaints may be occaſioned by exceſſive weakneſs, great fatigue, or a ſudden loſs of blood; but in perſons of weak nerves, or delicate conſtitutions, they may ariſe from various other cauſes; ſuch as fear, grief, and other violent paſſions of the mind; a ſudden tranſition from cold to heat, or breathing air deprived of its proper elaſticity, as happens in crowded aſſemblies, where the apartment is not duly ventilated.

When a perſon is ſeized with a fainting fit, his hands and face ought immediately to be ſprinkled with vinegar or cold water, and his temples rubbed with ſtrong vinegar or brandy. He ought likewiſe to be made to ſmell to vinegar, or volatile ſalts or ſpirits; and if he can ſwallow a little wine, or ſome other cordial, it ſhould be poured into his mouth. If he ſhould not recover by theſe means, and was not before exceſſive weak, it will be proper to draw ſome blood, and afterwards give a clyſter, but bleeding is not adviſable where the perſon is of a delicate conſtitution.

If the patient be a perſon ſubject to hyſteric fits, caſtor, aſſafœtida, or burnt feathers, ſhould be applied to the noſe, as directed in the treatment of the hyſteric diſeaſe.

After recovering from a fainting fit, if it had been produced by great fatigue, long faſting, or other obvious cauſes of accidental weakneſs, the patient muſt be ſupported by generous cordials, ſuch as wines, jellies, and the like; which muſt at firſt be given in ſmall quantities, and gradually increaſed as the patient is able to bear them. Freſh air ſhould be admitted into his apartment, where he ſhould be allowed to lie quite ſtill and eaſy upon his back, with his head rather low.

## *Low Spirits.*

Perſons of weak nerves are ſubject to this diſtreſſing complaint, which generally proceeds from a relaxed ſtate of the ſtomach, and bowels. Nothing tends more to produce it than grief and anxiety long continued. It is very apt to be increaſed by flatulence; and is ſometimes occaſioned by a ſuppreſſion of the menſtrual or hæmorrhoidal flux.

Cure.—This complaint is to be treated entirely in the ſame manner as nervous diſorders, of which it may be conſidered as a ſymptom. If there be a load at the ſtomach, or any collection of acrid humours, which may be known either from a ſour or bitter taſte accompanying eructations or belchings, it will be proper to excite gentle vomiting by a moderate doſe of ipecacuanha, or an infuſion of chamomile-flowers. This being done, the patient ſhould next clear the inteſtines with ſome gentle purgative. To anſwer this purpoſe, he may take a drachm of ſal polychreſt, diſſolved in half a pint of warm water, two or three mornings ſucceſſively. If this doſe gives him two ſtools in the day, it will be ſufficient; and he may afterwards take it occaſionally, increaſing or diminiſhing the quantity according to its operation. He ought then to take the Peruvian bark, with ſtomachic bitters, and ſome of the preparations of iron, as before directed. But the cure is chiefly to be effected by exerciſe on horſeback, with a well regulated diet, agreeable company, and amuſements. The depreſſing paſſions in particular ought to be avoided; and a glaſs of generous wine, if it agrees with the ſtomach, may be taken at any time when the perſon feels himſelf languid. On ſuch occaſions, he may alſo take thirty or forty drops of the following mixture in a table-ſpoonful of water. Take of the tincture of aſſafœtida, caſtor, compound ſpirit of lavender, and dulcified ſpirit of nitre, each two drachms. Mix them together.

When the diſorder proceeds from a ſuppreſſion of either of the fluxes above mentioned, theſe evacuations ought to be reſtored, or others ſubſtituted in their room, ſuch as iſſues, ſetons, &c. But nothing has ſo immediate good effects in this caſe as bleeding.

Perſons afflicted with low ſpirits are apt to ſeek for a mitigation of their complaint in the ſolace of wine, or ſtrong liquors; but in this reſource they ſhould be careful never to exceed the bounds of temperance: for though the moderate uſe of wine, and even of ſpirituous liquors occaſionally, may prove beneficial, the abuſe of either, and eſpecially the latter, is pernicious, and augments the diſeaſe.

## CHAP. XXIV.

### *Palſy.*

THIS is a deprivation or diminution of ſenſe or motion, or of both, in one or more parts of the body; and is more or leſs dangerous, according to the importance of the part affected. When one ſide is affected, it is called *hemiplegia;* and when it ſeizes all the parts below the head, or the lower half of the body, it is termed *paraplegia.* If confined to any particular limb, or muſcle, it is a palſy of that part. In the *hemiplegia,* convulſions often take place in the ſound ſide, with the cynic ſpaſm or involuntary laughter, and other diſtortions of the face. Sometimes the whole paralytic part of the body becomes livid, or even mortifies before the patient's death; and ſometimes the paralytic parts gradually decay and ſhrivel up, ſo as to become much leſs than before.

Many perceptible varieties occur in the form of this diſeaſe. Sometimes there is a total loſs of ſenſe, while motion remains entire: in others a total loſs of motion, with very ſlight or even no affection of ſenſe; and, in ſome caſes, while a total loſs of motion takes place in one ſide, a total loſs of ſenſe has been obſerved in the other; but the caſe that moſt commonly occurs, is a loſs of voluntary motion, while feeling remains.

Causes.—The immediate cauſe of a palſy is any that prevents the uniform exertion of the nervous power upon a particular part of the body. The occaſional and prediſpoſing cauſes are of various kinds; ſuch as intemperance; ſuppreſſed evacuations; a retroceſſion of external eruptions; ſcorbutic acrimony; ſudden fear; preſſure upon the brain or nerves; and wounds of thoſe parts; ſpaſmodic colic; old age, and debility of the nervous ſyſtem, &c.

When the part affected feels cold, is inſenſible, or waſtes away, or when the faculties of the mind begin to fail, there is little hope of recovery; though death does not immediately follow even the moſt ſevere paralytic attacks. In a *hemiplegia,* it is not uncommon for the patient to live ſeveral years; and even in the *paraplegia,* if death do not enſue within two or three weeks, it may not take place for a conſiderable time. It is a favourable ſign when the perſon feels a ſlight degree of painful itchineſs in the part affected; and if a fever ſhould come on, there is a chance of its curing the palſy. When the ſenſe of feeling remains, there is much more room to hope for a cure than when this as well as the power of motion is extinct. Convulſions ſupervening on a palſy are a fatal ſign.

CURE.—If the person be young, and of a full habit of body, the palsy must be treated in the same manner as in the sanguineous apoplexy, by bleeding, blistering, sharp clysters, or purgative medicines. But when the disease comes on in old age, and proceeds from relaxation or debility, it will be necessary to pursue a quite contrary method of cure. The diet must be warm and strengthening, seasoned with spices or aromatic ingredients; and the drink must be generous wine, mustard-whey, or brandy and water. The first thing to be given is a laxative clyster, and afterwards a vomit, which should be repeated occasionally. Volatile and stimulating medicines are then to be administered. Take of ammonia prepared six grains; tincture of cardamoms one drachm; pennyroyal-water an ounce and an half; syrup of orange peel one drachm. Mix them for a draught to be taken every six hours.

Friction on the parts affected with a flesh-brush or warm cloths should be employed, as well as blistering-plasters and the volatile liniment. Electricity likewise is beneficial, moderately applied by a proper apparatus, and long persisted in.

The arnica-montana, or German leopard-bane, has been highly extolled in the cure of this disease by some foreign writers: but the trials made of it in this country have not proved equally successful. The leaves of the rhus toxicodendron have been found very efficacious in cases of palsy, and extreme debility, and even in the palsy of the lower extremities accompanied with distortion of the spine, but without caries. The powder of the dried leaves has been given from a third of a grain three times a day to one drachm; but as it is a deleterious medicine, and different parcels of the powder differ in their strength, great caution is necessary in its administration.

In a palsy of the tongue, the patient should frequently gargle his mouth with brandy and mustard; or hold in it a bit of sugar wet with the compound spirit of lavender, or the root of pellitory of Spain. In this case, the root of wild valerian is likewise of great advantage, taken either in powder or infusion: a table-spoonful of mustard-seed taken frequently is of great service.

A palsy of the lower extremities, arising from caries of the spine, and accompanied with a distortion of it, has been frequently cured by applying a large caustie on each side of the protuberant vertebræ, and keeping the ulcers open as issues. The eschar should be narrow, but long, according to the extent of the curve, just above which the upper end should reach; but perhaps setons are still preferable. Calcareous phosphat, or calcined bones, has of late years been recommended as a powerful auxiliary to this treatment.

When a palsy succeeds the rheumatism, scurvy, scrofula, lues venerea, or nervous colic, it will be neceſſary, in the cure, to advert to the primary diſeaſes, and adminiſter ſuch medicines as are reſpectively proper in thoſe different complaints.

Paralytic ſhakings or tremblings of the hands, or other parts, frequently follow upon hard drinking, or any other exceſſes in the non-naturals, and may, in general, be treated as a partial palſy, omitting the evacuations, which would, in theſe caſes, be injurious.

The medicinal waters both of Bath and Briſtol, under proper regulations, are adviſable in theſe circumſtances.

A perſon who labours under a paralytic complaint ſhould guard againſt cold and damp air; plethora; wear flannel next his ſkin; and regularly take ſuch exerciſe as he is able to bear.

## CHAP. XXV.

### *The Colic.*

THIS complaint of the bowels is diſtinguiſhed into ſeveral kinds, according to the different cauſes from which it proceeds. We ſhall conſider them in the following order, viz. the flatulent, or windy; the bilious; the hyſteric; and the nervous.

### *Of the Windy Colic.*

The moſt common of theſe is the windy colic, in which there is a wandering pain in the bowels, with rumblings, which abate on the expulſion of air, either upwards or downwards. The pain is not increaſed by preſſure; the thirſt not great; and the pulſe but varied little from its natural ſtandard.

This kind of colic is commonly occaſioned by unripe fruits, meats of hard digeſtion, flatulent vegetables, fermenting liquors, and other ſubſtances. It may likewiſe proceed from obſtructed perſpiration, and is moſt frequent with perſons of a delicate habit.

Cure.—When the diſorder is occaſioned by any thing of a flatulent nature, there is not a better remedy, on the firſt appearance of the ſymptoms, than a glaſs of brandy, or any other good ſpirits; and, indeed, it is the only colic in which any thing of a heating kind can be given with ſafety. Neither are theſe to be uſed unleſs at the very beginning of the complaint, and when there are no ſymptoms of inflammation. The patient, in the mean time, ought to keep his feet warm by the application of bricks, or whatever elſe may anſwer the purpoſe; and warm cloths ſhould be applied to his ſtomach and bowels.

Several kinds of food, ſuch as honey, eggs, &c. are apt to produce colics in ſome conſtitutions. The readieſt method of curing theſe is to drink plentifully of diluting liquors, as weak poſſet, water-gruel, toaſt and water, &c.

When a colic proceeds from exceſs and indigeſtion, it commonly goes of by ſpontaneous evacuation, which ought to be promoted by drinking plentifully of the liquids laſt mentioned. A doſe of ſome gentle purge ſhould afterwards be taken, to clear the bowels of any dregs that may remain.

If the complaint has been occaſioned by wet feet, or catching cold, the beſt remedy is bathing the feet and legs in warm water, which ought to be done immediately. The perſon ſhould then endeavour to promote perſpiration by drinking warm diluting liquors, ſuch as weak wine-whey, or water-gruel, with a ſmall quantity of rum or brandy in it.

## *Of the Bilious Colic.*

This ſpecies of colic prevails moſt in ſummer. It is attended with acute pain, ſometimes fixed about the region of the navel, ſometimes all over the abdomen, and at other times ſhifting from one part to another. There is likewiſe a pulſation, and ſenſe of cold, in the belly. The patient feels a bitter taſte in the mouth, with great heat; and is troubled with a vomiting of yellowiſh or greeniſh bile. He makes little or no urine, and is generally coſtive. The diſorder is accompanied with thirſt and fever, and frequently likewiſe with a hoarſeneſs.

Cure.—If the pulſe be full and frequent, it will be proper to bleed, and give an emetic; the patient drinking plentifully of an infuſion of chamomile, or the like, to work it off. Afterwards give opening emollient clyſters, and purgatives. The former may conſiſt of milk and water, with a table-ſpoonful of ſalt and moiſt ſugar, and two table-ſpoonfuls of ſweet oil, or ſome freſh butter. As a purgative, give two table-ſpoonfuls of caſtor oil, with fifteen drops of laudanum. Should it not operate in about an hour and a half, let the patient take one ſpoonful more of the oil, with a proportionable quantity of laudanum.

Vomiting is frequently a very urgent ſymptom in this diſorder, and no leſs difficult to reſtrain. The patient ſhould in this caſe drink mint-tea, or water in which ſome toaſted bread is boiled. If theſe ſhould not prove effectual, recourſe may be had to the ſaline draught, with a few drops of laudanum in it, and repeated as occaſion may require.

At the same time, some Venice-treacle, spread upon leather, may be applied to the pit of the stomach; and clysters, either with the same, or forty drops of laudanum, may be given and likewise frequently repeated. In this case columbo-root has been found particularly serviceable. A scruple, or upwards may be given in powder, in a cup of mint-tea, or any other vehicle.

The patient's belly, in the mean time, should be frequently fomented with cloths dipped in warm water; and, these not proving successful, he ought to be immersed up to the breast in the warm bath, and the opium to be repeated.

### *Of the Hysteric Colic.*

This species of colic bears a great resemblance to the preceding, in respect both of pain and vomiting; but the pain is about the region of the stomach, and the discharge generally of a greenish colour. Women of a lax and gross habit, and of an irritable disposition, are chiefly subject to this disorder. It is accompanied with great lowness of spirits, and difficulty of breathing, which are the characteristic symptoms of the disease. The pain goes off in a day or two, and frequently returns in a few weeks with equal violence. Sometimes it is accompanied with the jaundice; but this, for the most part, goes off spontaneously in a few days.

In this case both bleeding and purging are to be avoided, unless a full habit of body, or costiveness, should require any of these evacuations; and, with regard to the latter, it will be more advisable to employ clysters than purgatives. The stomach, however, should be cleared by drinking warm water, or chamomile-tea; after which, twenty, thirty, or thirty-five grains of opiate confection may be given; or, in place of it, fifteen, twenty, or twenty-five drops of laudanum, in a glass of cinnamon-water. Either of these may be repeated two or three times a day till the disorder abates; and the compound plaster of laudanum, spread upon soft leather, may, in the mean time, be applied to the region of the stomach.

When the complaint has ceased, the patient's strength ought to be recruited with the Peruvian bark, bitters, the preparations of iron, air, and excercise.

This disorder in men is named the hypochondriac colic, and should be treated in the same manner.

### *Of the Nervous or Painters' Colic.*

This disease prevails much among those who are employed in working about lead; and is likewise common in Devonshire, in particular; occasioned, as is supposed, by the drinking of cyder impregnated with that mineral, from the lead used for fastening the nails in the vats. It is, therefore, otherwise called the Devonshire colic. The colic of Poictou and the dry belly-ache in the West-Indies, are of the same nature.

Symptoms.—This disorder begins with a sense of weight or pain at the pit of the stomach, which extends itself down, with griping pains, to the bowels, attended with loss of appetite, yellowness in the countenance, a slight nausea, and costiveness. Soon after the stomach is distended, as with wind, and there are frequent retchings to vomit, without bringing up any thing but small quantities of bile and phlegm. Sometimes the intestines seem to the patient as if drawn to the spine; at other times they are drawn into hard lumps, which are plainly perceptible to the hand. In either case the complaint is attended with convulsive spasms; and the pain continues without remission for several hours together. The pulse is generally low, though sometimes a little quickened by the violence of the pain. The patient discovers a lowness of spirits. The extremities are often cold, and sometimes the violence of the pain occasions cold clammy sweats and fainting. The disease is often tedious, especially if improperly treated, insomuch that the patient will continue in this miserable state for three weeks or a month: instances have been known of its continuing for six months. In this case the pains at last become intolerable, and the patient's breath acquires a strong foetid smell At length when the pain in the bowels begins to abate, it is succeeded by a pain in the shoulder-joint, and adjoining muscles, with an unusual sensation and tingling along the spine of the back. This soon extends itself to the nerves of arm and legs, which become weak; and the weakness increasing, the limbs become paralytic, with a total loss of motion, though a small degree of feeling remain. Sometimes the brain becomes affected, and the nervous system is irritated to such a degree as to produce general convulsions, which are often followed by death. At other times, the peristaltic or natural motion of the intestines is inverted, and the true iliac passion is produced, which also proves fatal in a short time. Sometimes the paralytic affection of the extremities goes off, and the pain of the bowels returns with its former violence; and on the cessation of the pain in the intestines, the extremities again become paralytic, and in this manner the pain and palsy will alternate for a very long time.

Cure.—This disorder is so nearly allied to an inflammation of the bowels, in which it often terminates, that the same method of cure has generally been directed in both. But it is now the established practice to begin by cleansing the stomach with chamomile-tea; after which, the body is to be opened by mild purgatives, assisted by soft oily clysters. The best purgative in this case is castor oil, which may alſo be added to the clyſters; and, to mitigate the violence of the pain, fifteen or twenty drops of laudanum may be joined with the former, and double the quantity with the latter. In the mean time, the back and limbs ſhould be ſtrongly rubbed with the liniment of ammonia, camphorated ſpirits, and other hot liniments.

Dr. Percival has found alum very efficacious in this diſeaſe. It was given in the quantity of fifteen grains every fourth, fifth, or ſixth hour. But a yet more powerful remedy is blue vitriol, or vitriol of copper. Eight grains of it being diſſolved in half a pint of water, two or three table-ſpoonfuls are to be taken faſting for nine ſucceſſive mornings. For the firſt four or five days this medicine diſcharges much vitiated bile both ways; but the evacuation of this humour leſſens by degrees. During the uſe of this remedy, the patient ought to live upon broth made of lean meat, gruel, or panada; but about the ſeventh or eight day he may be allowed bread and boiled chicken. The moſt uſeful medicine in this diſeaſe is calomel, in doſes of eight or ten grains, every twelve hours, with a grain of opium; and twice that quantity in clyſters of caſtor-oil.

When the diſeaſe is over, the patient ſhould be ſtrengthened with the Peruvian bark and bitters, uſe a nouriſhing diet, and take exerciſe on horſeback. If the diſeaſe ends in a palſy, great benefit is generally found from the uſe of Bath waters.

## CHAP. XXVI.

### *Aſthma.*

THIS diſorder, which conſiſts of a difficulty of breathing, is moſt frequently in the decline of life, and more common to men than to women. It is diſtinguiſhed into two kinds, namely the moiſt and dry, or humoural and nervous; both which, however, appear to partake of a ſpaſmodic nature.

The paroxyſms or fits generally commence in the night-time, with a ſenſe of ſtraightneſs of the cheſt, difficulty of reſpiration, and a cough. The patient cannot lie in a horizontal poſture, and, if ſeized in that poſition, is obliged immediately to become erect. The difficulty of breathing increaſes, accompanied with a violent wheezing; and after continuing ſome hours, an expectoration of mucus or phlegm takes place, and the ſymptoms abate. They ſtill prevail, however, in a greater or leſs degree in the day-time, according to the weather and other circumſtances; but the fit returns next night, and often many nights ſucceſſively. There is frequently little variation of the pulſe; the urine at firſt is pale, but after a remiſſion it commonly becomes high coloured, and depoſits a ſediment. The complaint is for the moſt part attended with flatulence, and ſymptoms of indigeſtion.

CAUSES.—This diſorder may proceed from any cauſe that obſtructs the circulation of the blood through the lungs; ſuch as a ſtoppage of cuſtomary evacuations; the ſudden retroceſſion of the gout, or ſtriking in of eruptions; violent exerciſe; the fumes of metals or minerals received into the lungs, &c. Sometimes the diſorder is hereditary, or depends on a bad formation of the breaſt. In ſome perſons the fits are brought on by external heat, in others by cold.

This diſeaſe often occaſions a conſumption of the lungs in young perſons: when it continues a long time, it frequently terminates in a dropſy of the breaſt, or brings on an anueriſm of the heart, or great veſſels near it. A tremulous reſpiration, a palſy of the arms, and a diminition of the urinary ſecretion, are bad ſymptoms.

CURE.—During a violent fit of this diſeaſe bleeding is proper, unleſs in caſes of extreme weakneſs, or old age. A purging clyſter, with a drachm of aſſafœtida diſſolved in it, ſhould be immediately given, and, if neceſſary, repeated two or three times, the patient being generally coſtive. His feet and legs ſhould be put into warm water, and afterwards well rubbed with a dry cloth. If the violence of the ſymptoms ſhould not ſpeedily abate, it will be proper to apply a bliſtering-plaſter to the neck and breaſt.

To give a vomit in the height of a fit is not adviſable, as it would increaſe the accumulation of the blood in the veſſels of the head; but vomiting will often prevent a fit of the aſthma, eſpecially if the ſtomach happen to be foul. And aſthmatic perſons have generally ſome warning of the attack, from a langour, loſs of appetite, oppreſſion, and ſwelling of the ſtomach from flatulence, which precede the fit. Sometimes a vomit has good effect, even during the paroxyſm, and ſnatches the patient as it were from the jaws of death; but this will be more ſafe after other evacuations have been premiſed.

Coffee is recommended by Sir John Floyer, as the beſt abater of an aſthmatic fit that he had ſeen. It ought to be of the beſt Mocco, newly roaſted, and made very ſtrong immediately after grinding it. He commonly ordered an ounce for one diſh; which is to be repeated freſh after the interval of a quarter or half an hour, and taken without milk or ſugar.

In the moiſt aſthma, the patient ought to uſe ſuch medicines as promote expectoration; ſuch as gum-ammoniac, ſquills, and the like. Both in the moiſt and dry aſthma, the following pills will be found of great uſe. Take of gum-ammoniac, powdered, and aſſafœtida, each one drachm; balſamic ſyrup enough to make them into twenty-four pills; of which three to be taken twice a day. Or take an equal quantity of oxymel of ſquills, and cinnamon-water: mix them, and let the patient take a table-ſpoonful of the mixture three or four times a day.

The dry or nervous aſthma is beſt relieved by antiſpaſmodics and opiates; and ſometimes it is neceſſary to give very large doſes of the latter. The antiſpaſmodics moſt uſed are, aſſafœtida, caſtor, and valerian. A tea-ſpoonful of the following mixture may be taken with advantage two or three times a day. Take of the tincture of ſoot, one ounce; tincture of caſtor, and camphorated tincture of opium, each half an ounce: mix them. Two table-ſpoonfuls of vinegar, with an equal quantity of cold water, is often found effectual in relieving the fit.

To obtain permanent relief in the dry aſthma nothing is found to anſwer better than the powder of ipecacuanha in ſmall doſes. Three, five, eight, or ten grains, according to the ſtrength and conſtitution of the patient, given every other day, have produced the happieſt effects; acting ſometimes as an evacuant, pumping up the viſcid phlegm; at others, as an antiſpaſmodic or ſedative, allaying the irritation of the nerves. The Peruvian bark, in this caſe, by ſtrengthening the habit, is likewiſe found of great advantage. In both kinds of aſthma, iſſues are highly beneficial, and the uſe of them ſhould never be diſcontinued.

When the aſthma depends on ſome other diſeaſe, regard muſt always be had to the primary complaint. Thus in the arthritic aſthma, or that which proceeds from a gouty habit, ſinapiſms or warm poultices of muſtard ſeed powdered, and vinegar, muſt be applied to the feet, with bliſters to the legs or ancles, to bring on, if poſſible, a regular fit of the gout. Bliſters will alſo be neceſſary when the diſorder is occaſioned by the ſtriking in of any eruption; and when it proceeds from the dregs of an ague, recourſe muſt be had to the Peruvian bark.

People who are ſubject to the aſthma ought to avoid every thing in diet that is hard of digeſtion, or flatulent; and they ſhould uſe daily exerciſe, particularly riding on horſeback.

## CHAP. XXVII.

### *Jaundice.*

THE jaundice proceeds from an abſorption of the bile into the blood, which it renders of a vitiated quality. The diſeaſe begins with general laſſitude, and an obtuſe pain in the region of the liver, accompanied with weight and oppreſſion. The ſkin is dry, and affected with a troubleſome itching. The white of the eyes becomes yellow; and in a little time this colour is diffuſed over the body. The perſon feels a bitter taſte in his mouth. The ſtools are of a whitiſh or clay colour, and the urine ſo yellow, or rather reddiſh, as to communicate the ſame colour to linen. The diſeaſe is generally attended with coſtiveneſs, and ſometimes a degree of fever.

Causes.—The immediate cauſe of jaundice is an obſtruction to the paſſage of the bile into the inteſtines; and this may be effected in various ways. Catching cold, or the ſtoppage of cuſtomary evacuations, may produce the diſeaſe; as may likewiſe the bilious or hyſteric colic; violent paſſions; and the bites of ſome poiſonous animals. It is ſometimes the conſequence of obſtinate agues, when prematurely ſtopped by aſtringent medicines; and is frequently incident to pregnant women. It may alſo be occaſioned by ſtrong purgatives. It may likewiſe be occaſioned by gall-ſtones, or viſcid bile obſtructing the gall duct, or by the compreſſion of tumors in the neighbouring parts.

As the jaundice may ariſe from many different cauſes, ſome of which cannot be diſcovered during the patient's life, the iſſue of the diſeaſe cannot always be judged of with certainty. The only caſes which admit of a cure are thoſe depending upon biliary concretions, or obſtructions of the biliary ducts by viſcid bile, or ſpaſms of the duodenum; for the concretions are ſeldom of ſuch a ſize that the ducts will not let them paſs through, though frequently not without great pain. The coming on of gentle looſeneſs, attended with bilious ſtools, and a ceſſation of the pain, are ſigns of the diſeaſe being cured.

Cure.—In the beginning of the diſorder, if the patient be young, of a full habit of body, the degree of pain, and other ſymptoms, give reaſon to ſuſpect an inflammation of the liver, it will be neceſſary to bleed. A warm fomentation, made with chamomile-flowers, ſhould then be applied to the region of the liver; or the patient may ſit in the warm bath to the breaſt. The body ſhould be kept open with a mixture of Caſtile-ſoap, the powder of rhubarb, and tartarifed kali; which, with the addition of fimple fyrup, may be made into pills of a moderate fize, and two, three, or more of them taken twice a day, according to their effect on the bowels.

When the difeafe proceeds from any biliary concretion, or vifcid bile, obftructing the gall-duct, no remedy is better adapted than a vomit of ipecacuanha, which may be repeated once or twice at the interval of two or three days. If the pain, however, be violent, it will be proper to allay that fymptom by opium before the vomit is adminiftered.

If the jaundice be owing to fcirrhofity or fixed obftructions in the liver, which may generally be known from a weight in that part, of long continuance, and a darknefs of the complexion, little more can be done than to palliate the fymptoms. This is beft accomplifhed by fmall dofes of calomel and diuretics, which evacuate the bilious matter, and obviate the bad confequences that would enfue from its being retained in the blood. But even this artificial ftimulus is by no means equal to the common evacuation by ftool; nor can any attempt to fupply the want of bile in the inteftines, by bitters and other ftomachics, prove fufficient for accomplifhing the procefs of digeftion, and exciting the action of the bowels.

On all occafions, when the pain is violent, recourfe muft be had to opiates; and if very high coloured urine, or a difcharge of blood from any part, fhow that the blood has acquired a tendency to diffolution, recourfe fhould be had to the Peruvian bark, and other antifeptic medicines.

During the continuance of the difeafe the diet fhould be light, and chiefly of the vegetable kind. Many have been cured by living almoft entirely for fome days on raw eggs. The patient ought to take daily exercife, particularly on horfeback, where the motion increafes not the pain. Mineral waters, efpecially thofe of Harrowgate or Bath, are found beneficial. After the ceffation of the diforder, there can be no fecurity againft its return, when occafioned by biliary concretions in the gall-bladder; becaufe frefh concretions may be formed; and, accordingly, fome conftitutions are liable to frequent returns of the complaint. The beft preventive, however, is riding on horfeback; which, by fhaking the bowels, tends to diflodge thofe concretions before they have acquired fuch a fize as to render their paffage through the duct an object of difficulty.

## CHAP. XXVIII.

### *Dropſy.*

A DROPSY is a præternatural ſwelling of the whole body, or ſome part of it, occaſioned by a collection of watery humours, from a deficiency of urine or perſpiration. It is differently denominated, according to the part affected. When the water is lodged under the ſkin, it receives the name of *anaſarca*, or *leucophlegmatia*; when in the breaſt, *hydrops pectores*, or *hydrothorax*; when in the brain, *hydrocephalus*; and ſo of other parts: but the moſt common form of the diſeaſe is the *aſcites*, or dropſy of the belly. Of this there are two kinds; one in which the water floats round the inteſtines; and another, in which it is *ſaccated*, or contained in cyſts or bags.

CAUSES.—The dropſy is often the conſequence of a long continued jaundice, and frequently of a ſedentary life. It may likewiſe proceed from an abuſe of ſtrong liquors, which, by firſt affecting the liver, produce in the end this diſeaſe. Exceſſive evacuations, ſuch as frequent and copious bleedings, ſtrong purgatives often repeated, ſalivations, &c. may give riſe to it; it may alſo be occaſioned by the ſtoppage of cuſtomary evacuations, ſuch as the *menſes*, hæmorrhoids, &c. The diſeaſe may likewiſe be incurred by living in a damp ſituation, or uſing a crude watery diet; and ſometimes a diſpoſition to it is hereditary.

SYMPTOMS.—The *anaſarca* commonly begins with a ſwelling of the feet and ancles towards night, which for ſome time diſappears in the morning, after lying in bed. In the evening, the part, when preſſed with the finger, will pit, and then riſe ſlowly to its former fulneſs. The ſwelling gradually aſcends, and ſpreads over the trunk of the body, the arms, and the head. The body is generally bound, the perſpiration is greatly obſtructed, and the urine in ſmall quantity. The patient complains much of thirſt, and has a difficulty of breathing, accompanied with a troubleſome cough, and a ſlow waſting fever.

The *aſcites* is known by the ſwelling of the abdomen, and may be diſtinguiſhed from a tympany by the weight as well as the fluctuation of water; which will be felt by ſtriking the belly on one ſide, and laying the palm of the hand on the oppoſite.

When the dropſy ariſes from a ſcirrhus of the liver, or any other of the bowels, the event is always to be dreaded; as is the caſe likewiſe when it proceeds from diſorders of the lungs. Indeed an *aſcites* ſeldom admits of a radical cure; and the only reſource, on ſome occaſions, is to procure a temporary relief by tapping. When the diſeaſe, however, comes on ſuddenly, without any previous illneſs, and the patient is young, and apparently of a good conſtitution, there is reaſon to hope that an early uſe of medicine will be attended with ſucceſs.

CURE.—Towards effecting a cure, the patient muſt uſe a ſtimulating diet, ſuch as roaſted meats of eaſy digeſtion, and warm pungent vegetables; in which claſs are garlic, muſtard, raw onions, horſe-radiſh, &c. The diſeaſe has ſometimes been cured by living on hard biſcuit only, and rigidly abſtaining from all drink. But it is now found that this abſtinence is not neceſſary, and that a liquid diet may be uſed with ſucceſs. For this diſcovery we are indebted to the induſtrious inveſtigation of Dr. Milman, who condemns in the ſtrongeſt terms the practice of giving dropſical patients only dry, hard, and indigeſtible aliments. Theſe he obſerves, would oppreſs the ſtomach of the moſt healthy; and how much more muſt they do ſo to thoſe who are already debilitated by labouring under a tedious diſorder? He affirms, that unleſs plenty of diluting drink be given, the moſt powerful diuretics can have no effect; and this aſſertion he corroborates by an account of his practice in the Middleſex-Hoſpital.

According to the doctor's narrative, if the patient be not very much debilitated, he is ſometimes treated with the purging waters, and a doſe of jalap and calomel alternately. On the intermediate days he gets a ſaline mixture, with forty or ſixty drops of the vinegar of ſquills every ſixth hour; drinking with the purgatives oat-gruel and ſome thin broths. The doctor, that he might better aſcertain what ſhare the liquids given along with the medicines had in producing a copious flow of urine, ſometimes gave the medicines in the beginning of the diſeaſe without allowing any drink; but though the ſwellings were uſually diminiſhed a little by the purgatives, the urine ſtill continued ſcanty, and the patients were greatly weakened. Fearing, therefore, leſt by following this courſe, the ſtrength of the ſick might be too much reduced, he then began his courſe of diuretic medicines, giving large quantities of barley-water, with a little ſal diureticus or acetated kali; by which means, ſometimes in the ſpace of forty-eight hours after the courſe was begun, the urine flowed out in a very large quantity: but as the ſaline drinks are very diſagreeable to the taſte, a drink was compoſed purpoſely for hydropic perſons, of half an ounce of cream of tartar diſſolved in two pounds of barley-water, made agreeably ſweet with ſyrup, adding one or two ounces of French brandy.

The drink ought, at leaſt, not to be of the watery kind, or, if ſuch, ſhould be medicated by ſome ſtimulating ingredient. Muſtard-whey, in which ſome broom-aſhes are diſſolved, or broom-tops boiled, may be taken in a moderate quantity. For this purpoſe, the patient may alſo uſe Rheniſh-wine, or Spa-water, impregnated with the ſame or a ſimilar ingredient. The thirſt may likewiſe be allayed by acids, ſuch as the juice of lemons, oranges, &c.

It is of great importance in a dropſy that the patient take daily exerciſe, which promotes the abſorption of the ſerous or watery humours, and increaſes the excretions both by perſpiration and urine. Walking, as it affords a general exertion of the muſcles, is preferable to any other kind, and will tend more than any other to retard the increaſe of the diſeaſe; but if the patient's ſtrength will not admit of that expedient, he may ride on horſeback or in a carriage. Should he live in a damp ſituation, he ought to change the place of his reſidence, and betake himſelf, if poſſible, to a warmer climate. At all events, the air of his apartment ſhould be warm and dry; and, for promoting perſpiration, he ought to wear flannel next to his ſkin.

When the patient is under forty years of age, of a good conſtitution, and the diſeaſe has come on ſuddenly, the cure of an *aſcites* may commence with vomits and purgatives, frequently and alternately repeated, as being the moſt ſpeedy and effectual means of evacuating the collection of watery humours. The vomit may conſiſt of half a drachm of ipecacuanha for an adult, or half an ounce of oxymel of ſquills; and an infuſion of chamomile-flowers ſhould be drunk to promote their operation. Half a drachm of the powder of jalap, with five or ſix grains of calomel, will form a ſuitable purgative, and may be taken in the morning, made up into a bolus with ſome ſyrup. A grain or two of elaterium will commonly anſwer the purpoſe of an emetic and purgative of great efficacy in dropſy. In this caſe, as well as in the vomiting, nothing conſiderable ſhould be drunk.

On the days when the patient neither vomits nor purges, he ought to take ſuch medicines as promote either urine or perſpiration, combined with thoſe of a ſtrengthening kind. For promoting the diſcharge of urine, take an ounce of juniper-berries, and half an ounce of the tops of broom: boil them for a few minutes in a pint of water, and in the ſtrained liquor infuſe half an ounce of muſtard-ſeed; ſtrain again, and diſſolve in the liquor two drachms of the cryſtals of tartar. Of this the patient may take four table-ſpoonfuls every three or four hours in the day.

To excite perſpiration the patient may uſe at night the following draught: Take of the waters of ſpearmint, peppermint, and acetated ammonia, each half an ounce; compound ſpirit of lavender thirty drops; tincture of opium fifteen or twenty drops. Mix them.

During this courſe, the patient may take twice a day a glaſs of an infuſion of Peruvian bark, ruſt of iron, and orange-peel, in ſtrong white wine.

With regard to diuretics in general, it is to be remarked, that we cannot depend with certainty upon the operation of any of them. In particular conſtitutions, and at particular times, one will be found to ſucceed, after another, though commonly of much greater power, has been tried in vain. Various diuretics therefore are often uſed in ſucceſſion. Recourſe is particularly often had to dandelion and ſquills; the latter of which, eſpecially when combined with calomel, is often found to be a very powerful diuretic. The fox-glove alſo is ſtrongly recommended for the ſame purpoſe; but it is rough in its operation, and muſt therefore be given in exceeding ſmall doſes at firſt. An infuſion of tobacco is remarkably efficacious in this reſpect; and ſmoking has been found of great benefit. A table-ſpoonful of the juice of leeks, taken twice a-day, has been known to perform a cure.

Both in the anaſarca and aſeites frictions are of great advantage. They ought to be uſed two or three times a day for ſeveral minutes, and if with camphorated liniment they will be more efficacious.

When the diſorder ariſes from the too copious uſe of weak liquids, or obſtructed perſpiration, good effects may be expected from ſudorific medicines. If too free an uſe of ſtrong liquors has been the cauſe, riding on horſeback and the uſe of wine, or rather geneva diluted with water, in moderate quantity, will be ſerviceable. If the diſorder has come on after great loſs of blood, or from tedious fevers, purgatives ought not to be uſed too freely, but chalybeates, the Peruvian bark, and bitters, ſhould be the principal reſource. Some hoſpital-phyſicians in the metropolis are very ſucceſsful in the treatment of aſeites, &c. by directing mercurial friction to be employed till the mouth begins to be affected, and then commencing a courſe of diuretics and tonics, ſuch as have been above recommended.

In endeavouring to remove the *anaſarca*, it is a common reſource to ſcariſy the feet and legs, and by that means drain off the water: but in performing this operation, the inciſion muſt be made no deeper than to penetrate the ſkin; and care muſt be taken, by ſpirituous fomentations and proper digeſtives, to prevent a mortification of the part.

When an *aſcites* does not yield to purgative and diuretic medicines, recourſe muſt be had to tapping. But this ought to be performed before the texture of the bowels has ſuffered by a long immerſion in the water. If the bowels be ſound, this expedient generally proves ſucceſsful in effecting a radical cure; but if they be diſeaſed, it can act only as a palliative remedy.

## CHAP. XXIX.

### *Tympany.*

THIS diſorder is a flatulent diſtenſion of the belly, and is diſtinguiſhed into two ſpecies, namely, the inteſtinal, and abdominal. In the former the wind is pent up in the inteſtinal canal, chiefly the colon; and, in the latter, between the inteſtines and the membranes which line the muſcles of the belly. In the inteſtinal tympany the tumor of the belly is often unequal, and there is a frequent exploſion of wind, alleviating both the tenſion and pain; but in the other ſpecies the tumefaction is more equal, and the emiſſion of wind, which is leſs frequent, affords not ſuch evident relief. The diſorder is chiefly incident to thoſe who have been long troubled with flatulencies in the ſtomach and inteſtines.

CAUSES.—The abdominal tympany is generally the conſequence of an *aſcites*, and morbid affections of the liver; but the other may be produced by a variety of cauſes. It is frequently occaſioned by the unſeaſonable uſe of opiates in the dyſentery, or of the Peruvian bark in intermittent fevers. It may likewiſe be occaſioned by a ſuppreſſion of the menſtrual or hæmorrhoidal flux; and is ſometimes the conſequence of an abortion.

CURE.—The patient ought to abſtain from all flatulent vegetables, and fermented liquors. If no fever attends, the beſt diet is light animal food, and the moſt ſuitable drink geneva diluted with water.

If the diſorder be accompanied with fever, and a full pulſe, it will be proper to bleed. The body ſhould be kept open by gentle laxatives, joined with aromatics; but ſtrong purgatives muſt be avoided, as well as carminatives without laxatives. Take of rhubarb and ginger, powdered, each two drachms: mix, and divide them into twelve doſes; of which let the patient take one twice a day in a cup of chamomile-tea.

Clyſters with infuſion of tobacco have in this caſe been uſed with great benefit.

The belly ſhould be frequently rubbed, and ſwathed with flannel; and the patient ought to uſe exerciſe, particularly riding on horſeback.

When the tumor has begun to abate, the cure will be expedited, and the return of the complaint prevented, by a courſe of ſtrengthening medicines, conſiſting of Peruvian bark, ſome of the preparations of iron, bitters, and aromatics, ſuch as have been frequently

## CHAP. XXX.

### *Scurvy.*

THE term *ſcurvy* has been indiſcriminately applied to almoſt every kind of cutaneous eruption; but the diſeaſe here meant is the true ſea-ſcurvy, which, though frequent in many places at land, attains to its greateſt degree of virulence among ſailors, on long voyages, when expoſed to the want of freſh meat and vegetables. At land it prevails in cold countries, eſpecially thoſe where the air is moiſt, and the ſoil marſhy or damp.

Symptoms.—The firſt ſymptoms of this diſeaſe are heavineſs, laſſitude, and difficulty of breathing, particularly after motion. The face becomes ſallow and bloated, the breath offenſive, the gums ſpongy and putrid, and are apt to bleed on the ſlighteſt preſſure. Blood frequently iſſues likewiſe from the noſe and ſometimes from other parts. The patient feels commonly a dejection of ſpirits. The legs often ſwell into protuberances in different parts, and yellow, purple, or livid ſpots, reſembling bruiſe-marks, and flea-bites, appear upon the ſkin. The catching of the breath on motion, with the loſs of ſtrength, dejection of ſpirits, and putrid gums, are regarded as the diſtinguiſhing and characteriſtic ſymptoms of the diſeaſe.

Causes.—The ſcurvy is frequently the effect of a ſedentary or inactive life; cold, moiſt air; putrid, ſalted, or ſmoke-dried proviſions, and aliments hard of digeſtion. The depreſſing paſſions have a powerful influence in producing it; and it may likewiſe proceed from a ſuppreſſion of cuſtomary evacuations. Whatever vitiates the fluids either by introducing unwholeſome juices or bad air into the body, and relaxes the ſolids directly or indirectly; all tend to produce this diſeaſe, which is likewiſe ſometimes hereditary.

Cure.—The cure of the ſcurvy depends upon oppoſing the ſpecific cauſe which has produced it. If it has ariſen from cold, damp, or unwholeſome air, it will be proper that the patient remove to a more healthy ſituation. If a ſedentary life, and the indulgence of melancholy, be ſuppoſed to have brought on the diſeaſe, it can only be eradicated by means of exerciſe and cheerfulneſs.

When the ſcorbutic taint has been contracted by the long uſe of ſalted or putrid proviſions, the moſt obvious method of curing it is by adopting a courſe of diet conſiſting chiefly of freſh vegetables, and ſallads made of water-creſſes, ſcurvy-graſs, brook-lime, &c. The patient ought likewise to eat freely of acescent fruits, such as apples, oranges, *lemons*, cherries, and the like; and the less he is confined to animal food, for some time, it will be so much the better. But if his strength be greatly reduced, and a diet consisting entirely of vegetables disagree with the stomach, he may be indulged in some fresh animal food of the lighter kinds, always joining with it a sufficient quantity of vegetables; and when these cannot be obtained fresh, they may be used in the pickled or preserved state. It will likewise be proper to sharpen all the patient's food and drink with *lemon-juice* or its concrete acid, vinegar, or some other acid, such as cream of tartar, spirit of sea-salt, or elixir of vitriol.

Both in the land and sea-scurvy, the use of milk is highly beneficial, when it has not the effect of rendering the patient costive: but this inconvenience may be obviated by taking occasionally a little cream of tartar, or a drachm of sal polychrest dissolved in a sufficient quantity of water. Nothing more, however, is required, than to obviate costiveness: for large evacuations are always hurtful in this disease.

An excellent drink, in the scurvy, is whey, or butter-milk. In defect of these, the patient may use sound cyder, or spruce-beer. Great benefit has been received from the use of wort, which is particularly convenient at sea, as malt will keep sound during the longest voyage.

A moderate use of wine is serviceable in the scurvy, both as a strengthener and antiseptic; and the patient ought to take such exercise as he is able to bear without fatigue, which should always be avoided.

With regard to particular symptoms, when the gums are become soft, and liable to bleed on the least touch, the mouth ought to be frequently washed with the decoction of the Peruvian bark, or an infusion of red roses, with which a little of the tincture of myrrh is joined. In the case of swelled and indurated or hardened limbs, with stiffened joints, the parts ought to be fomented with warm vinegar, and relaxed by vapour-baths, confining the vapour to the parts by means of blankets spread over them. For ulcers of the legs, when such exist, the most proper application is likewise the decoction of Peruvian bark; avoiding all greasy and oily liniments, which are in this case injurious.

## CHAP. XXXI.

### *Gout.*

THE gout, though often a hereditary diſeaſe, may be acquired by various cauſes, and is chiefly incident to thoſe who take little exerciſe, and uſe a full diet of animal food. It is more frequent with men than women, ſeizes moſtly ſuch as have large heads, and are of a corpulent habit. It ſeldom attacks perſons employed in conſtant bodily labour, or thoſe who live much on vegetable aliment. In conſtitutions ſtrongly inclined to it by hereditary diſpoſition, it ſometimes makes its appearance early in life, but does not commonly attack men before the age of thirty-five, and generally at a later period.

Beſides a hereditary diſpoſition, and the two other cauſes above mentioned, the diſorder may be brought on by a deficiency of the cuſtomary diſcharges; too free an uſe of acidulated liquors; ſevere application of mind; grief; vexation; night-watching, &c.

SYMPTOMS.—A fit of the gout ſometimes comes on ſuddenly, but for the moſt part it is preceded by particular ſigns of its approach. Theſe are generally ſuch as accompany a relaxed ſtate of the ſtomach: viz. indigeſtion, belching of wind, a ſlight head-ach, and drowſineſs. The appetite is diminiſhed, and the body is affected with a degree of languor. In ſome there is an unuſual coldneſs of the feet and legs, accompanied with cramps, and frequently a numbneſs, alternating with a ſenſe of prickling along the whole of the lower extremities.

Theſe ſymptoms take place for ſeveral days, ſometimes for a week or two, before the fit comes on; but, commonly, upon the day immediately preceding the fit the appetite becomes keener than uſual.

Moſt commonly a paroxyſm or fit of the gout comes on in the ſpring, and ſooner or later according to the period at which the vernal heat ſucceeds the winter's cold, and according as the body may happen to be expoſed to the changes of temperature. The attack is ſometimes firſt felt in the evening, but more frequently about two or three o'clock in the morning. The fit begins with a pain affecting one foot, generally in the ball or firſt joint of the great toe, but ſometimes in other parts of the foot. This is uſually accompanied with more or leſs of a ſhivering; which abates by degrees as the pain increaſes, and is ſucceeded by a hot ſtage ſubſequently of the ſame duration with the pain. From the firſt attack, the pain uniformly increaſes, attended with great reſtleſſneſs of the whole body till the midnight following, after which it gradually declines; and a gentle ſweat coming on, the patient falls into a ſleep. In the morning, he finds the part affected with ſome redneſs and ſwelling, which, after continuing ſome days, gradually abate. The patient, however, is not yet entirely relieved from the paroxyſm. For ſome days, he experiences every evening a return of pain and feveriſhneſs, which continue for more or leſs violence till morning. After this courſe of variation for ſeveral days, the diſorder generally ceaſes, not to return till after a conſiderable interval.

At the beginning of the complaint, the returns of it are ſometimes only once in three or four years; but afterwards the intervals becoming ſhorter, at length the attacks are annual, and ſometimes ſo frequent in the courſe of a year, that the patient is ſcarcely ever free from ſome degree of it except perhaps for two or three months in ſummer.

In the progreſs of the diſeaſe different parts become affected. At firſt, it commonly affects one foot only, but in the ſubſequent fits, both feet in ſucceſſion; and frequently removes from one foot into the other. Beſides the feet it often ſeizes other joints, which it variouſly affects in the ſame fluctuating manner juſt deſcribed.

In many perſons, but not in all, after a frequent return of the complaint, concretions of a chalky nature are formed upon the outſide of the joints, and for the moſt part immediately under the ſkin; where it ſeems to be depoſited at firſt in a fluid ſtate, but afterwards become dry and firm; and contributes, with other circumſtances, to deſtroy the motion of the joint.

Regimen.—There being as yet no radical cure diſcovered for the gout, we can only recommend the directions proper to be followed during the fits of the diſeaſe and the intervals.

In a fit of the gout, if the patient be young and ſtrong, the beſt courſe he can adopt is to uſe a thin and cooling diet, with drinks of a diluting nature; but if the conſtitution be weak, and the patient accuſtomed to live high, it will be ſafeſt not to deviate much from his uſual manner of living, and that he take frequently a cup of ſtrong negus, or a glaſs of generous wine. A beneficial drink, in this caſe, is wine-whey, which promotes perſpiration, without much heating the body; and it may be rendered more efficacious, by mixing with it, twice a day, a tea-ſpoonful of ſpirit of hartſhorn. A good ſubſtitute for this medicine, at night, is the ſame quantity of the volatile tincture of *guaiacum*, given in a ſmall baſon of warm wine-whey.

During the continuance of the paroxyſm, the leg and foot ſhould be wrapped in ſoft flannel or wool, and the patient be kept quiet and eafy, with particular attention to avoid all difturbance of mind. There is danger in every external application to the parts affected during the inflammatory ftate; and all evacuations ought likewife to be ufed with caution, though it be generally beneficial to keep the body gently open by means of diet, or very mild laxative medicines, when the conftitution can bear them.

Opiates afford the moft certain relief from pain; but this refource, when employed in the beginning of gouty paroxyfms, has been thought to occafion a more violent return of the complaint. When the pain, however, is very great, and the patient reftlefs, thirty or forty drops of laudanum, more or lefs, according to the violence of the fymptoms, may be taken at bed-time, both with fafety and advantage; efpecially in the cafe of perfons advanced in life, and who have often been affected with the difeafe. When, after the ceffation of the fit, fome fwelling and ftiffnefs remain in the joints, recourfe fhould be had to the diligent ufe of the flefh-brufh. The patient may then take a gentle dofe or two of the bitter tincture of rhubarb, or wine of aloes. Stomachic bitters, with the Peruvian bark, either in infufion or tincture, will likewife be ferviceable. The diet fhould be light, but nourifhing, accompanied with gentle exercife on horfeback, or in a carriage.

Should the joints affected remain weak, recourfe may be had to the flefb-brufh, or flannels impregnated with frankincenfe, amber, or myrrh, by way of friction. Though ufing the joint affected, during the decline of the fit, may be painful, ftill the practice is advifable: for it prevents the too great relaxation of the ligaments from the flux and ftagnation of fluids in thefe veffels; gives them ftrength, and prevents the continuance of that debility, of which people fo much complain when the fit is quite over. The motion may at firft be gentle, and afterwards in proportion, as the parts recover ftrength.

Such is the treatment proper in a regular fit of the gout; but when the diforder is irregular, a very different procedure becomes neceffary. Of this kind of gout there are three fpecies: the atonic, the retrocedent, and the mifplaced.

In the atonic gout, or that which does not fix itfelf in the feet and hands, the cure mult be effected by carefully avoiding all debilitating caufes; and by employing, at the fame time, the means of ftrengthening the fyftem in general, and the ftomach in particular. For accomplifhing the former of thefe indications, the moft ufeful means are frequent exercife on horfeback, and moderate walking. Cold bathing is likewife very efficacious for anfwering the fame purpofe; and may be fafely employed, if it appear to be powerful in ftimulating the fyftem, and be not applied when the extremities are threatened with any pain.

For ſupporting the ſtrength of the ſyſtem in general, when threatened with the atonic gout, ſome animal food ought to be uſed, and the more aceſcent vegetables ſhould be avoided. In the ſame caſe, ſome wine alſo may be neceſſary; but it ſhould be in moderate quantity, and of the leaſt aceſcent kinds. But if every kind of wine ſhould be found to increaſe the acidity of the ſtomach, the patient muſt, inſtead of them, make uſe of ſpirituous liquors diluted with water. For ſtrengthening the ſtomach, bitters and the Peruvian bark may be employed; but they ought not to be continned for any conſiderable length of time without intermiſſion.

In the atonic gout, or in perſons liable to it, to guard againſt cold is a caution of great importance; and the moſt certain means of doing this is by repairing to a warm climate during the winter. In northern ſituations, it is of great conſequence for this purpoſe to wear fleecy hoſiery, or at leaſt flannel, next the ſkin. In the more violent caſes, bliſtering the lower extremities may be uſeful; but this remedy ſhould be avoided when any pain threatens thoſe parts. In perſons ſubject to the atonic gout, iſſues in the extremities have been found of great advantage.

The retrocedent gout is that kind in which the diſorder ſuddenly retires from the extremities, and attacks ſome internal part; ſuch as the ſtomach, lungs, head, &c. This happens when the moving powers are ſo weakened, as not to be able to throw the offending matter to the extremities, or, when there depoſited, to keep it in that ſituation. When it fixes upon the parts above mentioned, it is extremely hazardous, in proportion to the degree of violence; and every effort ſhould be made as expeditiouſly as poſſible to throw it out of the habit into the extremities, and particularly into the feet.

When the diſorder affects the ſtomach and inteſtines, relief is to be inſtantly attempted by the free uſe of ſtrong wines, joined with aromatics, and given warm. Peppermint-water, likewiſe, and even brandy or rum, may be adminiſtered on this occaſion. In this ſtate the patient ought to keep his bed, and endeavour to promote perſpiration, by drinking warm liquors, with ſome ſpirit of hartſhorn; and if he feel any inclination to vomit, he may promote it by drinking ſome infuſion of chamomile-flowers, mixed with wine.

In this caſe opiates are often highly beneficial. They may be uſefully joined with aromatics, or a volatile alkali and camphor. Twenty or thirty drops of laudanum, with a tea-ſpoonful of compound ſpirit of lavender, may be taken in a cup of warm wine.

If, in conſequence of a retroceſſion of the gout, the inteſtines be affected with a looſeneſs, this ought to be at firſt promoted by taking plentifully of weak broth; and, after the bowels are thus cleanſed, the irritation may be allayed by opiates: for example, by the doſe of laudanum above directed.

When the gout attacks the lungs, and produces a difficulty of breathing, the feet ought to be bathed in warm water, and ſtimulating cataplaſms or poultices applied to the ſoles. Theſe may conſiſt of the common ſinapiſm, made of crumbs of bread and the flower of muſtard-ſeed, with ſtrong vinegar; to all which may be added ſome bruiſed garlic. Bliſters ſhould be applied to the back or breaſt, and the calves of the legs. Here, likewiſe, opiates are of advantage; as are alſo aſſafœtida, caſtor, and muſk.

When the gout ſeizes the head, affecting it with pain, giddineſs, apoplexy, or palſy, the external applications mentioned in the preceding paragraph may be employed, and a bliſter applied to the head: beſides which, ten grains of ginger, and five grains of the ſalt of hartſhorn, ſhould be thrown into the ſtomach, if poſſible, in two or three table-ſpoonfuls of warm wine.

In perſons who never have had any regular fit of the gout, but whoſe conſtitution and manner of living ſeem favourable to the production of the complaint, and of an age when it commonly makes its appearance, great caution is neceſſary in treating any diſorder with which they may happen to be attacked. This remark holds particularly with reſpect to evacuations; in the regulation of which it will be proper to purſue ſuch a method of cure as that, whilſt adapted to the apparent diſorder, it may not prove injurious ſhould the real cauſe of the ſymptoms be the gout in diſguiſe.—In doubtful caſes of this kind, it can hardly ever be improper to bathe the feet in warm water. The caution here recommended will be ſtill more neceſſary if the perſon has formerly experienced a fit of the gout.

A conſiderable reſpite from the gout may often be obtained by the uſe of Bath waters, but neither theſe nor any medicines are calculated to eradicate the diſorder from the habit. For accompliſhing this purpoſe, there appears to be no other means than a ſtrict attention to regimen; in which, univerſal temperance, and daily exerciſe, or rather labor, mnſt form an indiſpenſable part. A vegetable diet, or a diet entirely of milk, has been ſtrongly recommended as the moſt certain preſervative from the gout, and many inſtances confirm its utility; but a change from the uſe of animal food, and ſtrong liquors, can only be adopted with ſafety by ſlow degrees. To uſe light ſuppers, to avoid night watching, and to riſe early, are objects of great importance; and a circumſtance no leſs beneficial is to guard againſt vexation of mind.

## CHAP. XXXII.

*Rheumatifm.*

THE rheumatifm is diftinguifhed into two kinds, namely, the acute, and chronic; the former of which is accompanied with fever. It is a difeafe more frequent in cold than in warm climates, and is moft common in autumn and fpring. It prevails moft among the peafantry who are ill-clothed, live in damp houfes, and feed upon crude and unwholefome diet.

CAUSES.—The rheumatifm often proceeds from obftructed perfpiration. Wet feet, wet clothes, and lying in damp beds, or on the damp ground, are all very apt to produce it. It may alfo be occafioned by the ftoppage of the cuftomary difcharges; or by exceffive evacuations, which debilitate the body. On the fame account, it may be the confequence of fevers, or other previous difeafes, which vitiate the humours; fuch as the fcurvy, lues venerea, &c.

Thefe caufes may affect perfons of all ages; but the acute rheumatifm appears neither in very young or elderly perfons, and moft commonly occurs from the age of puberty to the age of thirty-five; affecting chiefly perfons of a fanguine temperament.

SYMPTOMS.—The acute rheumatifm commonly begins with a cold ftage, attended with wearinefs and fhivering, which are foon after fucceeded by a quick pulfe, often full and hard, reftleffnefs, thirft, and often other fymptoms of fever. The patient then complains of unufual pains in different parts of the body, which, afterwards, particularly affect the joints, and for the moft part thefe alone. They frequently fhoot along the courfe of the mufcles, from one joint to another, and are always much increafed by the action of the mufcles. The joints moft frequently affected are thofe of the larger kind; fuch as the joints of the hip, knees, fhoulders, and elbows. The ancles and wrifts are alfo frequently affected; but feldom the fmaller joints. Sometimes the difeafe is confined to one part, but often to many parts at a time.

Sometimes the fever is formed before any pains are perceived; but, more commonly, pains are felt in particular parts before any fymptoms of fever occur. The pains do not ufually remain long in the fame joint, but frequently fhift from one to another, and having abated in one joint they become more violent in another. The fever attending thefe pains is perceptibly increafed every evening, and is moſt conſiderable during the night, when the pains alſo become more violent; and it is likewiſe at this time that the pains ſhift their place from one joint to another.

When a joint has for ſome time been affected with pain, there commonly enſues a ſwelling and redneſs of the part, which is painful to the touch; but, on the appearance of the ſwelling, the pain, if it ecaſe not entirely, moſt generally abates.

It is often difficult to diſtinguiſh the acute rheumatiſm from the gout; but in the former there in general occurs much leſs affection of the ſtomach, and more fever. The diſeaſe likewiſe commonly appears at an earlier period of life than the gout; it is not obſerved to be hereditary; and it may in general be traced to ſome obvious exiſting cauſe, particularly to the effect of cold upon the body.

CURE.—The treatment of the acute rheumatiſm is nearly the ſame as that of an inflammatory fever. Bleeding is neceſſary, and ought to be repeated according to the violence of the ſymptoms; but ſtill with caution, as very profuſe bleedings occaſion a ſlow recovery, and, if not abſolutely effectual, are apt to produce ehronic rheumatiſm

After bleeding from a vein, it will be of great advantage to apply leeches to the joints affected. Six or eight may be laid on at a time; and the ſame number next day, if the pain be ſtill very ſevere. The body ought likewiſe to be kept open by gentle purgatives, ſuch as tamarinds, cream of tartar, or ſenna, or partienlarly an infuſion of mountain flax, (linum catharticum.) Next to blood-letting, nothing is of ſo much ſervice in this diſeaſe as ſudorifie medicines, or thoſe which promote perſpiration. One of the moſt effectual for this purpoſe is the compound powder of ipecacuanba, known by the name of Dover's powder. Of this, ten grains may be taken every hour for three times, unleſs the firſt or ſecond doſe has proved ſudorific. The patient ſhould, in the mean time, take frequently a cup of warm barley-water, or gruel, to promote perſpiration.

Nitre joined with antimony is alſo an efficacious remedy in this diſeaſe. Fifteen grains of the former, with two of the latter, may be taken in a wine-glaſsful of water, and repeated every three or four hours while the fever and pain continue.

If, in the courſe of the diſeaſe, the extremities ſhould ſwell, and be much pained, leeches, as above directed, may be applied to the tumefied parts; as may likewiſe the following cataplaſm. Take of rye-meal, one pound; old yeaſt, four ounces; common ſalt, two ounces; warm water, a ſufficient quantity: let the whole be wrought into a paſte, and wrapped round the part affected as warm as can be; renewing it morning and evening.

It is not uncommon for this diſeaſe, after ſome days, to put on the appearance of an intermittent. In ſuch a caſe the Peruvian bark is the moſt effectual remedy; and even without the appearance now mentioned, when plentiful ſweats break out, and the urine depoſits a copious ſediment, the uſe of the bark is highly adviſable, and will tend greatly to ſhorten the diſeaſe. By the early uſe of this remedy, where a complete intermiſſion from pain is obtained, the neceſſity of repeated blood-letting and ſweating is often ſuperſeded: but where a complete remiſſion cannot be obtained, it has been ſuſpected by ſome to be hurtful. In theſe caſes, when bleeding and ſudorifics have been puſhed as far as may be thought prudent, without producing the deſired effect, great benefit has often been experienced from the uſe of calomel combined with opium. From one to five grains of the former, and from one fourth of a grain to one grain of the latter, in proportion to the age and ſtrength of the patient, is to be given every ſix, eight, or twelve hours, made into a bolus with any conſerve, or ſome crumbs of bread and a tea-ſpoonful of water. During the exhibition of this medicine, the patient muſt uſe plentiful dilution with barley-water, or any other weak drink.

In the *acute* rheumatiſm it is neceſſary that the diet be of the loweſt kind, and taken in very ſmall quantity. Water-gruel may conſtitute the whole of the patient's nouriſhment through the diſeaſe.

The *chronic* rheumatiſm is moſt common to people in the decline of life. It is generally confined to ſome particular part of the body, and ſeldom accompanied with any conſiderable degree of fever. Sometimes a ſwelling attacks the parts affected, but without much inflammation or redneſs. Sometimes there appear in different parts ſmall tumors, of a roundiſh figure, affecting chiefly thoſe of a full habit, and women who have not their menſes regularly.

In curing this ſpecies of rheumatiſm, in full habits, it may often be of advantage to bleed once; but the diſorder is beſt carried off by the natural diſcharges. A drachm of cream of tartar, taken twice a day in a cup of the decoction of burdock-root, made with half an ounce of the root to a pint of water, has been found of great ſervice in this complaint. The patient ſhould alſo take at night a tea-ſpoonful of the volatile tincture of guaiacum, in ſome wine-whey.

If, after uſing theſe remedies for a little time, the pain ſtill continues fixed, it will be proper to apply a bliſter to the part, and to take a table ſpoonful of white muſtard-ſeed two or three times a day in a glaſs of water or ſmall wine.

Every thing heating in diet ought to be avoided in this kind of rheumatiſm, as well as the acute. Vegetables and light puddings are the moſt ſuitable aliments. A diet of whey and bread has been ſtrongly recommended in this caſe. The patient ought to uſe exerciſe, wear flannel next the ſkin, and avoid as much as poſſible, all expoſure to night-air, wet clothes, and wet feet, which are particularly hurtful.

Cold-bathing, eſpecially in ſalt water, is a very efficacious remedy in this kind of rheumatiſm; as are likewiſe the warm baths of Buxton or Matlock in Derbyſhire. When the diſeaſe is accompanied with a ſcorbutic habit, the Harrowgate and Moffat waters, taken internally and uſed as a warm bath, are very beneficial.

In full habits ſubject to the rheumatiſm, iſſues are found to have good effect. When the pain affects the upper parts, the place moſt proper for an iſſue is the arm; but when ſeated in the loins, and the contiguous parts, as in the lumbago, and ſciatic or hip gout, it ſhould be put into the leg or thigh.

For the lumbago, juſt now mentioned, the following is an efficacious remedy. Take of camphor, two drachms: diſſolve it in an equal quantity of oil of turpentine; and add of baſilicon, an ounce; common black ſoap, half an ounce; and volatile ſal ammoniac, half a drachm. Let the mixture be ſpread upon leather, and applied to the part.

## CHAP. XXXIII.

### *Cholera Morbus.*

THE characteriſtics of this diſeaſe are a violent vomiting and purging of a bilious matter, accompanied with ſickneſs, gripes, and a flatulent diſtenſion of the belly. It is moſt frequent in autumn, and ſometimes comes on ſuddenly; but is commonly preceded by a diſorder at the ſtomach, and an uneaſy ſenſation in the bowels, producing in a ſhort time, an exceſſive evacuation both ways. The patient has great thirſt, with a ſmall unequal pulſe, and often a fixed acute pain about the region of the navel. In the progreſs of the diſeaſe he is frequently affected with violent contractions in particular parts of the body. The urine is obſtructed, and there is a palpitation of the heart. When the diſorder rages with great violence, it produces cold clammy ſweats, hiccup, convulſions, faintings, and the patient is ſometimes carried off in twenty-four hours. It is divided into two kinds; namely, the *ſpontaneous*, or that which ariſes after a hot ſummer, without any manifeſt cauſe; and the *accidental*, when it is not obviouſly the conſequence of the ſeaſon, but of improper food or of a ſickneſs.

CAUSES—It is in general occaſioned by a redundancy and acrimony of the bile; fat meats, and ſuch as become either rancid or acid on the ſtomach; too free an uſe of ſweat-meats, and cold fruits, ſuch as cucumbers and melons. It is ſometimes produced by a ſtoppage of perſpiration; ſtrong acrid purges or vomits; violent paſſions, &c.

CURE.—In this diſeaſe, there being much bile depoſited in the alimentary canal, particularly in the ſtomach, the firſt object is to counteract its effects, and promote an eaſy diſcharge of it. To accompliſh this end, we muſt aſſiſt the efforts of nature, by giving the patient a large quantity of warm water, or very weak broth; which ought not only to be drunk plentifully to promote the vomiting, but a clyſter of it given every hour to favour the diſcharge by the inteſtines.

When by theſe evacuations the acrimonious humours have been in great meaſure diſcharged, and the pains begin to abate, an infuſion of toaſted oat-bread, or of oat-meal made brown, may be drunk to ſtop the vomiting. For the ſame purpoſe an infuſion of mint-leaves, or good ſimple mint water, with a few drops of laudanum, is frequently very efficacious.

Sometimes the propenſity to vomit is ſo ſtrong, that no drink will ſit on the ſtomach. In this caſe it will be proper to give a ſaline draught every hour with ten drops of laudanum, till the vomiting ceaſes: but when the opiate cannot be retained in a fluid form, by the aid of any addition, it ſhould be given in the ſolid ſtate; for inſtance, half a grain or more of opium made into a pill with conſerve of roſes, or any other conſerve, and repeated as occaſion may require.

The evacuations in this diſeaſe are critical and ſalutary, and therefore, as long as they do not *weaken* the patient, they are rather to be promoted than reſtrained; but if the pulſe begin to ſink, and there be ſymptoms of great debility, it will be neceſſary to have recourſe to opiates, and to adminiſter them in ſuch quantity as may be requiſite for ſtopping the diſcharge.

In the mean time, ſtrong wine-whey, or brandy and water, &c. may be given to ſupport the patient's ſtrength, and excite perſpiration; with this intent Dover's powder may alſo be given with great advantage. His legs ſhould be bathed in warm water, and rubbed with flannel cloths. Flannels wrung out of warm fomentations, made with a decoction of wormwood and chamomile-flowers, with the addition of ſome brandy, or other ſpirituous liquor, ſhould likewiſe be applied to the region of the ſtomach.

To prevent a relapſe, and at the ſame time keep the inteſtines free from feculent matter, it will be proper to repeat the opiate at leaſt twice a day for a week; giving with it in the morning and at night eight grains of rhubarb, or fuch a quantity as will procure a ftool once in the twenty-four hours.

A difpofition to vomiting often remains for a confiderable time after the difeafe has ceafed. To allay this fymptom, and reftore the ftrength of the ftomach, it will be proper that the patient take twice a day a tea-fpoonful of the following powder, in a glafs of wine, or mint-tea. Take of the powder of Peruvian bark, half an ounce; of the powder of columbo-root, two drachms and a half; ginger, powdered, one drachm. Mix them.

The patient fhould ufe a light nourifhing diet, but taken in fmall quantity at a time, and alfo moderate exercife.

## CHAP. XXXIV.

### *Diarrhœa, or Loofenefs.*

A DIARRHŒA confifts in evacuations by ftool more frequent than ufual, and of a thinner confiftence. It is incident to people of all ages, and happens at any feafon of the year.

CAUSES.—It may be occafioned by a ftoppage of perfpiration, efpecially by cold applied to the feet; eating food hard of digeftion, or in too great quantity; the ftoppage of any cuftomary evacuation; acrid fubftances received into the ftomach; violent affections of the mind, &c.

CURE.—When the complaint proceeds from a ftoppage of perfpiration, it is to be treated as a cold. The patient ought to keep warm, drink plentifully of weak diluting liquors, and bathe his feet in warm water.

If it be owing to any load upon the ftomach, the proper remedy is a vomit of ipecacuanha. A day or two after, the patient fhould take a dofe of rhubarb, and repeat it two or three times if the diforder continues. The diet, in the mean time, fhould confift of light puddings and vegetable food; and the drink, of thin gruel or barley-water.

When the complaint arifes from the obftruction of any cuftomary difcharge, if the pulfe is full, bleeding may be neceffary; and an effort fhould be made to reftore the fuppreffed evacuation.

When a loofenefs is occafioned by acrid fubftances taken into the ftomach, the patient ought to drink largely of diluting and mucilaginous liquors, with oil and fat broths, both to fheath the acrid matter, and promote its difcharge by vomiting and purging; interpofing now and then fmall dofes of laudanum to abate the irritation.

If it proceed from acidity in the bowels, in which cafe the ftools are of a green colour, the cure muft be accomplifhed by abforbents. Take of the pureft chalk in powder, two ounces; gum-arabic, half an ounce; water, three pints: boil to one quart, and, after ftraining the decoction, add two table-fpoonfuls of brandy, and fweeten with fine fugar when ufed. Four table-fpoonfuls may be taken every two or three hours while the loofenefs continues.

When the diforder is occafioned by a retroceffion of the gout from the extremities, it ought to be promoted by gentle dofes of fome mild purgative, fuch as rhubarb, or fenna; endeavouring at the fame time to recall the gout to the extremities by warm fomentations and cataplafms. In this cafe, it will alfo be proper to encourage perfpiration by taking fome wine-whey, rendered more diaphoretic by fpirits of hartfhorn, or a few drops of the tincture of opium.

When a diarrhœa proceeds from violent affections of the mind, it requires to be treated in the gentleft manner, avoiding all irritation that might be excited either by vomits or purgatives; and on the contrary, by endeavouring to allay the commotion of the body and the agitation of mind. Thefe purpofes will be beft anfwered by giving ten or twelve drops of laudanum every eight or ten hours in a cup of barley-water, or linfeed-tea.

When a loofenefs is occafioned by worms, which may be fufpected from various fymptoms, fuch as pains of the belly, fudden ftartings, picking the nofe, &c. but clearly afcertained from decayed fragments of this inteftinal brood being mixed with flimy ftools; the patient fhould take twice a-day half a drachm of a powder made of equal parts of worm-feed* and tin, and every two or three days a dofe of rhubarb, with a few grains of calomel.

Sometimes the diforder proceeds from drinking bad water, in which cafe it is generally obferved to be epidemical. As foon as the caufe is difcovered, the water ought, if poffible, to be changed; or where this cannot be done, the noxious quality of the water fhould be corrected, by mixing with it fome lime, chalk, or alum.

When a diarrhœa is produced by a weaknefs of the ftomach and bowels, in which cafe the complaint is apt to become habitual, the patient may take twice a day half a drachm of a powder made of an ounce of Peruvian bark, and half an ounce of rhubarb, in a glafs of port wine; or ten grains of anguftura, with one or two of falt of fteel; decoction of logwood,† &c.

When a loofenefs, from whatever caufe it proceeds, requires to

* See *Appendix.* † Ibid

be checked, the diet ought to consist of rice boiled with milk, and flavoured with cinnamon; sago; and the lighter sorts of flesh roasted. Salted meats, pork, and all kinds of fish are unsuitable. The most proper drink is port wine diluted with water.

Those who are apt to be seized with a looseness upon catching cold, ought always to wear flannel next the skin. Where the disorder is frequent in its returns, we may justly suspect a weakness and irritability of the bowels: for obviating the effects of which, the person should be temperate in the quantity of aliments, and avoid meats hard of digestion, as well as such as are crude and unwholesome. To other objects of attention should be added tranquillity of mind, and the use of exercise on horseback. Chalybeate waters are also useful.

## CHAP. XXXV.

### *Dysentery.*

THIS disease affects chiefly persons of a bilious constitution, and is most frequent in autumn: in ships and camps it is likewise often contagious.

Causes.—It may be occasioned by a stoppage of perspiration, especially after hot weather; unwholesome food; bad air; wet clothes, &c. It is a frequent disease in camps, and other places where a number of men are assembled under circumstances favourable for its production.

Symptoms.—In many cases this disease comes on with chillness and other symptoms of fever, but more commonly without them; the patient being generally costive, and troubled with unusual flatulence in the bowels. Then commences a flux of the belly, attended with gripings and a frequent inclination to go to stool; all which increase in the progress of the disease. At first the stools are commonly greasy and frothy, afterwards more or less streaked with blood; though sometimes this symptom is absent, and at other times exists in a high degree. The natural fæces in the mean time are generally retained, or voided in small quantity, and in a compact hardened form. But in the course of the disease, the matter voided by stool is often various in its appearance, though commonly of a strong and unusually fœtid smell. There are often mixed with liquid matter some fragments resembling bits of skin, and frequently small lumps of a sebaceous or fatty appearance. When natural stools are voided, which, as has been already observed, are gene-

If it proceed from acidity in the bowels, in which case the stools are of a green colour, the cure must be accomplished by absorbents. Take of the purest chalk in powder, two ounces; gum-arabic, half an ounce; water, three pints: boil to one quart, and, after straining the decoction, add two table-spoonfuls of brandy, and sweeten with fine sugar when used. Four table-spoonfuls may be taken every two or three hours while the looseness continnes.

When the disorder is occasioned by a retrocession of the gout from the extremities, it ought to be promoted by gentle doses of some mild purgative, such as rhubarb, or senna; endeavouring at the same time to recall the gout to the extremities by warm fomentations and cataplasms. In this case, it will also be proper to encourage perspiration by taking some wine-whey, rendered more diaphoretic by spirits of hartshorn, or a few drops of the tincture of opium.

When a diarrhoea proceeds from violent affections of the mind, it requires to be treated in the gentlest manner, avoiding all irritation that might be excited either by vomits or purgatives; and on the contrary, by endeavouring to allay the commotion of the body and the agitation of mind. These purposes will be best answered by giving ten or twelve drops of laudanum every eight or ten hours in a cup of barley-water, or linseed-tea.

When a looseness is occasioned by worms, which may be suspected from various symptoms, such as pains of the belly, sudden startings, picking the nose, &c. but clearly ascertained from decayed fragments of this intestinal brood being mixed with slimy stools; the patient should take twice a-day half a drachm of a powder made of equal parts of worm-seed* and tin, and every two or three days a dose of rhubarb, with a few grains of calomel.

Sometimes the disorder proceeds from drinking bad water, in which case it is generally observed to be epidemical. As soon as the cause is discovered, the water ought, if possible, to be changed; or where this cannot be done, the noxious quality of the water should be corrected, by mixing with it some lime, chalk, or alum.

When a diarrhoea is produced by a weakness of the stomach and bowels, in which case the complaint is apt to become habitual, the patient may take twice a day half a drachm of a powder made of an ounce of Peruvian bark, and half an ounce of rhubarb, in a glass of port wine; or ten grains of angustura, with one or two of salt of steel; decoction of logwood,† &c.

When a looseness, from whatever cause it proceeds, requires to

* See *Appendix*. † Ibid

and windows; and the floor of it be frequently sprinkled with vinegar, or some other acid.

After the evacuations which have been mentioned, it will be proper to give two or three grains of the powder of ipecacuanha three times a day in a table-spoonful of the syrup of poppies, in order to impel the fluids towards the surface of the body. At the same time the intestines are to be defended by mucilaginous medicines, and the flux of humours towards them checked by gentle astringents; interposing occasionally a moderate dose of laudanum to allay irritation.

For defending the intestines, an ounce of gum-arabic may be dissolved in a pint of barley-water, and two or three table-spoonfuls of it taken frequently; while, for the same purpose, the patient may drink linseed-tea. For this intention spermaceti is also a proper medicine. Half a drachm of it dissolved with a little of the mucilage of gum-arabic, may be taken three or four times a day in a cup of barley-water.

During the use of these remedies, clysters ought also to be administered, both for restraining the discharge, and abating the tenesmus or continual desire of going to stool, which is one of the most distressing symptoms of this disease. The clysters may be made of half a pint of fat mutton broth, with thirty or forty drops of laudanum, given twice every day. Or, for the same purpose, half an ounce of powdered starch may be dissolved in a half a pint of barley-water, and given with the laudanum as now mentioned.

The violent griping is generally relieved by the free use of mucilaginous liquors; and may be likewise much abated by frequently applying to the belly flannel cloths wrung out of a decoction of chamomile-flowers.

When the disease proves tedious, or terminates in a lingering looseness, the wearing flannel next the skin will be found of great advantage.

When it is complicated with an intermittent, and protracted chiefly from that circumstance, recourse should be had to the Peruvian bark: but this is not to be practised in the earlier periods of the disease. In hot climates, small doses of calomel and opium frequently repeated are found successful.

Besides the diarrhoea and dysentery, there are other fluxes of the belly, such as the lientery and cœliac passion, in which the aliments pass too rapidly through the intestines. They are generally of a chronic nature, and to be cured by the use of chalk and astringents, in the same way as a looseness. In these, however, the Peruvian bark, with bitter stomachic medicines, and riding on horseback, ought generally to be administered; and indeed the same regimen should be adopted, for completing the cure, and restoring the tone of the bowels, after every flux of the belly.

## CHAP. XXXVI.

### *Costiveness, and the Hæmorrhoids, or Piles.*

BY costiveness is here understood, not those astrictions of the belly which accompany some diseases of the bowels, but that retardment of the alvine discharge which exceeds the common standard of most constitutions in a healthy state, and may prove the cause of different complaints.

Costiveness may be either constitutional or accidental. When the latter it may be occasioned by food too much seasoned with spiceries, or by crude insipid aliments, which do not sufficiently stimulate the intestines; drinking hard water, rough red wines, or other astringent liquors; too much exercise, especially on horseback; a sedentary life. Sometimes it proceeds from too inert a state of the bile, or its not descending into the intestines, as happens in the jaundice: sometimes from a torpidity of the bowels, and it may also be occasioned by a laxity of the abdominal muscles, which sometimes occurs in women who have borne several children.

When costiveness is constitutional, it may be suffered without any sensible inconvenience for an almost incredible length of time; but when the complaint is occasional, it is apt to produce pains of the head, vomiting, colics, and different disorders of the bowels. There is a species of costiveness incident to persons much relaxed, and which is attended with great pain at the fundament; the fæces being so extremely hardened that the person is unable to protrude them. In this case, the best remedy is a small clyster of linseed-oil, or oil of olives; which, by lubricating the passage, will facilitate the discharge.

As the frequent use of purgatives tends to weaken the bowels, it is better to obviate costiveness by means of diet than medicine. Those, therefore, who are subject to it, should avoid all astringent food and drink, and chiefly confine themselves to aliments of a moistening and laxative kind, such as veal-broth, boiled meats, apples roasted or boiled, stewed prunes, raisins, currants, &c.—Butter, honey, and sugar, especially the moist kind, are likewise suitable articles of diet; as are also soft pot-herbs, such as spinnage and leeks, with the roots of turnip and parsnip. The best bread for such constitutions is brown bread, or that which is made of a mixture of wheat and rye.

The drink ought likewise to be of an opening quality. Malt liquor of a moderate strength, and not much hopped, is well adapted;

as are likewiſe whey, butter-milk, and other watery liquors that have nothing in them of an aſtringent nature. Spirituous liquors, as well as rough wines, are improper.

Beſides diet there are other circumſtances to which perſons of a coſtive habit ſhould be attentive, they ought to uſe moderate exerciſe, and neither to keep the body too warm nor lie too long in bed, as both theſe practices increaſe the complaint by too much promoting perſpiration. Another circumſtance of great importance towards acquiring a proper regularity of bowels, eſpecially among females and ſedentary perſons, is never to neglect the ſolicitations of nature.

## *Of the Hæmorrhoids, or Piles.*

Theſe are painful tumors about the lower part of the ſtraight-gut diſtinguiſhed into the *external* and *internal*, according to their ſituation, either without or within the anus. They are alſo diſtinguiſhed into the *bleeding* piles, and the *blind* piles; in the former of which there is a diſcharge of blood, but in the latter, though very painful, no diſcharge.

Sometimes theſe tumors appear without any previous indiſpoſition, but more frequently they are preceded by various affections in different parts of the body; ſuch as head-ache, vertigo, or dizzineſs, difficulty of breathing, ſickneſs, colic pains, and ſometimes a conſiderable degree of feveriſhneſs; beſides which ſymptoms there is a ſenſe of fullneſs, heat, itching, and pain, about the anus.

The quantity of blood diſcharged in this complaint is variable on different occaſions. Sometimes it flows only when the perſon goes to ſtool, and commonly follows the diſcharge of fæces. In other caſes, it flows without any diſcharge of fæces; and then generally in conſequence of the diſorders above mentioned, when it is alſo commonly in larger quantity. Sometimes the complaint returns at ſtated periods; and in the decline of life, when the hœmorrhoidal flux ceaſes to flow where it formerly had been frequent, the perſon is generally attacked with an apoplexy or palſy.

The piles are moſt incident to perſons of a full habit of body, who live high, and take but little exerciſe. In general, men are more liable to this complaint than women; but the latter are often ſubject to it during the advanced ſtate of pregnancy; and there are few women who have had children, that are afterwards entirely free from the piles.

Causes.—The diſorder may be occaſioned by too great a quantity of blood, drinking freely of ſweet wines, much riding on horſeback, ſtrong aloetic purges, great coſtiveneſs, and a ſtoppage of cuſtomary evacuations. Sitting on damp ground will ſometimes give riſe to it; as will likewiſe the changing from thick breeches to thin.

It has been a generally received opinion, that the hæmorrhoidal flux is a ſalutary diſcharge, which prevents many diſeaſes that would otherwiſe have happened, and that it even contributes to longevity. But Dr. Cullen is of a contrary opinion. He maintains that we can never expect to reap much benefit from this flux, which at firſt is purely topical; and granting that it ſhould become habitual, it is never, he thinks, proper to be encouraged. It is a diſagreeable diſeaſe, ready to go to exceſs, and thereby to prove hurtful, and ſometimes even fatal. At beſt it is liable to accidents, and thus to unhappy conſequences. He is therefore of opinion, that even the firſt approaches of the diſeaſe are to be guarded againſt; and that, though it ſhould have proceeded for ſome time, it ought always to be moderated and the neceſſity of it ſuperſeded.

Cure.—The queſtion, whether the bleeding piles be ſalutary to the conſtitution, can only be determined by conſidering the ſtate of the body at the time. If there exiſt any diſeaſe, the cure of which may be favoured by diminiſhing the quantity of blood, the hæmorrhoidal flux muſt in that caſe be regarded as advantageous; and it may, in the ſame manner, prevent the return of any ſimilar diſeaſe to which the conſtitution is ſubject. But abſtracted from theſe two conſiderations, it is doubtleſs a waſte of the vital fluid, and ought to be prevented from becoming habitual to the conſtitution.

When the piles exiſt in the ſtate of tumor, the principal objects are to counteract the inflammation, and promote a diſcharge of blood from the part. When it is in the ſtate of evacuation, the chief intentions of cure are to diminiſh the impetus or force of the blood at the part affected, and to increaſe the reſiſtance to the paſſage of blood through the ruptured veſſels.

When the cauſe of the piles is evident, it ought, if poſſible, to be immediately removed. Of this kind none is more frequent than coſtiveneſs, which, if it cannot be ſufficiently obviated by diet, muſt be oppoſed by gently laxative medicines. For this purpoſe the patient may uſe the following electuary, in the quantity of a tea-ſpoonful, three or four times a day, according as it produces the effect of keeping the belly open. Take of the electuary of ſenna, two ounces; flowers of ſulphur, one ounce; with as much ſimple ſyrup as will mix them into a proper conſiſtence. Or, inſtead of this compoſition, he may take as often, if neceſſary, the ſame quantity of a mixture made of equal parts of flowers of ſulphur and cream of tartar.

When the diſcharge from the piles has continued long, or is in ſo great a quantity as to weaken the perſon, it muſt be moderated by a cooling diet and aſtringent medicines. Half a drachm of the powder of Peruvian bark, with ten or fifteen drops of the elixir of vitriol, may be taken three or four times a day in a glaſs of red port.

When the bleeding piles return periodically, once in three weeks or a month, as ſometimes happens, they may be conſidered as a diſcharge beneficial to the conſtitution, by unloading it of a redundancy of blood, and ought therefore not to be ſtopped, unleſs they become exceſſive: in which caſe, beſides the uſe of the Peruvian bark and elixir of vitriol above mentioned, the anus may be fomented with a decoction made with half an ounce of powdered galls, boiled for a few minutes in ſomewhat more than half a pint of ſmiths' forge-water, and applied cold. Vinegar, in which a little alum is diſſolved, may be uſed for the ſame purpoſe; as may even cold water, frequently applied with a linen rag.

During a flux of blood from the piles, the perſon ſhould lie in a horizontal poſture on a hard bed, and avoid external heat.

In the *blind* piles, bleeding is commonly of ſervice. The ſame cooling diet is proper here as in the other ſpecies of the complaint; and the belly muſt in the ſame way be kept open. If the piles be internal, ſoftening clyſters are of advantage, when an aſtriction of the anus does not prevent their being admitted. When, on the contrary, they are external, and the veins painful and ſwelled, but diſcharge nothing, the patient ought to ſit over the ſteams of warm water, and afterwards apply to the part a little of the following ointment. Take of ſimple ointment half an ounce; laudanum a tea-ſpoonful. Mix. But if the part be much ſwelled, the moſt effectual remedy is to apply leeches. If theſe, however, ſhould not fix, the piles may, with great eaſe and ſafety, be opened with a lancet.

Much exerciſe during the piles is both inconvenient and improper, but at other times very advantageous; and, for preventing the return of the complaint, it is particularly uſeful to guard againſt a plethoric ſtate of the body, or that in which the veſſels abound too much with blood. A ſedentary life, therefore, a full diet, and intemperance in the uſe of ſtrong liquors, ought all to be avoided by thoſe who are ſubject to the diſorder.

## CHAP. XXXVII.

*Of the Diabetes, and other diſorders relative to the Urinary Diſcharge.*

A DIABETES is an exceſſive diſcharge of urine, with ſymptoms different from that which takes place in the hyſteric or hypochondriac diſeaſe. It ſeldom attacks young people, but frequently perſons in the decline of life, eſpecially thoſe who are employed in laborious occupations, and have been uſed to drink freely of ſtrong liquors.

SYMPTOMS.—In this diſeaſe the urine is ſo copious that it commouly exceeds in quantity all the liquids which the perſon conſumes. It is clear, pale, commonly ſweet to the taſte, and has, generally, an agreeable ſmell. The patient is moleſted with a continual thirſt, his mouth is clammy and dry, and he frequently diſcharges from it a frothy ſpittle. There is likewiſe a heat of the bowels; with a fullneſs of the loins, teſticles, and feet. The pulſe is ſmall and quick. Sometimes there is an extraordinary appetite; but in the progreſs of the diſeaſe this ſymptom totally ceaſes, and the patient becomes weak and emaciated.

CAUSES.—A diabetes may proceed either from too diſſolved a ſtate of the blood, or ſome fault of the ſtomach or kidneys, whether a relaxation of thoſe organs, or a morbid ſtimulus applied to them. It is ſometimes the conſequence of acute diſeaſes, in which the patient's ſtrength has been reduced by exceſſive evacuations. It may not only be occaſioned by hard drinking, as intimated above; but by too free an uſe of ſtrong diuretic medicines; as it may likewiſe by long-continued riding on a hard trotting horſe; carrying heavy burdens, and other violent exertions of the body.

This diſeaſe, when taken at the beginning, generally admits of a cure; but when it has continued ſo long as greatly to weaken the conſtitution, little hope is to be entertained of a recovery.

CURE.—For leſſening the ſecretion of urine by the kidneys, it is of advantage to ſupport the natural diſcharge of the watery part of the blood by the other outlets of the body. If, therefore, the patient be not too much weakened by the continuance of the diſeaſe, he ought to take every day ten grains of the powder of rhubarb, more or leſs, according as may be neceſſary to keep the body gently open; ſupporting, at the ſame time, the perſpiration by wearing flannel next the ſkin, and taking, every other night, twelve or fifteen grains of the compound powder of ipecacuanha.

Aſtringent and ſtrengthening medicines are next to be given. Of equal parts of gum-kino, catechu, alum, and gum-arabic, all powdered and mixed together, the patient may take two ſcruples three or four times a day; drinking after it a cup of lime-water, in a quart of which ſix drachms of oak-bark has been infuſed. Alum-whey is likewiſe highly beneficial, if the ſtomach can bear it along with the powder now mentioned. It is made by boiling over a ſlow fire two quarts of milk with three drachms of alum, till the curd ſeparates. Opiates are found beneficial in this diſeaſe, by allaying the irritation of the kidneys: on which account, the patient may take, three or four times a day, ten drops of laudanum in a cup of his drink, notwithſtanding he may reſt well without it.

As a ſtrenthening remedy in this diſeaſe, no medicine is preferable to the Peruvian bark; of the powder of which the patient may take two ſcruples or a drachm in a glaſs of red port two or three times a day, adding, to each doſe, fifteen drops of the elixir of vitriol, or eight drops of the ſulphuret of ammonia.

During this diſeaſe the patient's diet ought to be entirely of the ſolid kind. Jellies, ſago, and ſhell-fiſh, are alſo proper; but all vegetables muſt be avoided. The drink ſhould be Briſtol-water, or, where that cannot be procured, lime-water with an infuſion of oak-bark, as above directed. For the ſame purpoſe, the White Decoction mentioned in the Appendix, is alſo ſuitable. The patient ought to take daily exerciſe, but ſuch as not to fatigue him; and he ſhould lie upon a hard bed or mattreſs.

## *Incontinency of Urine.*

In this diſorder, the water paſſes off, involuntarily, by drops, but does not exceed the uſual quantity. It is a complaint moſt frequent with people in the decline of life, and is rather troubleſome than dangerous. It proceeds from a relaxation of the ſphincter of the bladder, and is often the effect of a palſy. Sometimes, however, it is produced by a continued uſe of ſtrong diuretics, or by hurts received about the neck of the bladder in conſequence of bruiſes, violent labours, &c.

Cure.—All ſtrengthening medicines, ſuch as the Peruvian bark, uva urſi, the preparations of iron, elixir of vitriol, and balſam of copaiba, are the remedies moſt proper for this complaint. The cold-bath, likewiſe, is of great advantage, where nothing prohibits the uſe of it; but the ſpeedieſt and moſt effectual remedy yet known, and the utility of which has been confirmed in various inſtances, is the application of a bliſter to the *os ſacrum*, or lowermoſt part of the back-bone. It commonly produces the deſired effect in twenty-four hours.

An incontinence of urine frequently occurs to children, otherwiſe healthy, when aſleep. It is often merely the effect of lazineſs, and may be checked by proper correction; but ſometimes it is a real infirmity, and proceeds from a weakneſs of the ſphincter of the bladder.

## *Of a Suppreſſion of Urine.*

A ſuppreſſion of urine may proceed from a variety of cauſes, and it differs in its ſymptoms according to the parts which are the original ſeat of the diſorder. It may be occaſioned by an inflammation of the kidneys or bladder; gravel or ſmall ſtones obſtructing the urinary paſſages; a ſpaſm or contraction of the neck of the bladder; hard fæces lying at the bottom of the rectum; a diſtenſion of the hæmorrhoidal veins; pregnancy, &c.

When the cauſe of the ſuppreſſion exiſts in the kidneys, there is a pain and uneaſy ſenſation of weight in the region of the loins, unaccompanied with a fullneſs about the bladder, or any deſire of making water. When the ureters are the part affected, there is a ſenſe of pain or uneaſineſs in the courſe of thoſe ducts, with the ſame exception as in the preceding caſe. When the complaint proceeds from the bladder, there is a tumor or diſtenſion of the lower part of the belly, attended with pain of the neck of the bladder, and a frequent deſire to make water. When the cauſe of the ſuppreſſion is in the urethra, there is a pain in ſome part of that paſſage, accompanied with the ſymptoms laſt mentioned.

When there is not a total ſuppreſſion of urine, but it is diſcharged in drops, accompanied with pain, the diſeaſe is called a ſtrangury. This likewiſe may proceed from various cauſes, ſuch as inflammation about the neck of the bladder, preſſure, a ſtone in the bladder, diſcharge of mucus, or ſlimy matter, &c.

Cure.—In all ſuppreſſions of urine, bleeding is proper, ſo far as the patient's ſtrength will bear it. The body ſhould alſo be kept open by gentle purgatives, ſuch as manna, ſenna, the electuary of ſenna, and the like; or rather by ſoftening clyſters, which, at the ſame time that they keep the body open, have the effect of an internal fomentation, and tend greatly to alleviate the ſpaſms of the bladder and the contiguous parts, which, if not the primary cauſe, always greatly aggravate a ſuppreſſion of urine.

The patient having been bled, warm fomentations, made with mallows and chamomile-flowers, ought to be frequently applied, or the perſon be put into a warm bath up to the middle of the body.

In moſt of the ſuppreſſions of urine, a ſpaſm or conſtriction of the urinary paſſages is either an original or acceſſory ſymptom, and in both caſes the uſe of opiates is of advantage.

In ſuppreſſions of extreme urgency, the laſt reſource is the catheter for drawing off the water; but the management of this inſtrument requiring ſurgical dexterity, a more proper expedient for general uſe is a hollow bougie, which may be introduced into the urethra more eaſily.

During this complaint the diet ſhould be of a light kind, and taken in ſmall quantities. The drink may be weak broth, linſeed-tea, or a decoction of marſh-mallows; and to whatever of this kind is uſed, a tea-ſpoonful of the ſpirit of nitrous æther ſhould frequently be added.

## *Gravel and Stone.*

Theſe are calculous concretions, to which, in many conſtitutions, the urinary paſſages are ſubject. When ſmall ſtones or ſand are diſcharged with the urine, the perſon is ſaid to have the gravel. But if any of theſe, by long retention in the bladder, acquire ſuch a ſize as to be incapable of expulſion, the complaint receives the name of the ſtone.

They are both moſt frequent to perſons in the decline of life, eſpecially thoſe who have been long afflicted with the gout.

Causes.—High living, and a ſedentary life, with the free uſe of ſtrong aſtringent wines, are frequently the cauſes both of the gravel and ſtone. They may alſo be occaſioned by a continual uſe of water impregnated with earthy or ſtony particles; aſtringent aliments; and lying on too ſoft a bed, or too much upon the back, by which means the kidneys ſuſtain a preſſure injurious to the regularity of their function.

Symptoms.—The exiſtence of ſmall ſtones or gravel in the kidneys gives riſe to a pain in the loins, ſickneſs, vomiting, and, ſometimes, bloody urine. When the ſtone deſcends into the ureter, and is too large to paſs with eaſe through that canal, all theſe ſymptoms are increaſed; the pain extends along the courſe of the duct towards the bladder; the thigh and leg of the affected ſide are benumbed; the teſticles are drawn upwards, and the urine is obſtructed in its paſſage.

A ſtone in the bladder is known from a weight in that part, and a pain at the time as well as before and after making water; from the urine being diſcharged in drops, or ſtopping ſuddenly in the midſt of the evacuation. There is alſo pain in the neck of the bladder upon motion, eſpecially on horſeback, or in a carriage on a rough road; in conſequence of which the urine is often bloody. There is likewiſe frequently a white, thick, and copious ſediment in the urine, an itching at the top of the yard, and an inclination to go to ſtool during the diſcharge of the urine. The patient paſſes his urine more eaſily when lying than in an erect posture. The existence of a stone in the bladder may also be known from a kind of convulsive motion occasioned by a sharp pain in discharging the last drops of urine; and it may be fully ascertained by sounding, or searching, with the catheter.

Cure.—In a fit of the gravel, as it is called, which is occasioned by the difficult passage of a small stone or sand from the kidneys down to the bladder, the patient must be bled, softening clysters administered, and warm fomentations applied to the part affected, with the use of diluting and mucilaginous liquors. But this subject has been already treated under the articles of inflammation of the kidneys and bladder, to which the reader is referred.

A late celebrated physician and professor of medicine, Dr. Whyte, recommends to persons who are subject to frequent fits of gravel in the kidneys, but have no stone in the bladder, to drink every morning, two or three hours before breakfast, an English pint of cockle-shell lime-water. In support of this advice, he observes, that though this quantity might be too small to have any sensible effect in dissolving a stone in the bladder, yet it may very probably prevent its enlargement.

When a stone is formed in the bladder, the same eminent author advises the use of Alicant soap, and oyster, or cockle-shell lime-water, to be taken in the following manner: The patient must swallow every day, in any form that is least disagreeable, an ounce of the internal part of Alicant soap, and drink three or four English pints of oyster or cockle-shell lime-water. The soap is to be divided into three doses; the largest to be taken fasting in the morning early; the second at noon; and the third at seven in the evening; drinking, after each dose, a large draught of the lime-water; the remainder of which he may take any time betwixt dinner and supper, instead of other liquors.

The person should begin with a smaller quantity of the lime-water and soap than that mentioned above; at first, an English pint of the former, and three drachms of the latter, may be taken daily. This quantity, however, he may increase by degrees, and ought to persevere in the use of these medicines, especially if he finds any abatement of his complaints, for several months; nay, if the stone be very large, for years.

The medicine now chiefly used for the stone, is the caustic alkali, or soap-lees; which may be prepared by mixing two parts of quick-lime with one of pot-ashes, and suffering them to stand till the lixivium be formed, which must be carefully filtrated before it is used. If the solution does not take place readily, a small quantity of water may be added to the mixture. This medicine being of an acrid nature, it ought to be given in some mucilaginous liquor, such as linseed-tea, a decoction of marsh-mallow roots, or a ſolution of gum-arabic. It is proper that the patient begin with ſmall doſes of the lees, ſuch as thirty or forty drops, and increaſe, by degrees, as far as the ſtomach can bear it.

An objection generally made to the uſe of ſoap-lees is the acrimony with which it is endowed, and the bad effects which may therefore reſult to the conſtitution from the long continued uſe of it. When this conſideration weighs much with the patient, he may have recourſe to other means, which are found in many caſes highly ſerviceable. Great benefit has been experienced from an infuſion of the ſeeds of the *darcus ſylveſtris*, or wild carrot, ſweetened with honey, in caſes where the ſtomach could not bear any thing of an acrid nature. The leaves of the *uva urſi*, known in this country by the name of bear's whortleberry, or trailing arbutus, which, though inferior to the ſoap and lime-water, is leſs diſagreeable, and has in many inſtances proved uſeful. It may be taken either in powder or infuſion. The doſe of the powder is commonly from half a drachm to a whole drachm, two or three times a day; but it may be uſed in larger quantity. In the other form, three drachms of the leaves may be infuſed for ſome hours in a pint of boiling water, and, after ſtraining, the patient may take a wine-glaſsful two or three times a day. The doſe of this may alſo be increaſed. A decoction of raw coffee-beans, taken morning and evening, in the quantity of half a pint, or upwards, with ten drops of dulcified ſpirit of nitre, has been found efficacious in diſcharging by urine large quantities of earthy matter in flakes. Honey, likewiſe, taken in gruel, marſh-mallow tea, or any other way more agreeable to the patient, is aſcertained to be of conſiderable advantage. The muriatic acid, or ſpirit of common ſalt, taken in doſes of from 12 to 16 drops in any agreeable vehicle, has lately been found an efficacious remedy: ſo has the aërated ſoda-water; or ſoda in any form.

Thoſe who are afflicted with the gravel or ſtone ſhould be attentive to their manner of living. They ought to avoid aliments that are hard of digeſtion, flatulent, or of a heating nature. Mutton, veal, or lamb, are preferable to beef or pork. Fiſh, in general, may conſtitute a proper article of their diet; and all the vegetables which promote the ſecretion of urine, and keep the belly open, ſuch as artichokes, aſparagus, ſpinnage, parſley, ſuccory, celery, onions, leeks, &c. are ſerviceable. The moſt proper drinks are whey, milk and water, barley-water; decoctions or infuſions of the roots of marſh-mallows, liquorice, linſeed, &c. Malt liquors, if not ſtale, may likewiſe be uſed, but all wines and ſpirituous liquors are hurtful. If any thing of this kind may be uſed with ſafety, it is gin and water, which, when not too ſtrong, may prove of advantage by its diuretic quality.

Gentle exercife is in thefe complaints advifable; but violent motion ought to be avoided, on account of its tendency to occafion bloody urine. It is common for perfons habitually fubject to the gravel to pafs a great number of ftones after riding on horfeback, or in a carriage; but thefe kinds of exercife can feldom be endured by thofe who have a ftone in the bladder. A fedentary life, however, ought not to be indulged where there is any degree of tendency to thefe complaints.

## CHAP. XXXVIII.

### *Bleeding at the Nofe, Vomiting of Blood, and Bloody Urine.*

SPONTANEOUS difcharges of blood frequently happen from various parts of the body, but moft commonly from thofe cavities which communicate with the external air. They are, however, not always to be regarded as dangerous: for, on feveral occafions, they not only carry off both acute and chronic difeafes, but preferve the conftitution from others, which perhaps might prove fatal. People ought, therefore, to be cautious of immediately ftopping the difcharges, efpecially fuch as are periodical. It is only when they are immoderate, or continue fo long as to weaken the perfon, that they ought to be reftrained.

One of the moft frequent hæmorrhages is bleeding at the nofe, which is particularly common in the early period of life. It is generally p [illegible] by a flufhing in the face, heavinefs in the head, dimnefs of fight, pulfation of the temporal arteries, with heat and itching of the noftrils.

To thofe who have a redundancy of blood, this evacuation may be ferviceable; frequently curing a diforder of the head, and fometimes an epilepfy. It is often particularly beneficial in fevers, where there is a great determination of blood towards the head. In inflammations of the liver and fpleen it is alfo advantageous; as likewife in the gout and rheumatifm. And what fhows the fuperiority of nature in curing difeafes, a fpontaneous difcharge of blood from the nofe is of more fervice than the fame quantity let with a lancet, where bleeding is neceffary.

From what has been faid, it will readily be thought a point of confequence to determine, on any fuch emergency, whether a bleeding of the nofe fhould be ftopped. When this difcharge happens in an inflammatory difeafe, there is reafon to hope that it may prove falutary; and it will therefore be prudent to let it proceed while the patient is not thereby weakened.

When this bleeding happens to perſons in perfect health, and who abound with blood, it ought not to be ſuddenly checked, left fatal effects might enſue, by the rupture of ſome internal blood-veſſel, or an extravaſation in the brain. But when the diſcharge continues till the pulſe becomes weak, the lips pale, and the patient complains of being ſick or faint, it ought to be inſtantly ſtopped.

In this caſe, the patient ſhould be placed nearly upright, with his head a little reclined, and both his legs and hands put into water, of the natural heat of the body, or that of milk when it flows from the veſſel of the cow. His garters ought to be tied a little tighter than uſual; and ligatures, likewiſe, with nearly the ſame degree of tightneſs, applied to the arms, as practiſed in bleeding with the lancet. Theſe are to be gradually ſlackened as the blood begins to ſtop, and removed entirely as ſoon as the evacuation ceaſes.

Cold metal, or cold water, applied to the back of the neck, or genitals, will frequently, ſtop the diſcharge. Sometimes dry lint put up the noſtrils will produce the ſame effect. When this does not ſucceed, doſſils of lint, dipped in brandy or ſtrong vinegar, may be uſed for the ſame purpoſe. Other applications, frequently uſed, are blue vitriol diſſolved in water, white vitriol in the ſame manner, or a tent dipped in the white of an egg, well beat up, and rolled in a powder, either ſingly or jointly, of white ſugar, burnt alum, and white vitriol, and put up the noſtril from which the blood iſſues.

In a ſpontaneous and violent bleeding of the noſe, the neceſſity of an immediate ſtoppage does not admit a recourſe to aſtringent medicines taken internally, as their ſlow operation would render them ineffectual on ſo urgent an emergency. It may, however be proper that the patient take a cooling purgative conſiſting of half an ounce, or ſix drachms, of Glauber's ſalts, and the ſame quantity of manna diſſolved in warm water. Half a ſcruple of nitre may alſo be taken in a glaſs of cold water and vinegar, every hour, or oftener if the ſtomach will bear it. If a ſtronger medicine be required twenty or thirty drops of the diluted vitriolic acid may be taken every hour in a tea-cupful of the roſe infuſion. From ten to twenty drops of the oil of turpentine in a little water, given frequently, has a powerful effect in reſtraining hæmorrhages of this kind. Where things cannot be procured, the patient may drink a mixture of equal parts of water and vinegar, or water in which a little common ſalt is diſſolved.

It ſometimes happens that, when the diſcharge of blood is ſtopped outwardly, it forces its way through the noſtril into the top of the throat, and endangers ſuffocation, eſpecially if the patient falls aſleep, to which he is very liable after loſing a great quantity of blood. In this ſituation, to prevent the blood from getting into the throat, the paſſages ſhould be ſtopped by drawing threads up the noſtrils, and bringing them out at the mouth, afterwards faſtening pieces of ſponge, or ſmall rolls of linen cloth, to their extremities; then drawing them back, and tying them on the outſide ſufficiently tight. The moxa, brought from the Eaſt Indies, is a powerful ſtyptic, and ſo is the ſpirit of turpentine, externally applied. Of all internal remedies to reſtrain hæmorrhagy, none is ſo powerful as acetated ceruſſe, which may be given in doſes of a grain, with three grains of opiate confection, every four hours, for ſix times.

When the bleeding is ſtopped, the patient ought to be kept eaſy, and as free from diſturbance as poſſible, lying with his head a little raiſed; and he ſhould not pick his noſe, nor remove the tents, or clotted blood, till they fall off of their own accord.

Thoſe who are ſubject to frequent bleeding at the noſe ought particularly to avoid getting cold or wet in the feet; or, if by accident they have incurred it, they ought to bathe their feet in warm water. The collar of their ſhirt, their ſtock, or cravat, ſhould all be eaſy on the neck, and they ſhould never view any object obliquely; as ſuch an attitude obſtructs the return of the blood from the head, and thereby favours a renewal of the hæmorrhage, if not a ſtill more dangerous effect. If they be of a ſanguine conſtitution, and liable to a redundancy of blood, they may abate this diſpoſition by a vegetable diet, and the occaſional uſe of ſome cooling purgative.

Sometimes hæmorrhages proceed from a thin diſſolved ſtate of the blood; in which caſe the diet ought to be rich and nouriſhing, conſiſting of light animal food, with mild vegetables, lemons, jellies, tapioca, &c. with the moderate uſe of wine. Milk, if it agrees with the ſtomach and bowels, is in ſuch conſtitutions beneficial. In reſpect of medicine, the uſe of the Peruvian bark, in any form leaſt unpalatable to the patient, with elixir of vitriol, will be found of advantage.

## *Vomiting of Blood.*

This diſcharge is generally preceded by pain of the ſtomach, and ſickneſs, with great anxiety, and frequent fainting fits; but with no cough where the ſtomach alone is concerned. It is an accident more common to women than men, and generally owes its origin to obſtructed catamenia. When it occurs in men, a ſuppreſſion of the hæmorrhoidal diſcharge is uſually the prelude. It is often the effect of obſtructions in the liver, or ſome of the other bowels; and may be occaſioned both by any thing acrid taken into the ſtomach, and by external violence. However alarming this ſymptom may appear, it is not only frequent with hyſteric women, but ſeems even not to be dangerous.

The patient's food ſhould be weak broths, taken cold in ſmall quantity, mixed with the expreſſed juice of the leaves of plantain, and the infuſion of red roſes. Drinking cold water alone has ſometimes been found of great ſervice, but it will prove more effectual when ſharpened with the diluted vitriolic acid. Opiates may be uſeful, but muſt be given in ſmall doſes; ſuch as four or five drops of laudanum twice or thrice a day, or the acetated ceruſſe with opium. This diſorder might be obviated at the very beginning by immediately letting blood from the arm; but after a conſiderable diſcharge from the ſtomach, the patient's ſtrength hardly admits of the expedient. When the diſcharge has ceaſed, a few gentle purges will be proper, to alleviate the gripes which commonly ſucceed, and may be ſupported by the acrimony of the putrid blood remaining in the inteſtines.

## *Bloody Urine.*

In this complaint the blood may iſſue from any part of the urinary paſſages below the veſſels which ſecrete the urine in the kidneys. When pure blood is voided ſuddenly, without either pain or interruption, it may be judged to proceed from a dilatation of the veſſels of the kidneys. But if the diſcharge be in ſmall quantity, of a dark colour, and accompanied with heat and pain about the bottom of the belly, there is every reaſon for thinking that it iſſues from the bladder. If the complaint be attended with a ſharp pain in the back, between the region of the kidneys and the bladder, we may preſume that it is occaſioned by a rough ſtone deſcending through the duct named the ureter. When bloody urine is attended with an acute pain about the bladder, and a previous ſtoppage of urine, there is ground for concluding that the coats of the bladder have been hurt by a ſtone.

Bloody urine may likewiſe proceed from a ſtone lodged in the kidneys, from ulcers in the bladder, or from ſharp diuretic medicines, particularly cantharides. It may alſo be occaſioned by venereal exceſſes, falls, bruiſes, hard riding, or carrying of heavy burdens. Sometimes this diſcharge proceeds from a redundancy of blood, accumulated by repletion, or the ſtoppage of ſome other evacuation. The complaint is never entirely void of danger, but the reſult of it is moſt to be apprehended when the urine is mixed with purulent matter, as this evinces the exiſtence of an ulcer in the urinary paſſages.

If the diſorder be accompanied with a plethora, or fulneſs of blood, either with or without ſymptoms of inflammation, bleeding will be neceſſary. The body muſt at the ſame time be kept open by ſoftening clyſters, or cooling purgative medicines, ſuch as cream of tartar, manna, rhubarb, or ſenna.

When the cauſe of bloody urine is a diſſolved ſtate of the blood, the complaint is the effect of a general indiſpoſition of the habit, which requires to be corrected. The cure, in this caſe, depends on the free uſe of the Peruvian bark and acids.

When the diſorder is owing to a ſtone in the bladder, there is no other method of affording relief but by performing the operation of lithotomy, which is the buſineſs of a ſurgeon.

Where the ſymptoms juſtify a ſuſpicion that there is an ulcer in the urinary paſſages, the patient muſt uſe a cool diet of the vegetable kind, and his drink ſhould be of a ſoft balſamic quality, ſuch as decoctions of marſh-mallow roots, with liquorice, linſeed-tea, ſolutions of gum-arabic, &c. Two ounces of marſh-mallow roots, and half an ounce of liquorice, may be boiled in three Engliſh pints of water to a quart; diſſolving in the ſtrained liquor half an ounce of gum-arabic, and three drachms of nitre. Of this the patient may take a tea-cupful every three hours during the day.

An early uſe of aſtringent medicines is not adviſable in this complaint, as the diſcharge being ſtopped before the veſſels are relieved from a ſuperabundance of fluids, the grumous blood thence ariſing may produce inflammations, abſceſs, and ulcers. In great urgency, however, recourſe may be had to gentle aſtringents. The patient may take thrice a day half gill of lime-water with a table-ſpoonful of the tincture of the Peruvian bark.

## CHAP. XXXIX.

### *Menſtrual Diſcharge, with the Obſtruction and immoderate Flux of it.*

It is ordained by nature, that females, when they reach the age of puberty, ſhould generate more blood than is neceſſary for the ſupport of their own bodies, as a proviſion for the *fœtus* during its continuance in the womb. But it is neceſſary for the preſervation of their health that the overplus be periodically diſcharged. Such, therefore, is the ſource of menſtruation, which, commencing about the age of fifteen, and terminating towards fifty, makes its appearance uſually every month during that period, unleſs when pregnancy ſuſpends the diſcharge. About the firſt appearance of this evacuation the conſtitution undergoes a conſiderable change, generally for the improvement of the health, but sometimes operating otherwise. It is an important epoch in the life of females, and upon their conduct at this period the state of their health afterwards in a great measure depends. Indeed an attention to the management of themselves is not only necessary in the first menstruation, but in all its subsequent returns.

At this critical time of life, if a girl be confined to the house, kept constantly sitting, and employed in no active business which promotes the circulation of the blood, she becomes relaxed, the natural functions are impaired or obstructed, and the whole of her appearance shows a manifest declension of health—the fatal consequences of inactivity and imprudent indulgence, at a time when the process of nature required to be assisted by exercise and the invigorating quality of fresh air.

Besides the pernicious effects of indolence, whether voluntary or constrained, unwholesome food is particularly hurtful to girls at this period of life. Nor is this often so much the effect of necessity, as of their own inclination; indulging themselves in all manner of trash, by which their digestion is impaired, and, instead of wholesome chyle to afford proper nourishment to the body, the fluids are every day more corrupted by the accession of crude humours. Hence ensues not only an obstruction of the *menses*, that important discharge so intimately connected with health, but a train of evils, general and local, which never fail to accompany this event.

One practice, which formerly proved extremely injurious to young females, is now happily abolished; I mean that of tight lacing, by which their stomach and bowels were squeezed to a degree that impeded their natural functions; but as the present interdiction proceeds only from fashion, than which nothing is more variable or capricious, it is uncertain whether the rising generation may not yet experience the baneful effects of that obsolete practice which proved detrimental to the health of their mothers and grand mothers.

The flow of the menses is generally preceded by symptoms which announce its approach. These are, a sense of heat, weight, and dull pain in the loins; distension and hardness of the breasts; lassitude, loss of appetite, paleness of the countenance, head-ach, and sometimes a slight degree of fever. On the appearance of these symptoms about the age at which the menstrual flux usually begins, every thing which may obstruct that salutary evacuation should be carefully avoided, at the same time that endeavours should be diligently used to promote it. Wholesome diet, not flatulent, exercise, and cheerfulness, are all conducive to this purpose; and if she sit frequently over the steams of warm water, and foment the belly with a decoction of chamomile flowers, and the leaves of penny-royal, the process of nature will be facilitated.

When the expected discharge has made its appearance, great care should be taken to avoid every thing by which it might be checked, or the stomach and bowels disordered. All meats of hard digestion, fish, acid and austere fruits, butter-milk, whatever is liable to sour upon the stomach, or chill by its coldness, must be particularly guarded against; as well as every thing else which, from experience, is found to disagree with the individual.

An object likewise of great importance at this time, is to avoid catching cold; such an accident being attended with great danger. All great affections of the mind, such as sudden surprizes, frights, violent passions, particularly grief and anger, are also extremely prejudicial; and nothing, on the contrary, is more favourable at this period than cheerfulness.

When, unfortunately, the discharge is obstructed, exclusive of the state of pregnancy, all the means above recommended, respecting diet, exercise, &c. should be carefully observed; and if the person be feeble and languid, some generous liquor ought to be taken to invigorate the efforts of nature. But if this regimen prove ineffectual for recalling the discharge, it will be necessary to employ the aid of medicine.

When obstructions are occasioned by a relaxed habit of body, the proper remedies are those which brace the solids, promote digestion, and give force to all the powers by which the natural functions are conducted. The preparations of iron, the Peruvian bark, and bitter stomachic medicines, are the best adapted for this purpose, and may be taken in various forms, as is most agreeable to the patient. The following composition will in this case be used with great advantage. Take of filings of iron, two ounces; Peruvian bark roughly powdered, and the outer rind of Seville oranges, each one ounce; infuse them for a week or ten days in a quart of Lisbon-wine, and then filter the tincture. About half a wine-glassful of it may be taken twice a day.

In women of a gross and full habit of body, and where the obstruction proceeds from a viscid state of the fluids, it is necessary to bleed, to give once in three or four days a gentle purge of Glauber's salts or senna, and in the intervals such medicines as attenuate the humours. In this case, a tea-spoonful of the tincture of black hellebore, taken twice a day in a cup of pennyroyal-tea, is generally productive of good effect. The patient ought to take sufficient exercise, and to bathe her feet frequently in warm water; living at the same time on a spare thin diet, and avoiding the use of strong liquors.

When obstructions proceed from violent transports, or great

affections of the mind, they, never can be removed before the return of tranquillity. To forward this purpose, a change of place, amusements, and cheerful company, are of great importance; and every soothing means should be used to allay the inordinate emotion.

Though an obstruction of the *menses* proceeds for the most part either from constitutional causes, or accidents, yet it is frequently the effect of other disorders, the removal of which is necessary, previous to any efforts for promoting the sexual discharge. In this case, the method of cure will fall under some concomitant malady different from obstruction, but the nature of which can only be ascertained from examining the state of the patient.

In obstinate obstructions of the *menses*, small doses of calomel, or other mercurials, are frequently of great use; as is likewise electricity, directed in the form either of sparks or small shocks about the region of the womb. Another efficacious remedy, particularly in a difficulty of the first menstruation, is, after taking a vomit of ipecacuanha, to sit, during its operation, in a warm bath, where the water comes up to the middle of the body. It ought to be observed, that, in general, the artificial efforts to restore or promote the menstrual flux are most successfully made at the approach of its expected return.

## *Immoderate Flux of the Menses.*

The quantity of the menstrual discharge depending in general upon that of the blood, it is different in different women, but may, at an average, be estimated about two ounces. When the quantity therefore is much beyond this proportion, especially if the discharge returns more frequently than it ought, or the duration of it exceeds the usual period, the flux may be considered as immoderate. In this case, the patient becomes weak and pale, her digestion, as well as appetite, is impaired, and an œdematous swelling gradually occupies her feet and legs.

The period at which women are most exposed to this disorder is betwixt the age of forty-five and fifty, when the menstrual evacuation usually ceases. The disorder may proceed from relaxation, or a dissolved state of the blood; from a sedentary life, or excessive fatigue; a full diet, especially of salted or high seasoned food; the use of spirituous liquors; violent affections of the mind, &c.

The treatment of this complaint, in particular cases, must depend upon the cause which produces it; and this being fully ascertained, the patient must adopt such a course as is directly calculated to oppose its operation. In the mean time she must lie in an horizontal posture, with her head low, and be kept perfectly quiet, both in body and mind.

She muft likewife ufe a cool flender diet, fuch as veal or chicken broths, with bread; and take every three hours a cupful of a decoction of tormentil root, in which an ounce and a half of the root powdered is boiled in three pints of water to a quart. This, when ftrained, may be rendered more palatable by the addition of a little fugar. If coftivenefs attend, it ought to be removed by gentle laxatives, fuch as the electuary of fenna, taken in the quantity of a nutmeg two or three times a day.

If this courfe fhould not prove effectual, recourfe may be had to other aftringent remedies. Take of gum-kino, half a drachm; alum, one drachm and a half; gum-arabic, two drachms: powder them all together, and divide the whole into eight dofes; of which the patient may take one every four hours, with a cup of the infufion of rofes; taking likewife, two or three times a day, ten drops of laudanum, if there appear any figns of irritability, or the acetated ceruffe with opium.

If the alum, even in the moderate quantity above mentioned, fhould difagree with the ftomach, the patient may take, inftead of that compofition, half a drachm of the powder of Peruvian bark, with ten drops of the elixir of vitriol, in a glafs of red wine four times a day.

Aftringents may likewife be ufed externally in the way of fomentation; and large compreffes of linen, dipped in cold water and vinegar, may be applied to the belly and loins, and frequently renewed.

In full plethoric habits, bleeding may fometimes be proper in an immoderate flux of the menfes, but is feldom neceffary. If the diforder arifes from a cancerous ftate of the womb, which may be conjectured from a long continuance of the complaint, a darting deep-feated pain about that part, and a bearing down, the cafe is attended with great danger. If any thing can here afford relief, it is the ufe of hemlock, as formerly recommended in the treatment of fuch a difeafe.

It was obferved above, that the commencement of menftruation is an important period in the life of a female; and the fame may be faid of the term at which it finally ceafes. So much is the health affected by the fuppreffion of a long accuftomed difcharge, that many women either fall into chronic difeafes, or die about this time. But if they furvive it without contracting any tedious ailment, their health becomes more ftationary, and they acquire a degree of conftitutional ftrength that fubfifts to a very advanced age. The alternative is more or lefs critical in proportion as the ceffation of the difcharge is fudden or gradual. When the former is the cafe, in women of a full habit of body, they ought to retrench a little their ufual quantity of food, efpecially the more nourifhing kind, ſuch as fleſh, fiſh, eggs, jellies, &c. They ſhould alſo take daily ſufficient exerciſe, and keep the body open, by the occaſional uſe of a few grains of rhubarb or aloes. Five grains of either of theſe may be made into pills with an equal quantity of Caſtile ſoap, and taken at bed-time.

In women of a groſs habit of body, the ceſſation of the menſes is frequently followed by ſwellings in the legs, and other parts, which uſually become ulcerous. Theſe diſcharges ought either to be left open, or iſſues ſubſtituted in their place: for ſome acute or chronic diſeaſe is generally the conſequence of ſuppreſſing them.

## CHAP. XL.

### *Fluor Albus or Whites, Pregnancy, Child-birth, and Barrenneſs.*

THIS is a diſcharge of matter, variable both in colour and conſiſtence, from the womb and vagina; and is moſt incident to women of relaxed conſtitutions, who have borne many children. It is diſtinguiſhed into two kinds; one which ariſes from a general weakneſs of the ſolids, and another in which the debility is confined to the womb, in conſequence of a ſuppreſſion or immoderate flux of the *menſes*, frequent miſcarriages, hard labours, or a ſtrain of the back or loins.

When this diſeaſe has continued for any conſiderable time, it produces general debility, loſs of appetite, indigeſtion, faintneſs, palpitation of the heart, and, commonly, a pain in the loins. If, however, it be moderate, it may be borne a long time without much inconvenience; though in ſome women it occaſions barrenneſs, and in others a propenſity to miſcarriage.

When the diſeaſe ariſes from a general relaxation of the body, we muſt endeavour to ſtrengthen it by diet, exerciſe, and medicines. The food ſhould be ſolid and nouriſhing, but of eaſy digeſtion; and the moſt proper drink is red port wine, mixed with Tunbridge, Pyrmont, or Briſtol water, or with lime-water. A milk diet alone has often been found of great advantage; but it is more efficacious when mixed with a fourth part of lime-water. The patient ſhould abſtain from tea, as well as lying too long in bed; and ought to ride daily on horſeback. Dancing, however, is hurtful; as is alſo much walking, and a ſtanding poſture of body long continued.

In reſpect of medicines, the Peruvian bark, with elixir of vitriol, is preferable to every other remedy. Half a drachm of bark may be taken twice a day in a glaſs of port wine: premiſing, however, a gentle puke, if the ſtomach be foul. In ſummer, ſea-bathing, or bathing even in freſh water, is highly advantageous.

When the diſorder is occaſioned by a partial, rather than a general weakneſs, aſtringent remedies may be applied to the part affected, by means of a womb-ſyringe. For this purpoſe, the patient may uſe green tea, filtered ſmiths' forge-water, or common water, in half a pint of which two drachms of alum are diſſolved. It will be proper likewiſe, in this caſe, to apply a ſtrengthening plaſter to the ſmall of the back. Cold ſpring-water pumped on the loins, or a bliſtering-plaſter applied to the bottom of the ſpine or back, are both very powerful in their effects, and have ſometimes ſucceeded after other remedies had been tried in vain.

As women, from motives of falſe delicacy, often entruſt themſelves to the management of empirics, who are equally bold and ignorant in their practice, it is a circumſtance of the utmoſt importance to diſtinguiſh a freſh venereal infection, called gonorrhœa, from the *fluor albus*, or whites; for if one be miſtaken for the other, the moſt pernicious conſequences may enſue.* The following are the ſureſt ſigns for aſcertaining this neceſſary diſtinction.

In the gonorrhœa the diſcharge chiefly proceeds from the parts contiguous to the urinary paſſage, and continues whilſt the *menſes* flow; but in the whites it iſſues from the cavity of the womb and its paſſage, and then the *menſes* are ſeldom regular.

In gonorrhœa, an itching, inflammation, and heat of urine, are the fore-runners of the diſcharge; the orifice of the urinary paſſage is prominent and painful, and the patient is affected with a frequent irritation to make water. In the whites, the discharge is attended with pains in the loins, and loſs of ſtrength; and if any inflammation or heat of urine follow, they happen in a leſs degree, and only after a long continuance of the diſcharge, which, becoming ſharp and acrimonious, excoriates the ſurrounding parts.

In gonorrhœa, the diſcharge appears ſuddenly; but in the whites it comes on more ſlowly, and is often produced by irregularities of the *menſes*, frequent abortion, ſtrains, or long-continued illneſs.

In gonorrhœa, the diſcharge is uſually greeniſh or yellow, leſs in quantity, and not attended with the ſymptoms of weakneſs. In *fluor albus*, it is alſo often of the ſame colour, eſpecially in bad habits of body, and after long continuance; but is uſually more offenſive, and redundant in quantity.

During this diſeaſe, coſtiveneſs ſhould be prevented by taking occaſionally eight or ten grains of rhubarb, or three tea-ſpoonfuls of caſtor oil.

* See the Chapter on the Venereal Disease.

## *Pregnancy.*

This, though not a disease, is apt to be attended with a variety of complaints, which sometimes require the use of medicine. Women during pregnancy are often subject to the heart-burn, the treatment of which has been mentioned in a former chapter.* In the more early stage of pregnancy, they are likewise often troubled with sickness and vomiting, especially in the morning, immediately after getting out of bed. This is owing partly to the change of posture, but more to the emptiness of the stomach; and may generally be prevented by taking some light breakfast in bed. The propensity to vomiting, in the state of pregnancy, is commonly cured by keeping the body gently open. Bleeding, if used, ought to be in small quantities at a time, and the purgatives should be only of the mildest kind, such as manna, senna, or its electuary, stewed prunes, &c. If the vomiting still continue, a saline draught, taken in the act of effervescence, is of remarkable efficacy in stopping it, it may be compounded as follows, and repeated every two hours, if necessary. Take of the salt of tartar or wormwood, half a drachm; lemon-juice, two table-spoonfuls; mint-water, and simple cinnamon-water, each two table-spoonfuls; with a bit of loaf sugar.

Both the head-ach and tooth-ach are also very frequent with pregnant women; besides several other complaints, for the treatment of which we refer to the respective articles.

## *Abortion.*

Abortion is an accident to which every pregnant woman is more or less liable, and it ought to be more carefully avoided, not only as it weakens the constitution, but is apt to introduce a habit by which a future pregnancy may terminate in the same way. Abortion may happen in any period of gestation, but is more frequent in the second or third month. If it happens within the first month, it usually receives the name of a false conception; if after the seventh month, the infant may often be kept alive by proper care. Abortions are seldom dangerous in the first five months; but a repetition of them, by weakening the system, lays the foundation of chronic diseases of the most obstinate and dangerous nature.

The usual causes of abortion are violent exercise; jumping, or stepping from an eminence; violent coughing; blows on the belly; superabundance of blood; living too high or too low; indolence; relaxation; the death of the child; violent passions, &c.

* See Chap. XVI. page 215.

The approach of abortion may be known from a pain in the loins, or about the bottom of the belly, with a dull heavy pain along the inside of the thighs, a slight shivering, sickness, and palpitation of the heart. The breasts subside, and become flaccid or soft, the belly sinks, and there ensues a discharge of blood, or watery humours from the womb.

As soon as any signs appear which threaten an abortion, the woman ought to be laid on a mattrass, with her head low; where she should be kept as quiet and comfortable as possible, but not too hot; nor should she take any thing of a heating nature. Her food ought even to be cold, and of a kind the most remote from exciting any agitation in the body; such as broths, jellies, gruel, rice-milk, and the like; and her drink should be barley-water, sharpened with the juice of lemon.

If her strength be able to bear it, eight or ten ounces of blood should be drawn from her arm; but no medicines need to be given, unless to obviate particular symptoms. Thus, if she should be seized with a violent looseness, she ought to use the decoction of hartshorn as common drink. If with a vomiting, she may take the saline draught above recommended, every two hours. In this case, ten drops of laudanum may likewise be given three or four times a day; especially if the cause of the complaint has been any violent agitation of the mind.

Women of a sanguine constitution, who are liable to miscarry at a certain time of pregnancy, ought always to be bled a few days before the period arrives. They ought likewise to live sparingly, and be kept quiet until that term has elapsed.

If a pregnant woman be weak, delicate, and nervous, she will find great benefit from a light infusion of Peruvian bark and the outer rind of Seville oranges in white wine. The use of Tunbridge water, or other such chalybeate, will also prove serviceable. The most effectual remedy, in relaxed habits disposed to miscarriage, is the cold or shower-bath, which, however, must not be indiscriminately used in the pregnant state. But when the patient has been accustomed to it, she may safely continue it for some months after conception.

## *Child-birth.*

Most labours, being natural, child-birth is commonly effected with safety; but improper treatment after delivery may give rise to various disorders. During actual labour, the woman ought to take nothing of a heating nature; confining herself for food to panada, and for drink to plain toast and water. If the labour prove tedious and difficult, it will be proper to bleed, for the purpoſe of preventing inflammation. An emollient clyſter ought likewiſe to be frequently adminiſtered, and the patient ſhould ſit over the ſteams of warm water. The paſſage ought to be gently anointed with a little ſoft pomatum or freſh butter, and cloths wrung out of warm water applied over the belly. If the patient be much exhauſted with fatigue, ſo that nature ſeems to ſink, a draught of generous wine, or ſome other cordial, may be given, but only in ſuch circumſtances.

After delivery, the woman ought to be kept as quiet and eaſy as poſſible. Her food ſhould be light and thin, ſuch as gruel, panada, and the like; and her drink weak and diluting. But to this general rule there are many exceptions: for to ſome women in child-bed it is neceſſary to adminiſter a glaſs of wine, and a little of the lighteſt animal food, ſuch as a chicken. Much depends, in this caſe, upon the preſent circumſtances, and the former habits of the patient.

Sometimes a flooding, or great diſcharge of blood, happens after delivery. In this caſe, the patient ought to be laid with her head low, kept cool, and be treated in the ſame manner as for an exceſſive flux of the *menſes*.* She may take every two hours two table-ſpoonfuls of the following mixture. Take of pennyroyal-water, ſimple cinnamon-water, and ſyrup of poppies, each two ounces; elixir of vitriol, a drachm. Mix them. At the ſame time linen cloths, wrung out of a mixture of equal parts of vinegar and water, or red-wine, ſhould be applied to the belly, the loins, and the thighs, Theſe muſt be changed as they grow dry, and the uſe of them diſcontinued as ſoon as the flooding abates.

If the delivery be ſucceded by violent pains, the patient ought to drink plentifully of warm diluting liquors; and take every two hours a drachm of ſpermaceti in a cup of them; to which, if ſhe be reſtleſs, a table-ſpoonful of the ſyrup of poppies may be added. Should ſhe be hot or feveriſh, a ſcruple or half a drachm of nitre, if her ſtomach will bear it, may likewiſe be taken every four hours.

Child-bed women are ſometimes attacked with an inflammation of the womb after delivery. This is a dangerous diſeaſe, and requires the moſt ſpeedy application. The exiſtence of it may be aſcertained by pains in the lower part of the belly, which are greatly increaſed upon touching; a conſtant fever, with a weak and hard pulſe, great weakneſs, ſometimes inceſſant vomiting, an inclination to go frequently to ſtool, a heat, and ſometimes a total ſuppreſſion of urine.

This diſeaſe is to be treated, like other inflammations, by bleeding and plentiful dilution; taking frequently through the day a

* See page 299.

ſcruple or half a drachm of nitre, as recommended above. Clyſters of warm milk and water ſhould be given every four or five hours; and cloths wrung out of warm water be applied to the belly.

In the ſame manner muſt be treated the milk-fever, and a ſuppreſſion of the *lochia*, or uſual diſcharge after delivery. Plentiful dilution, gentle evacuations, and fomentations of the parts affected, are in all theſe caſes the ſafeſt and moſt proper means of cure. In the milk-fever, the breaſts may be anointed with a little warm linſeed oil. The child likewiſe ſhould be often put to the breaſt, or it ſhould be drawn by ſome other perſon; and, in thoſe women who do not ſuckle their own children, this practice ſhould be continued at leaſt for a month after delivery.

When an inflammation happens in the breaſt, the practice is common to apply emollient and anodyne fomentations, and poultices to the part affected, both to give caſe to the patient, and to haſten the formation of matter. But this method begins to be rejected by practitioners the moſt converſant with the treatment of women in child-bed. Inſtead of it, Dr. John Clarke, in particular, recommends the uſe of a ſolution of lead, conſtantly applied cold to the part inflamed, even though it ſhould be the whole of the breaſt. What he adviſes is a ſolution of acetated ceruſſe, or ſugar of lead, in two ounces of diſtilled vinegar; to which may be added an ounce of rectified ſpirit of wine, and five ounces of diſtilled water.

In an inflammation of the breaſt, if the patient be of a ſtrong conſtitution, and the ſymptoms of fever run high, bleeding from the arm will be neceſſary, and alſo evacuation by purging, ſo as to procure two or three ſtools every day; at the ſame time that the patient's diet muſt be of the loweſt and moſt cooling kind. Blood ſhould likewiſe be taken away from the breaſt by the application of three or four leeches to the part.

Theſe evacuations having been made, the ſolution of lead ought to be applied; the advantages of which are the following:

1. The cold repels the blood from the part, which is farther aſſiſted by the aſtringent quality of the lead, and hence the inflammation is leſſened.

2. The breaſt is not weakened; ſo that if an abſceſs ſhould be formed, it will ſooner be filled up with healthy granulations.

3. If the inflammation ſhould be diminiſhed, the woman will ſuffer leſs pain, and the conſtitution will be leſs affected.

4. Matter will either be not formed at all, or, if formed, it will be in leſs quantity, which will ſhorten the duration of the diſeaſe.

If there should be much pain, it will be proper to give fifteen or twenty drops of laudanum in a saline draught, every six hours.

If this plan be adopted at an early period, and pursued with punctuality, the inflammation will often be altogether suppressed; but if it be practised too late to produce a complete resolution, the extent of the suppuration will be very much lessened.

When the nipples are tender or chapped, they may be anointed with a mixture of oil of olives and bees'-wax; or, what is frequently used, a little powdered gum-arabic may be sprinkled on them.

The most fatal disorder consequent upon delivery is the puerperal or child-bed fever: but this having been the subject of a former chapter, we shall say nothing farther of it in this place; observing only, in general, that with respect to child-bed women, nothing is of greater importance than to avoid catching cold.

One other circumstance deserves to be particularly mentioned. A practice is still very prevalent among persons in the middle and lower stations of life; which is that of taking during labour a variety of substances rendered stimulating by being impregnated with spices, wine, or spirits. Nothing can be more false in principle, nor more destructive in its tendency. If a labour be going on well, there can be no occcasion for them, and if ill, they are much more likely to do harm than good. If they do any thing, they will most certainly increase the action of the heart and arterial system beyond that degree which the mere exertions of labour will produce; and this increased action will not subside when the woman is delivered. If there were any previous disposition to fever in her body, nothing is so likely to bring it into activity; and though the labour alone might not stimulate the constitution beyond what it could bear,—or, in other words, though the increased circulation arising from the exertions of the womb might gradually go off after delivery,—yet if such means have been employed as tend still farther to increase the action of the vascular system, a fever may be the consequence; and how dangerous this will prove to the life of the woman it is unnecessary to say.

## *Barrenness.*

Though this may be regarded rather as a negative than a positive affection, yet it implies a disposition of body distinct from that of health; and, in fact, we find that most married women, who have no children are generally subject to complaints. Where barrenness arises from any natural defect of the womb, it may not admit of a cure: but it seems to proceed most commonly from general relaxation, which may be occasioned by indolence, high living, debilitating passions, unwholesome air, and other circumstances.

That one of the most powerful causes of barrenness is high living, appears to be confirmed, not only by the general fecundity of women in the lower stations of life, but by the prolific effects of a change of diet upon the constitutions of those of rank and fortune. Were we, therefore, to prescribe the method of living most favourable to procreation, it would be to use a diet consisting chiefly of milk and vegetables; to take sufficient exercise in the open air; to preserve the mind as much as possible in a state of tranquillity and cheerfulness; to make use of an infusion of the Peruvian bark; and to drink of some chalybeate waters, such as those of Bath, Spa, and Tunbridge. But a partial, as well as general, relaxation being often the cause of sterility, nothing proves more effectual for removing it than the use of the cold or shower-bath, which in this case particularly should always be used in the morning.

## CHAP. XLI.

### *Disorders of the Senses.*

TO enter upon a minute description of the organs of sense could not afford any useful information to the reader. It will therefore be sufficient to give a concise account of the diseases to which they are most liable, and point out the means by which these may be best prevented or removed.

### *The Eye.*

The curious and complicated mechanism of the eye renders this organ subject to a variety of diseases extremely difficult to be cured; and it is affected by causes, respecting the influence of which no other part of the body is susceptible. Certain modes of life conduce greatly to weaken and wear out the eyes, or at least to render them too irritable. This is particularly observable among those classes of people who are employed in sedentary occupations, are much exposed to dust, or who work by candle-light, &c.

The eyes are hurt by looking too much at bright and luminous objects; the effluvia from acrid or volatile substances; a long-continued use of bitters; an immoderate use of the cold-bath; excessive venery; head-ach, and various other disorders; but, above all, by night-watching, and candle-light lucubrations. Excefs of every kind is prejudicial to the fight, particularly the immoderate ufe of ftrong liquors. Long fafting is another circumftance hurtful to the eyes; as is likewife the ftoppage of any cuftomary evacuation; with frequent and fudden tranfitions from darknefs, or obfcure degrees of light, into that of funfhine, or the glare of a number of candles.

In all difeafes of the eyes, the food fhould be of eafy digeftion; and the drink, water, whey, or fmall beer. Spirituous liquors ought to be carefully avoided; and all irritation from fmoke of every kind; the vapours of onions, garlic, muftard, and horfe-radifh; or from vivid lights and glaring colours.

For preventing diforders of the eyes, iffues or fetons are of great advantage; infomuch that perfons whofe eyes are tender ought never to be without one of thefe, at leaft, in fome part of the body; but the arms, or fuperior parts, are moft advifable. To keep the body gently open is alfo ufeful.

The difeafe of the eye called a *gutta ferena* or *amaurofis*, is a deprivation of the light without any perceptible fault or imperfection in the eyes. When this arifes from a decay of the optic nerve, it admits of no cure; but when it proceeds from a compreffion only of the nerves by a redundancy of fluids, there may be a poffibility of draining thefe off, and confequently reftoring the patient's light. In this cafe the body ought to be kept open by fome gentle laxative; and if the patient be young, and of a fanguine habit, he may be bled. Cupping, with fcarifications on the back part of the head, will likewife be advifable. A draining of the humours by the nofe may be promoted by volatile falts or fpirits, ftimulating powders, &c. But the moft promifing means of evacuation are iffues or blifters on the back part of the head, behind the ears, or on the neck, kept open for a long time.

If thefe means fhould not fucceed, a trial may be made of the effects of falivation by mercury; and likewife of electricity. In the mean time, the patient may take two or three times a day a cup of an infufion of the root of wild valerian.

A *cataract* is an opaque fubftance obftructing the pupil; in fuch a manner as either to impair or totally deftroy the fight. This blemifh is generally owing to an opacity of the cryftalline humour. In the early ftage of a cataract, the means to be ufed for relief are the fame as in the gutta ferena; and they will fometimes produce the defired effect. But when every hope of fuccefs is fruftrated, recourfe may be had to the extraction of the cataract, after it has become fufficiently firm to admit of that operation.

*Specks* or *fpots* on the eyes are frequently the confequence of inflammation. Thefe often appear after the fmall-pox, the meafles, or violent opthalmias, and are very difficult of cure. If the fpecks, however, are foft and thin, they may fometimes be removed by gentle canfties and difcutient applications. In this cafe, the common remedy is white vitriol. When fuch means prove of no benefit, the only remaining expedient is a furgical operation, extremely nice in the performance, and no lefs doubtful in the iffue.

A *blood-fhot* eye may be occafioned by external violence, or by vomiting, coughing, &c. and occurs moft frequently in fcrofulous or fcorbutic habits. It goes off for the moft part fpontaneoufly, changing gradually into a yellowifh colour, and foon after totally difappears. If it fhould prove obftinate, the patient may be bled, and the eye fomented with warm milk; then applying to the part a foft poultice of bread and milk. In the mean time, the body fhould be kept open by fome gentle laxative.

The *watery* or *weeping eye* proceeds from a relaxation of the glandular parts of that organ, which therefore require to be ftrengthened. For this purpofe the eye may be wafhed with common water fharpened with brandy; or with rofe-water in which a very fmall quantity of white vitriol is diffolved. Gentle purgatives are here alfo proper, as well as blifters on the neck kept open for fome time. This complaint, no lefs than the blood-fhot eye, is attendant on a fcrofulous habit. When it proceeds from an obftruction of the lachrymal duct, the natural paffage of the tears into the nofe, it receives the name of a *fiftula lachrymalis*, for which the only remedy is a furgical operation.

A *ftrabifmus*, or *fquinting*, proceeds from a contraction of the mufcles of the eye, in confequence either of a nervous affection, or a vicious habit; but when owing to the former, it is feldom uniform, or of long duration. Children often contract this habit by having their eyes unequally expofed to the light; and they may likewife acquire it by imitation from a fquinting nurfe or play-fellow, &c. Perhaps the only expedient for correcting it is to furnifh the child with a mafk, which will only permit him to fee in a ftraight direction.

The *myopia*, or *fhort-fightednefs*; and the *prefbyopia*, or *feeing only at a great diftance*; are diforders which depend on the original conformation of the eyes, and are therefore incurable. They may both, however, be in fome meafure remedied by the help of proper glaffes; the former by means of a concave, and the latter of a convex glafs. All glaffes ufed to affift vifion are thought to require fome effort of the eyes; and, unlefs they be indifpenfably neceffary, it is better not to employ them at an early period of life.

*The Ear.*

The ear, like the eye, is admirably conſtructed for the function to which it is deſtined; but cannot be exempted, any more than the other, from diſorders incident to every organized body. It may be injured by wounds, inflammations, ulcers, or any thing that greatly affects its ſubſtance. The ſenſe of hearing may likewiſe be hurt by various cauſes, ſuch as fevers, violent colds in the head, exceſſive noiſe, too great a degree of moiſture or dryneſs of the organ, and hard wax, or other ſubſtances obſtructing the cavity of the ear. Some degree of deafneſs is incident to moſt people in an advanced age; but when it exiſts from the birth, it is owing to an original defect in the ſtructure of the ear, and is commonly incurable. Several perſons, however, have lately been reſtored to, and others prevented with, the ſenſe of hearing, by an operation on the tympanum, or drum—firſt, I believe, recommended by Mr. Aſhley Cooper.

The deafneſs ariſing from old age is difficult of cure, as is, likewiſe, that which is the conſequence of wounds or ulcers. When it is the effect of a fever, it commonly goes off with the diſeaſe. If it be occaſioned by wax ſticking in the paſſage of the ear, the offending matter may be removed by dropping into the ear a little oil of ſweet almonds, and afterwards ſyringing with warm milk and water. But the moſt frequent cauſe of deafneſs is cold in the head. In this caſe, the patient ſhould be careful to keep his head warm, eſpecially in the night. He ought, likewiſe, to keep his feet warm, and bathe them frequently in tepid water at bed-time; taking occaſionally ſome gentle purgative to keep the body open.

When the ears abound too much with moiſture, it may be drained off by an iſſue, or ſeton, which ought to be put as near as poſſible to the part affected. In this caſe, likewiſe, it is proper to keep the body open.

When deafneſs proceeds from a deficiency of moiſture in the ears, which may be known from looking into the paſſage, a few drops of a mixture made of two parts of oil of ſweet almonds, and one part of the compound tincture of caſtor, may be put into them every night at bed-time, ſtopping them afterwards, with a little cotton or wool.

A noiſe in the ears is a frequent complaint, and, when it proceeds not from cold in the head, may be conſidered as a nervous affection, and treated accordingly. It may, however, be frequently relieved by conveying into the ears, through a funnel, the vapours of aromatic plants, ſuch as thyme and ſweet margoram, &c. infuſed for a quarter of an hour in hot water. Or, inſtead of this, introduce into the ears a few drops of a mixture made of equal parts of oil of ſweet almonds, compound tincture of lavender, and tincture of caſtor.

A variety of applications has been recommended for the cure of deafneſs, none of which can prove uſeful againſt every cauſe of that complaint, and many of them may even be prejudicial. In all caſes of deafneſs, however, it is of importance to keep the head warm, and likewiſe the feet.

### *Taſte and Smell.*

There is ſo great an affinity between theſe two ſenſes, that whatever hurts one of them generally affects the other; and both are liable to be impaired by exceſſive gratification. The principal organ of taſte is the tongue, which is provided with innumerable nerves, terminating in *papillæ*, or eminences, of different ſizes and figures; ſome of them pointed, ſome oblong, and others of a fungous texture.

The different degrees of taſte depend on the greater or leſs ſenſibility of the nervous papillæ, above mentioned, as well as on the quality of the ſaliva, in a more or leſs healthy ſtate of the body.

When this ſenſibility is blunted by too ſtrong and highly ſeaſoned food, or by the copious uſe of ſpirituous liquors, the ſenſe of taſte no longer exiſts in its former and orginal perfection.

The ſenſe of ſmell is exerciſed by the noſe, and chiefly by the mucous membrane, which lines that organ. The whole inſide of the noſe is covered with this membrane, which is a continuation of the general integuments of the body, but much ſofter and porous, full of veſſels exquiſitely ſenſible, and covered with hair towards the lower part of the noſtrils, to prevent any impurities or noxious particles from aſcending too far.

In many animals the ſenſe of ſmelling is more acute than in man, who would probably be much incommoded by too refined a perception of this kind. But it may be much improved by exerciſe, or depraved by neglect. Hence, the American Indian, it is ſaid, can diſcover the footſteps of a man or other animal by ſmell alone; while perſons who live in a bad and fœtid atmoſphere are ſcarcely ſenſible of the difference between the moſt fragrant and offenſive ſubſtances. This ſenſe is much injured by taking great quantities of ſnuff.

Both theſe ſenſes, when habitually ſtimulated by fragrant and poignant diſhes, become in the end incapable of reliſhing the gratifications of luxury; but when impaired by other cauſes than exceſſive indulgence, they may by proper means recover their former acuteneſs.

The *taſte* may be diminiſhed by filth, mucus, aphthæ, &c. covering the tongue: it may be depraved by a fault of the ſaliva, or by impure effluvia from the ſtomach or lungs; and it may be entirely deſtroyed by local injuries, and nervous affections of the tongue and palate. A violent cold in the head will vitiate or aboliſh for a time both the ſenſes of taſting and ſmelling.

When the taſte is obſtructed by filth, mucus, &c. the tongue ought to be wiped with a linen cloth, and frequently waſhed with ſome detergent application, ſuch as a mixtue of water, vinegar, and honey. But when it is depraved by any fault of the ſaliva, that circumſtance muſt be corrected. If there be a bitter taſte, which affords reaſon to ſuſpect the exiſtence of bile in the ſtomach, it muſt be evacuated by vomits and purges. A nidorous taſte, ariſing from putrid humours, muſt be oppoſed by acids, ſuch as the juice of oranges, lemons, and citrons. An acid taſte is deſtroyed by abſorbents and alkaline ſalts, ſuch as magneſia, ſoda, kali, and chalk, &c. And a ſalt taſte may be extinguiſhed by ſufficient dilution with watery liquors.

When the nerves which actuate the organs of taſte are impaired in reſpect of ſenſibility, the chewing of ginger or other ſtimulating ſubſtances, is adviſable; but this expedient will prove moſt ſucceſſful where the perſon has not been much accuſtomed to the uſe of ſpiceries.

When the ſenſe of ſmelling is obſtructed by mucus in the noſe, the cauſe may frequently be removed by a plug of tobacco, or the ſteam of hot vinegar received up the noſtrils.

When the noſe abounds with moiſture, the complaint is beſt cured by keeping the body open, and ſupporting the natural perſpiration.

If there be reaſon to think that the defect proceeds from a torpid ſtate of the nerves which ſupply the organs of ſmelling, volatile ſalts, ſtrong ſnuffs, and whatever excites ſneezing, may be applied to the noſe.

## *Of the Touch.*

While all the other ſenſes have each its appropriate organ, that of *touch* is univerſally diffuſed over the ſurface of the body. In order to underſtand more clearly the means by which this ſenſe is conducted, it may not be improper to give here a conciſe deſcription of the external integuments of the human body.

Theſe integuments conſiſt of three different layers; the uppermoſt of which, the epidermis, or ſcarf-ſkin, is the thinneſt, and is nearly tranſparent. It envelops the whole body, both externally and internally. This covering is of eſſential ſervice to the whole frame, by protecting the parts encloſed from external injury, by preventing them from adhering internally, and by keeping every thing in the body in its proper ſituation. It is deſtitute of ſenſation, but possessed of the property, that it is very quickly renewed after it has been destroyed by accident or disease.

Immediately under this covering their lies a second reticular and mucous membrane, termed by anatomists *rete mucosum*. It is in most parts of the body extremely thin, but on the heels and palms of the hands it is considerably thicker.

This second envelopment merits particular attention, as being the seat of the colour of different nations; though the cause of this diversity remains yet undiscovered. In the Negroes it is black; in the American Indians nearly of copper-colour; and in the Europeans generally white. That the colour of the human body is contained in this second or middle skin is sufficiently ascertained; for not only the third or true skin of the negroes is as white as in the Europeans, but the uppermost, or scarf-skin, likewise though rather of a greyish tint, is scarcely darker in blacks than in white people; and in the latter also the middle skin is frequently of a yellowish, brown, or blackish colour; in which case the whole external skin exhibits a similar appearance.

The third and innermost of the integuments of the body is the *cutis vera*, or true skin, which immediately covers the fat and the muscles. It is of a cellular texture, very compact and smooth on its upper surface; of a white colour in all nations; loose or pliable on its inner surface, and furnished with more or less fat. It is not only endowed with a considerable degree of expansibility and contractility, but is provided with enumerable pores. Its thickness varies in different individuals. It is traversed by a great number of fine arteries interwoven in the form of a net; with an equal number of veins, and delicate absorbent vessels.

From the many nerves which pervade the true skin, it possesses an uncommon degree of sensibility, especially in those parts where the *papillæ* of the nerves are perceptible. In some places, as the lips, they are not unlike flakes, though they generally resemble little warts. They are most visible on the ends of the fingers in delicate persons: they can be traced with the naked eye, by the spiral lines terminating almost in a point, and are protected and supported by nails growing out of the skin. It is in these papillary extremities that every external impression is most distinctly and forcibly perceived, on account of the number of nerves lying almost exposed to view in these places.

When the nervous papillæ are pressed against external objects, the nerves receive a kind of vibration, which is communicated to their branches, and thence to the brain. Thus we are enabled to feel the hardness, roughness, figure, size, and other sensible qualities of bodies. But that this feeling may not become painful, nature has provided another cover, namely, the scarf-skin, which ſerves the important purpoſes of excluding the air from the true ſkin, and preventing the body from being too much dried. The nails increaſe the energy of touch, and render the ſenſe of it more acute, by reſiſting the preſſure of external ſubſtances.

The ſenſe of touching, being ſeated at a greater diſtance from the brain than the other ſenſes, is more liable to experience an obſtruction of the nervous influence from external cauſes. It may therefore be affected by preſſure, extreme cold, bruiſes, inflammations, &c. It may alſo ſuffer from two great a degree of ſenſibility; which renders its functions not only indiſcriminate, but painful. When there exiſts no evident cauſe of the defect, it may juſtly be aſcribed to ſome latent diſorder affecting the origin of the nerves; and ought to be treated in nearly the ſame manner as a palſy, of which it may, in fact, be conſidered as a modification. After opening the body by ſome gentle purgative, the ſtimulaing medicines and outward applications recommended for the palſy may be uſed. Warm bathing likewiſe, eſpecially in the natural hot baths, is adviſable.

## CHAP. XXXVII.

### *Of the Itch.*

THIS diſeaſe generally appears in the form of ſmall watery puſtules, firſt about the wriſts or between the fingers; afterwards affecting the arms, legs, thighs and other parts. The ſource of it, originally, is want of cleanlineſs, which produces animalcula, or very ſmall inſects, in the ſkin; and theſe, by irritating the fibres, in the places where they are lodged, occaſion the violent itching which gives name to the diſeaſe.

The itch is communicated by infection; either from the animalcula themſelves getting from the affected to the ſound perſon, from touching any ſoft ſubſtance where they may be lodged, or from the perſon receiving upon the ſkin ſome of the *ova* or eggs, which being rubbed into the furrows, and lying there ſome time, may produce animalcula.

The itch is ſeldom a dangerous diſeaſe, unleſs it be neglected or treated improperly; but, if ſuffered to continue, it may vitiate the whole maſs of humours; and, if ſuddenly repelled, or driven in without proper evacuations, it may give riſe to fevers, inflammations of ſome of the bowels, or other internal diſorders.

For the cure of this diſeaſe different remedies are recommended, ſuch as the vitriolic acid, and ſome preparations of quickſilver; but experience confirms that nothing is preferable to ſulphur. This ought to be uſed both externally and internally. Two ounces of the flowers of ſulphur may be made into an ointment with four ounces of hog's lard, or butter, and two drachms of crude ſal ammoniac, or the root of white hellebore. If half a drachm of the eſſence of lemon, or oil of bay-berries, be added, it will entirely take away the ſulphureous ſmell, which to delicate people is offenſive. Of this ointment, about the bulk of a nutmeg may be rubbed upon the arms, legs, and thighs, at bed-time every night. If any other parts be affected with the diſeaſe, they likewiſe may be rubbed; but it is ſeldom neceſſary to apply the ointment to the whole body. If the patient be of a full habit, it will be proper to bleed, or take one or two purges before the application of the ointment; during the uſe of which, it will alſo be proper to take, every night and morning, as much of the flowers of ſulphur and cream of tartar, equally mixed, as will keep the body gently open. This laxative mixture may be taken in a little treacle, or new milk. The patient ſhould beware of catching cold while he uſes the ointment, ſhould be more thickly covered than uſual, and take every thing warm. Except the linen, it will be better to wear the ſame clothes daring the uſe of the ointment; and ſuch clothes as have been worn while the patient was under the diſeaſe muſt not be uſed again until they are fumigated with brimſtone, and thoroughly cleanſed. The quantity of ointment mentioned above will generally be ſufficient for the cure of one perſon; and when this is completed, he ought to waſh his body with ſoap and water; or, if it be ſummer, to bathe in a river for that purpoſe.

Some eruptive diſorders, to which children are liable, have a great ſimilarity to the itch; but care ſhould be taken not to treat them in the ſame manner; for, thoſe eruptions being often ſalutary, the application of greaſy ointments might be productive of pernicious effects.

Few perſons eſcape ſome cutaneous eruption, or affection of the ſkin, either in ſpring or autumn; and young ladies are often induced to employ various waſhes, lotions, and coſmetics; by which many excellent conſtitutions have been irreparably injured. The only innocent coſmetics, or beautifiers of the ſkin, care exerciſe in the open air, the warm bath, Harrogate-bath, a decoction of the dulcamara or bitter-ſweet, or the inner bark of the elm, an ounce to a pint of water; or, laſtly, ſoap and water.

# CHAP. XLIII.

## *Surgery.*

IT would be inconſiſtent with the plan of a work of this nature to deſcribe the various operations of ſurgery. All that is required is to give a conciſe and clear account of the proper treatment of ſuch caſes as may be managed without profeſſional education for the purpoſe, and which may occur where the aſſiſtance of a ſurgeon cannot readily be obtained.

### *Bleeding.*

The moſt common operation of ſurgery is that of bleeding; the knowledge of rightly performing which, is only to be acquired by example. Were we to judge of this operation by the frequency and facility with which it is practiſed, we ſhould be apt to conclude that it was a matter of very little importance; whereas, in fact, there is none that more affects the conſtitution, and even life itſelf, according as it is either neglected on one hand, or carried to exceſs on the other.

This operation is proper at the beginning of all inflammatory fevers, ſuch as pleuriſies, peripnuemonies, &c. It is alſo proper in all topical inflammations of internal parts, ſuch as thoſe of the ſtomach, inteſtines, &c. and likewiſe in the apoplexy, aſthma, rheumatiſms, coughs, violent head-achs, and other diſorders, proceeding either from too great a quantity of blood, or an impediment to its circulation. Bleeding is no leſs neceſſary after falls, blows, bruiſes, or any violent hurt received, externally or internally; as it is likewiſe in caſes of ſuffocation from foul air, ſtrangulation, &c. But in all diſorders proceeding from a relaxed habit of body, and a vitiated ſtate of the fluids, bleeding is injurious.

In topical inflammations bleeding ought to be performed as near the part affected as poſſible; and, in general, the beſt method of doing it is by a lancet: but where a vein cannot be found, recourſe muſt be had to the application of leeches, or cupping.

### *Leeches.*

Previous to the application of leeches, the ſkin ſhould be carefully cleanſed from any foulneſs, and moiſtened with a little milk, by which means they faſten more readily, and this farther promoted by allowing them to creep upon a dry cloth, or a dry board, for a few minutes before application. The moſt effectual method to make them fix upon a particular ſpot, is to confine them to the part by means of a ſmall wine glaſs. As ſoon as the leeches have ſeparated, the uſual method of promoting the diſcharge of blood is, to cover the parts with fine linen cloths wet in warm water. But if the blood ſhould continue to flow from the orifice made by a leech, longer than is deſired, as has happened, in ſome inſtances, to children, who have been nearly loſt by the inability of the attendants to ſtop the diſcharge; after carefully waſhing off the blood, the point of the finger ſhould be preſſed moderately upon the orifice, and afterwards a compreſs be kept upon it for a little time.

## *Cupping.*

When, either from the ſeverity of a local fixed pain, or from any other cauſe, it is judged proper to evacuate blood directly from the ſmall veſſels of the part affected, inſtead of opening any of the larger arteries or veins, it is uſual, beſides leeches, to employ ſcarification and cupping. Slight ſcarifications may be made with the ſhoulder or edge of a lancet; or by means of an inſtrument termed a *ſcarificator*; in which ſixteen or twenty lancets are commonly placed, in ſuch a manner that, when the inſtruments is applied to the part affected, the whole number of lancets contained in it are, by means of a ſtrong ſpring, puſhed ſuddenly into it, to the depth at which the inſtrument has been previouſly regulated. This being done, as the ſmaller blood-veſſels only, by this operation, are intended to be cut, and as theſe do not commonly diſcharge freely, ſome means or other becomes neceſſary for promoting the evacuation. Various methods have been propoſed for this purpoſe; glaſſes fitted to the form of the affected parts, with a ſmall hole in the bottom of each, were long ſince contrived; and theſe being placed upon the ſcarified parts, a degree of ſuction was produced by a perſon's mouth ſufficient for nearly exhauſting the air contained in the glaſs. This method accordingly increaſed the evacuation of blood to a certain extent; but as it was attended with a good deal of trouble, and did not always prove effectual, an exhauſting ſyringe was at laſt adapted to the glaſs, by means of which the contained air was extracted. The application of this inſtrument however, for any length of time, is very troubleſome; and it is difficult to preſerve the ſyringe always air-tight.

The application of heat to the cupping-glaſſes has been found to rarefy the air contained in them to a degree ſufficient for producing a very confiderable fuction; and this expedient, therefore, is now employed inftead of the fyringe.

Different methods have been practifed for applying heat to the cavity of the glafs. By fupporting the mouth of it for a few feconds above the flame of a taper, the air may be fufficiently rarefied; but if the flame be not kept exactly in the middle, but allowed to touch either the fides or bottom of the glafs, the latter is very apt to be cracked. A more certain, as well as an eafier method of applying the heat is, to dip a piece of foft bibulous paper in fpirit of wine, and, having fet it on fire, to put it into the bottom of the glafs; and, on its being nearly extinguifhed, to apply the mouth of the inftrument directly upon the fcarified part. This degree of heat, which may be always regulated by the fize of the piece of paper, and which, it is evident, ought to be always in proportion to the fize of the glafs, if long enough applied, proves fufficient for effectually rarefying the air, and at the fame time, if done with any manner of caution, never injures the glafs in the leaft.

The glafs having been thus applied, if the fcarifications have been properly made, they inftantly begin to difcharge freely; and, fo foon as the inftrument is nearly full of blood, it fhould be taken away. This may eafily be done by raifing one fide of it fo as to admit the external air. When more blood is defired to be taken, the parts fhould be bathed with warm water; and, being made perfectly dry, another glafs, exactly the fize of the former, fhould be inftantly applied in the fame manner. Thus, almoft any neceffary quantity of blood may be obtained. It fometimes happens, however, that the full quantity intended to be difcharged cannot be got at one place. In fuch a cafe, the fcarificator muft be again applied on a part as contiguous to the former as poffible; and, this being done, the application of the glaffes muft alfo be renewed as before.

When it is wifhed to difcharge the quantity of blood as quickly as poffible, two or more glaffes may be applied at once on contiguous parts previoufly fcarified; and, on fome occafions, the quantity of blood is more quickly obtained by the cupping-glaffes being applied for a few feconds upon the parts to be afterwards fcarified. The fuction produced by the glaffes may poffibly have fome influence in bringing the more deep-feated veffels into nearer contact with the fkin; fo that more of them will be cut by the fcarificator.

A fufficient quantity of blood being procured, the wounds made by the different lancets fhould be all perfectly cleared of blood; and a bit of foft linen, or charpie, dipped in a little milk or cream, applied over the whole, is the only dreffing that is neceffary. When dry linen is applied, it not only occafions more uneafinefs to the patient, but renders the wounds more apt to suffer than when it has been previously wetted in the manner directed.

Dry-cupping consists in the application of the cupping-glasses directly to the parts affected, without using the scarificator. By this means a tumor is produced upon the part; and where any advantage is to be expected from a determination of blood to a particular spot, it may probably be more easily accomplished by this means than by any other.

When the part from which it is intended to produce a local evacuation of this kind is so situated, that a scarificator and cupping-glasses can be applied, this method is greatly preferable to any other; but in inflammatory affections of the eye, nose, and other parts of the face, &c. the scarificator cannot be properly applied to the parts affected. In such cases, therefore, the common recourse is to leeches, which can be placed upon almost any spot whence we would wish to discharge blood.

## *Issues.*

These are a kind of artificial ulcers, formed in different parts of the body, for the purpose of procuring a discharge of purulent matter, which is frequently of advantage in various disorders. Practitioners were formerly of opinion that issues served as drains to carry off noxious humours from the blood; and therefore they placed them as near the affected part as possible. But as it is now known that they prove useful merely by the quantity of matter which they produce, they are generally placed where they will occasion the least inconvenience. The most proper parts for them are, the nape of the neck; the middle, outer, and fore part of the shoulder; the hollow above the inner side of the knee; or either side of the back-bone; or between two of the ribs; or where-ever there is a sufficiency of cellular substance for the protection of the parts beneath. They ought never to be placed over the belly of a muscle; nor over a tendon, or thinly covered bone; nor near any large blood-vessel. The issues commonly used are, the blister-issue, the pea-issue, and the seton or cord.

When a blister-issue is to be used, after the blister is removed, a discharge of matter may be kept up by dressing the part daily with an ointment mixed with the powder of cantharides, or Spanish flies, or savin ointment. If the discharge be too little, more of the powder may be used; if too great, or if the part be much inflamed, the issue-ointment may be laid aside, and the part dressed with basilicon, or with common cerate, till the discharge be diminished, and the inflammation abated.

It is sometimes most proper to use the issue-ointment and a mild one alternately.

A pea-iſſue is formed either by making an inciſion with a lancet, or by cauſtic, large enough to admit one or more peas; though ſometimes, inſtead of peas, kidney-beans, gentian-root, or orange-peas are uſed. When the opening is made by an inciſion, the ſkin ſhould be pinched up and cut through, of a ſize ſufficient to receive the ſubſtance to be put into it. But when it is to be done by cauſtic, the common cauſtic, or lapis infernalis of the ſhops, anſwers beſt. It ought to be reduced to a paſte with a little water or ſoft ſoap, to prevent it from ſpreading; and an adheſive plaſter, with a ſmall hole cut in the centre of it, ſhould be previouſly placed, and the cauſtic paſte ſpread upon the hole. Over the whole an adheſive plaſter ſhould be placed, to prevent any cauſtic from eſcaping. In ten or twelve hours the whole may be removed, and in three or four days the eſchar will ſeparate, when the opening may be filled with peas, or any of the other ſubſtances above mentioned.

The ſeton is uſed when a large quantity of matter is wanted, and eſpecially from deep-ſeated parts. It is frequently uſed in the back of the neck for diſeaſes of the head or eyes, or between two of the ribs in affections of the breaſt.

When the cord, which ought to be made of threads of cotton or ſilk, is to be introduced, the parts at which it is to enter and paſs out ſhould be previouſly marked with ink; and a ſmall part of the cord being beſmeared with ſome mild ointment, and paſſed through the eye of the ſeton-needle, the part is to be ſupported by an aſſiſtant, and the needle paſſed fairly through, leaving a few inches of the cord hanging out. The needle is then to be removed, and the part dreſſed. By this method matter is produced in quantity proportioned to the degree of irritation applied; and this can be increaſed or diminiſhed by covering the cord daily, before it is drawn, with an irritating or mild ointment.

## *Inflammations and Abſceſſes.*

All inflammations, from whatever cauſes they proceed, can terminate only in three ways, viz. by diſperſion, ſuppuration, or gangrene. It is impoſſible to foretel with certainty in which of theſe three ways any particular inflammation will terminate, yet a probable conjecture may be formed with regard to the event, from a knowledge of the patient's age and conſtitution. Slight inflammations from cold, and without any previous indiſpoſition, will moſt probably be diſperſed; thoſe which immediately ſucceed a fever, or happen to perſons of a groſs habit of body, will generally ſuppurate; and thoſe which attack very old people, or perſons of a dropſical habit, will have a ſtrong tendency to a gangrene.

When the inflammation is ſlight, and the conſtitution ſound, the treatment ſhould always be adapted to produce a diſperſion. The beſt means of promoting this end is the uſe of a ſlender diluting diet, ſufficient bleeding, and repeated purges. The inflamed part ſhould be fomented with a decoction of wormwood and chamomile flowers; anointing it afterwards with a mixture of three-fourths of ſweet oil, and one-fourth of vinegar, and covering it with a piece of cerate, or wax-plaſter.

By means of theſe applications, in the courſe of three or four days, and ſometimes in a ſhorter ſpace of time, the diſperſion or reſolution of the tumor will in general begin to take place: at leaſt before the end of that period it may for the moſt part, be known how the inflammation will terminate. If the heat, pain, and other attending ſymptoms abate, and eſpecially if the tumor begin to decreaſe, without the occurrence of any gangrenous appearances, we may then be almoſt certain that by a continuance of the ſame plan a total reſolution will in time be effected.

If, on the contrary, all the ſymptoms rather increaſe, eſpecially if the tumor grow larger, and ſomewhat ſoft, with an increaſe of throbbing pain, we may then with tolerable certainty conclude that ſuppuration will take place. The means which were uſed for diſperſion muſt now be laid aſide, and endeavours be exerted to promote ſuppuration.

For this purpoſe, flannels wrung out of any emolient fomentation ought to be applied to the part as warm as the perſon can bear them, continued half an hour at a time, and repeated every three or four hours.

Immediately after the fomentation is over, a large emolient poultice ſhould likewiſe be applied warm, and renewed after every fomentation. Of all the forms recommended for emolient cataplaſms, a common milk and bread poultice, with a ſmall portion of freſh butter or oil, is perhaps the moſt eligible, as it not only poſſeſſes all the advantages of the others, but can in general be more eaſily obtained.

Onions, either roaſted or raw, garlic, and other acrid ſubſtances, are frequently made uſe of as additions to ripening cataplaſms or poultices. When there is not a due degree of inflammation in the tumor, the addition of ſuch ſubſtances may be of ſervice; but when ſtimulants are neceſſary in ſuch caſes, a ſmall proportion of ſtrained galbanum, or of any of the warm gums, diſſolved in the yolk of an egg, and added to the poultices, is a more effectual application.

When the ſwelling is come to maturity and matter is formed, which may be known by a re-miſſion of all the ſymptoms, and generally likewiſe by a fluctuation, unleſs the abſceſs be thickly covered with mufcles, it may be opened in the moft prominent part either with a lancet, or by means of cauftic, or feton. The firft, however, feems preferable. In many cafes nature will do the work herfelf, and abfceffes, when fuperficially feated, will certainly burft of themfelves; but where the matter lies deep, we are by no means to wait for this fpontaneous opening; as before the purulent matter can break through the integuments, it may acquire fuch an acrimony as will prove prejudicial to health. It is, however, a general rule not to open abfceffes till a thorough fcparation has taken place: for when laid open before that period, and while any confiderable hardnefs remains, they commonly prove more troublefome, and feldom heal fo kindly.

The laft way in which an inflammation terminates, is in a gangrene or mortification, which makes known its approach by the following fymptoms. The inflammation, from being red, affumes a dufkifh or livid colour; the tenfion of the fkin goes off, and it feels flabby; little bladders filled with a thin acrid fluid of different colours fpread all over it; the tumor fubfides, and at length becomes black. The pulfe at this period is quick and low, cold clammy fweats break forth, and death in a fhort time enfues.

On the firft appearance of thefe fymptoms, the part ought to be embrocated with a folution of fal ammoniac in vinegar and water: a drachm of the falt to two ounces of vinegar and fix of water, forms a mixture of a proper ftrength for every purpofe of this kind; but the degree of ftimulus can be eafily either increafed or diminifhed, according to circumftances, by ufing a larger or fmaller proportion of the falt. In this cafe the patient muft be fupported with generous wines, and the Peruvian bark adminiftered in as large dofes as the ftomach will bear. If the mortified parts fhould feparate, the wound will become a common ulcer, and muft be treated accordingly.

## *Wounds.*

It is a prevailing, though erroneous opinion, that particular and fpecific applications are neceffary for the cure of wounds; while, in fact, neither herbs, ointments, nor plafters, contribute to this purpofe in any other way than by keeping the parts foft and clean, and defending them from the influence of the external air. Dry lint alone, therefore may be as ufefully employed for producing the defired effect as any of the moft extolled applications in the province of furgery.

Medicines taken internally are no lefs inadequate to accomplifh the cure of wounds than thofe externally applied. It is nature alone that conducts the curative procefs in every divifion or lofs of ſubſtance incidental to the ſolid parts of the human body; and medicines can only promote that object by removing whatever might obſtruct or impede her ſalutary operations.

When a perſon has received a wound, the firſt thing which claims attention is to examine whether any foreign ſubſtance, ſuch as lead, iron, glaſs, bits of cloth, or the like, be lodged in it. Theſe, if poſſible, ought to be extracted, and the wound cleaned before any dreſſings be applied. But when the patient's weakneſs or loſs of blood will not admit of the extraction immediately, the ſubſtances muſt be ſuffered to remain in the wound till he can bear their removal with more ſafety.

In wounds which ſeem to threaten the loſs of life, the aſſiſtance of a ſurgeon is indiſpenſable; but ſometimes the diſcharge of blood is ſo great, that, if ſomething be not done immediately to ſtop it, the perſon may expire before ſuch aſſiſtance can be procured. It is therefore of importance to know what ought to be done in an emergency of this kind. If the wound be in any of the limbs, the application of a tight ligature or bandage round the member a little above the wound may generally ſtop the bleeding. To accompliſh this object, the beſt expedient is to put a ſtrong broad garter round the part, but ſo ſlack as eaſily to admit a ſmall piece of ſtick to be put under it; which muſt be twiſted, in the ſame manner as is practiſed by countrymen to ſecure their loading with a cart-rope, till the bleeding ſtops. But when this is effected, the garter muſt be twiſted no longer, as ſtraining it too much might produce an inflammation of the parts, and endanger a gangrene.

In parts where ſuch a bandage cannot be applied, recourſe muſt be had to other methods of ſtopping the hæmorrhage. Cloths dipped in ſtyptic water, or in a ſolution of blue vitriol, may be applied to the wound. When theſe cannot be obtained, ſtrong ſpirits of wine may be uſed for the purpoſe. The application of even common writing-ink might be of advantage. The agaric of the oak has been deſervedly recommended for this purpoſe. The part to be uſed is that which lies immediately under the outer rind; and the only preparation it requires, is to be beat well with a hammer till it becomes ſoft and very pliable. A ſlice of it, of a proper ſize is to be applied directly over the bleeding veſſels. Where the agaric cannot be had, ſponge may be uſed in its ſtead. Whether the agaric or ſponge be employed, it ought to be covered with a good deal of lint, above which a bandage may be applied ſo tight as to keep it firm upon the part.

In ſlight wounds, which do not penetrate much deeper than the ſkin, nothing better can be applied than the common black ſticking-plaſter. By keeping the ſides of the wound together, this prevents the admiſſion of air, which is all that is required for promoting the cure. But when a wound penetrates deep, its lips muſt not be kept too cloſe, as this would retain the matter, and might occaſion a feſtering of the part. In ſuch a caſe, the beſt method is to fill the wound with charpie or caddis, which, however, ought not to be ſtuffed in too hard. This application may be covered with a cloth dipped in oil, or ſpread with the common wax-plaſter; and the whole muſt be retained by a proper bandage.

The firſt dreſſing ſhould be allowed to remain for at leaſt two days; after which it may be removed, and freſh caddis or charpie be applied as before. If any part of the firſt dreſſing adheres ſo cloſe as not to be removed without occaſioning pain and violence to the wound, it may be allowed to continue, and ſome freſh materials of the ſame kind, dipped in ſweet oil, be laid over it. It will by this means be ſo much ſoftened, as to come off eaſily at the next dreſſing. The wound may afterwards be dreſſed twice a day in the ſame manner till it be quite healed. Thoſe who conſider this method as too ſimple, may, after the wound is become very ſuperficial, dreſs it with the ointment called yellow baſilicum; and if any funguous or proud fleſh, as it is termed, ſhould riſe in the wound, it may be reduced by mixing with the ointment a little burnt alum, or red precipitate of mercury.

When a wound is much inflamed, the beſt application is a poultice of milk and bread, with a little ſweet oil, or freſh butter; which ſhould be renewed every four hours.

In large wounds, and where there is reaſon to apprehend an inflammation, the patient ought to be kept on a low diet; abſtaining from fleſh, ſtrong liquors, and every thing of a heating nature. If he be of a full habit of body, and has loſt but little blood from the wound, he muſt be bled; and that too a ſecond time, ſhould the ſymptoms prove urgent. But if, on the contrary, he has been much weakened by a great diſcharge of blood from the wound, it would not be adviſable to bleed him, even though a fever ſupervened: for, without ſufficient ſtrength, the powers of nature could not long maintain the ſtruggle againſt the violence of the diſeaſe.

Perſons labouring under ſevere wounds ought always to be kept, as much as poſſible, quiet and eaſy. Every thing that diſcompoſes the mind is highly prejudicial; and nothing is more pernicious than an indulgence in venery. The patient's body, during the cure, ſhould be kept gently open, either by clyſters, or ſuch articles in diet as prove laxative: for example, ſtewed prunes, boiled ſpinnage, roaſted apples, and the like.

## *Burns and Scalds.*

Various remedies are recommended for the treatment of these accidents; and it happens fortunately for the pressure of such an emergency, that some of the most common things are also the most useful on the occasion. The pain of burns and scalds may be instantly abated by immersing the part affected in cold water, or indeed in any cold fluid, or in spirits of wine. An excellent application likewise is vinegar, with or without powdered chalk in it. If the injury be on the fingers or hands, the application may be made by immersion; but if in any part where this would be inconvenient, the vinegar may be applied by means of linen rags dipped in it. In slight injuries, the vinegar, if early and assiduously applied, will of itself soon effect a cure; but should any degree of pain return, the immersion or fomentation must be repeated.

In recent burns or scalds, attended with large blisters, excoriations, or loss of substance, the vinegar ought to be applied till the pain nearly ceases, which generally happens within eight hours. Many practitioners recommend spirits of turpentine instead of vinegar; or lime-water and linseed-oil. The vinegar need not be employed longer than twelve hours, except on the outside of the sores, which, while they continue to be swelled or inflamed, should be fomented for a minute or two before they are dressed.

For dressing the sores which arise from burns or scalds, one of the best applications is a poultice of bread, water, and sweet oil. This should be removed in six hours, when the sores are to be covered with chalk finely powdered, till it has absorbed the matter, and appears quite dry. A fresh poultice must be laid over the whole, which, with the sprinkling of the chalk, is to be repeated morning and evening till the sores are healed.

After the second or third day, if the sores be on a part of the body where it is difficult to keep the poultice from shifting, a plaster of cerate, thickly spread, may be used as a substitute in the day-time.

When there are large blisters upon the part they should be opened with a lancet before the application of the vinegar; and the water they contain be pressed out with a linen cloth, that the vinegar may act more closely upon the burnt flesh, which in this case it does efficaciously. In severe cases, and in cold weather, the vinegar should be nearly blood-warm.

If the patient will not suffer the vinegar to be applied immediately to the surface, on account of the pain it excites, a linen rag soaked in sweet oil may be previously laid on the part, covering the whole with cloths dipped in vinegar; and these applications are to be occasionally repeated till the pain and inflammation be entirely removed; after which the parts ſhould be dreſſed, or, if the burning be very deep, with a mixture of *that* and yellow baſilicon.

When the burn or ſcald is violent, or has produced a high degree of inflammation, ſo that there is reaſon to be apprehenſive of a gangrene, the ſame method of cure becomes neceſſary as in other violent inflammations. The patient, in this caſe, muſt be put upon a low diet, and drink plentifully of weak diluting liquors. He muſt likewiſe be bled, and his body be kept open. But if the burnt parts ſhould become livid or black, with other ſymptoms of mortification, it will be neceſſary to apply to them camphorated ſpirits of wine, tincture of myrrh, and other antiſeptics or correctors of putrefaction, mixed with a decoction of the Peruvian bark. In this caſe, the bark muſt likewiſe be taken internally; the patient at the ſame time uſing a more generous diet, with wine, ſpiceries, &c.

When burns are occaſioned by the exploſion of gun powder, ſome of the grains of the powder are apt to be forced into the ſkin. At firſt they produce much irritation; and, if they be not removed, they commonly leave marks which remain during life. They ſhould therefore be picked out as ſoon as poſſible after the accident; and to prevent inflammation, as well as to diſſolve any powder which may remain, the parts affected, ſhould be covered for a day or two with emollient poultices,

A ſtrong ſolution of ſoap in water has long been in uſe with artificers employed in any buſineſs expoſing workmen to very bad ſcalds. This is allowed to be an excellent remedy. But, as the ſoap would take ſome time in diſſolving, and the ſolution ſome time in cooling, Dr. Underwood recommends a mixture of ſix ounces of oil to ten of water, with two drachms of the ley of kali; or potaſh. This quantity may be ſufficient for a burn on the hand or foot, which is to be immerſed, and kept about half an hour in the liquor, which will remove the injury, if recourſe to it immediately be had; but muſt be repeated, as the pain may require, if the ſcald or burn be of ſome ſtanding.

The moſt uſeful application, we are told, with which families can be provided againſt any emergency of this kind, is a ſtrong brine, made by placing ſliced potatoes and common ſalt in alternate layers in a pan, allowing them to remain until the whole of the ſalt is liquified; which muſt be then drained off, and kept in bottles, properly labelled, ready for immediate uſe.

## *Bruiſes.*

As bruiſes exiſt in various degrees, they are to be treated accordingly. In ſlight caſes it will be ſufficient to foment the part with warm vinegar, to which may be added occaſionally a little brandy or rum, and to keep conſtantly applied to it cloths wet with this mixture. But when a bruiſe is very violent, the patient ought immediately to be bled. His diet ſhould be light and cool, conſiſting chiefly of vegetables; and his drink weak, and of an opening nature, ſuch as whey ſweetened with honey, cream of tartar whey, decoctions of tamarinds, &c. The bruiſed part muſt be fomented with warm vinegar and water; applying to it, afterwards, a poultice made by boiling crumb of bread, elder-flowers, and chamomile-flowers, in equal quantities of vinegar and water. This poultice may be renewed two or three times a day, and is particularly proper when the bruiſe is attended with a wound.

When a bruiſe is attended with a violent pain, twenty-five or thirty drops of laudanum may be given, and repeated in a few hours, if neceſſary.

## *Ulcers.*

An ulcer is a ſolution of the continuity in any of the ſofter parts of the body, diſcharging pus, ſanies, or any other matter. They may happen in conſequence of wounds, bruiſes, or impoſthumes improperly treated; and may likewiſe proceed from a bad habit of body, in which the humours are depraved, by poor living, or a want of ſufficient exerciſe.

When an ulcer diſcharges matter of a mild kind, and a good conſiſtence, called laudable pus, it is in a fair way of healing in a ſhort time; but if it be of long duration, the humour watery and acrid, and the edges callous or hard, the cure of it is generally extremely difficult and tedious. In fact, as ulcers of this deſcription proceed from a bad habit of body, or venereal taint, it is more ſafe to refrain from attempting to heal them, until the conſtitution be improved by a proper regimen, or medicines; and when ſuch a change has taken place, they will be diſpoſed to heal of their own accord.

Ulcers which have been occaſioned by malignant fevers, or other acute diſeaſes, may for the moſt part be ſafely healed after the patient's health is entirely re-eſtabliſhed; though even then he muſt obſerve a proper regimen, and his body be kept open by gentle purgatives. The ſame caution muſt likewiſe be uſed, in reſpect to ulcers which accompany chronical diſeaſes. It may be laid down as a general rule, that if during the continuance of an ulcer the perſon otherwiſe enjoys good health, it ought not to be healed, eſpecially if it be of long ſtanding; but if, on the contrary, the patient's ſtrength ſenſibly declines, the cure of it ſhould be promoted with all poſſible ſpeed.

A ſtrict attention to regimen is in no caſe more neceſſary than in the cure of ulcers. To promote it, the patient muſt be temperate in eating and drinking; muſt live chiefly on cooling laxative vegetables, avoid all high ſeaſoned food, and ſtrong liquors; and for drink uſe butter-milk, or whey ſweetened with honey. He ought alſo to take moderate exerciſe, and cultivate a cheerful diſpoſition.

When the edges or any part of an ulcer are hard and callous, they may be ſprinkled twice a day with a little red precipitate, and afterwards dreſſed with the yellow *baſilicum* ointment. This is likewiſe done by touching them a few days with the lunar cauſtic. Some practitioners cut them off with a knife; but this is a painful operation, and not more efficacious.

Lime-water is often of great efficacy in the cure of obſtinate ulcers: for which purpoſe it may be uſed in the ſame manner as directed with regard to the ſtone and gravel; and in all caſes of obſtinate ulcers, the Peruvian bark, plentifully adminiſtered, will be found of great advantage.

When ulcers are attended with great pain and inflammation, bleeding, and opening the body with purgatives, will often be ſerviceable; but, above all things, reſt, and a horizontal poſture; which laſt circumſtance is of ſo great importance to the cure of ulcers in the legs, that, unleſs the patient ſtrictly conform to it, the ſkill of the ſurgeon, however well directed, will often prove abortive: for, as the indiſpoſition of theſe ſores is in ſome meaſure owing to the gravitation of the humours downwards, it will be much more beneficial to lie along than ſit upright, though the leg be laid on a chair; ſince even in this poſture they will deſcend with more force than if the body was reclined.

## CHAP. XLIV.

### *Diſlocations, and Sprains or Strains.*

WHAT is termed the diſlocation or luxation of a bone, is the ſtate in which that part of it which forms a joint is moved out of its place. When a bone is forced entirely out of a cavity, the diſlocation is called *compleat;* when this is not the caſe, it is *partial* or *incompleat.* That a bone is diſlocated may be known from the inability to move the injured limb, or by comparing it with the same joint on the other side. The accident is likewise attended with pain, tension, and a deformity in the part affected; sometimes with inflammation, twitcings of the tendons, and fever: but these three last are greater in partial dislocations.

In whatever part a dislocation happens, it is of great consequence that it should be reduced as soon as possible, because the operation becomes extremely difficult, if indeed practicable, after the swelling and inflammation have come on. If any thing, therefore, calls for the immediate interference of a person not a professed surgeon, it is an accident of this kind; and there needs only common resolution to interpose with happy effect.

A recent dislocation may generally be reduced by extension, or simple pulling, alone, which must vary in degree, according to the strength of the muscles which move the joint, the age, vigour, and other circumstances of the patient. If the bone has been dislocated any considerable time, and a swelling or inflammation has come on, it will be necessary to bleed the patient, and, after fomenting the part with warm vinegar, to apply soft poultices to it, for some time before the reduction is attempted.

After reduction, there is seldom any difficulty in retaining the bone in its place, unless it has often been dislocated before. All that is necessary is to apply cloths dipt in vinegar or camphorated spirits of wine to the part, to place the limb in a relaxed posture, and keep it perfectly easy. If any degree of inflammation remain, the use of leeches is the best remedy.

To keep the limb in an easy posture, is a matter of the utmost consequence: for their seldom happens any dislocation without the ligaments and tendons of the joint being stretched, and sometimes otherwise injured. While these are kept easy till they recover their strength and tone, the amendment gradually advances; but if the parts be irritated by too frequent an exertion, they may remain debilitated ever after.

## *Dislocation of the Jaw.*

The lower jaw may be luxated by yawning, blows, falls, chewing hard substances, or the like. This accident may be known to have taken place, from the patient's being unable to shut his mouth, or to eat any thing. The chin, likewise, either hangs down, or is wrested to one side; and the patient is neither able to speak distinctly, nor to swallow without considerable difficulty.

The common method of reducing a dislocated jaw is to place the patient upon a low stool, in such a manner that an assistant may hold the head firm by pressing it against his breast. The operator is then to push his two thumbs, protected with linen-cloths that they may not be bitten when the jaw slips into its place, as far back into the patient's mouth as he can, and then, with his fingers applied to the outside of the angle of the jaw, endeavour to bring it forward till it move a little from its situation. He should then press it forcibly downwards and backwards, by which means the elapsed heads of the jaw will immediately slip into their place.

In some parts of the country, the peasants perform this operation in the following manner; which, though sometimes successful, is doubtless attended with danger. One of them puts a handkerchief under the patient's chin; then, turning his back to that of the patient, pulls him up by the chin so as to suspend him from the ground.

## *Dislocation of the Neck.*

This part of the body may be dislocated by falls. A complete dislocation of the neck is immediately followed by death; but for the most part the accident is only partial. In this dislocation, the patient is immediately deprived of all sense and motion; his neck swells; his countenance appears bloated; his chin lies upon his breast, and his face is generally turned towards one side.

To reduce this luxation, the unfortunate person should immediately be laid upon his back on the ground, and the operator must place himself behind him, in such a manner as to be able to lay hold of his head with both hands, while he makes a resistance by placing his knees against the patient's shoulders. In this posture he must pull the head with considerable force, gently twisting it at the same time, if the face be turned to one side, till he perceives that the joint is replaced. This may be known from the noise which the bones generally make upon reduction, the patient's beginning to breathe, and the head remaining in its natural posture. After the dislocation is reduced, the patient ought to be bled, and should be suffered to rest for some days, till the parts recover their proper tone.

## *Dislocation of the Ribs.*

The articulation of the ribs with the back-bone being extremely firm, a dislocation of this part is happily a very rare occurrence. When it does, however, take place, either upwards or downwards, in order to replace it, the patient should be laid upon his belly on a table, and the operator must endeavour to push the head of the bone into its proper place. If this method should not fucceed, the arm of the diflocated fide may be fufpended over a gate or ladder, and, while the ribs are thus ftretched afunder, the heads of fuch as are out of place may be thruft into their former fituation.

Thofe diflocations in which the heads of the ribs are forced inwards, are not only more dangerous, but the moft difficult to reduce, as no means can be applied internally to direct the luxated heads of the ribs. Almoft the only thing that can be done is to lay the patient upon his belly over a calk, or fome fuch body, and to move the forepart of the rib inward towards the back, fometimes fhaking it. By this means the heads of the luxated ribs may flip into their former fituation.

## *Diflocation of the Shoulder.*

The humerus or upper bone of the arm is the molt fubject to diflocation of any in the body, and may be luxated in various directions: the accident, however, happens moft frequently downwards, but very feldom directly upwards. This diflocation may be difcovered by the patient's inability ro raife his arm, as well as by violent pain in attempting it, and by a depreffion or cavity on the top of the fhoulder. When the diflocation is downward or forward, the arm is lengthened, and a ball or lump is perceived uuder the arm-pit; but when it is backward, there appears a protuberance behind the fhoulder, and the arm is thrown forwards toward the breaft.

The ufual method of reducing a diflocation of the fboulder is to feat the patient upon a low ftool, and to caufe an affiftant to hold his body firm, while another lays hold of the arm a little above the elbow, and gradually extends it. The operator then puts a napkin under the patient's arm, and caufes it to be tied behind his own neck. By this, while a fufficient extention is made, he lifts up the head of the bone, and with his hands directs it into its proper place. In young and delicate perfons, an operator may generally reduce this diflocation by extending the arm with one hand, and thrufting in the head of the bone with the other. In making the extenfion, the elbow ought always to be a little bent.

## *Diflocation of the Elbow.*

The bones of the fore-arm may be diflocated in any direction, but moft commonly upwards and backwards. In this luxation, a protuberance may be obferved on that fide of the arm towards which the bone is pufhed; from which circumftance, joined to the patient's inability to bend his arm, a luxation at the elbow may be known.

For reducing a dislocation at the elbow, two assistants are for the most part necessary: one of them must lay hold of the arm above, and the other below, the joint, and make a pretty strong extension, while the operator returns the bones into their proper place. The arm must afterwards be bent, and suspended for some time with a sling about the neck.

Dislocations of the wrist and fingers are to be reduced in the same manner as those of the elbow, viz. by making an extension in different directions, and thrusting the head of the bone into its place.

## *Dislocation of the Thigh.*

When the thigh-bone is dislocated forward and downward, the knee and foot are turned out, and the leg is longer than the other; but when it is displaced backward, it is usually pushed upward at the same time, by which means the limb is shortened, and the foot is turned inward.

When the thigh-bone is displaced forward and downward, the patient, in order to its reduction, must be laid upon his back, and made fast by bandages, or held by assistants, while by others an extension is made by means of slings fixed about the bottom of the thigh a little above the knee. While the extension is made, the operator must push the head of the bone outward till it gets into the socket. If the dislocation be outward, the patient must be laid upon his face, and, during the extension, the head of the bone must be pushed inward.

Dislocations of the knees, ancles, and toes, are reduced much in the same manner as those of the upper extremities, viz. by making an extension in opposite directions, while the operator replaces the bones. In many cases however, the extension alone is sufficient, and the bone will slip into its place merely by pulling the limb with sufficient force. It is not hereby meant, that force alone is sufficient for the reduction of dislocations. Skill and dexterity will often succeed better than force; and one man who possesses them has been able to perform what the united force of many was found inadequate to accomplish.

# CHAP. XLV.

## *Broken Bones, or Fractures.*

TO reduce fractured bones properly demands, doubtless, the skill and dexterity of an expert surgeon; but where this cannot be obtained, the next object is, that the person who undertakes such a task should be furnished with such information as may prove useful in assisting him how to perform it. A few hints for this purpose may therefore not be improper.

When a large bone is broken, the patient's diet ought, in all respects, to be the same as in an inflammatory fever. He should likewise be kept quiet and cool, and his body open, either by means of emollient clysters, or food of a laxative quality, such as stewed prunes, boiled spinnage, &c. Persons, however, who have been accustomed to live high, must not be reduced all of a sudden to a very low diet; as such a transition might be attended with the most pernicious effects.

In general it is proper to bleed the patient immediately after a fracture, especially if he be young, of a full habit, or has, at the same time, received any considerable bruises; and if he continue feverish, the operation may be repeated next day. Blood-letting is peculiarly necessary when several ribs are broken.

If any of the large bones which support the body are broken, the patient must keep his bed for several weeks. There is, however, no necessity that he should lie all that time, as usual, upon his back; which is a situation extremely irksome and incommodious. After the second week he may be gently raised up, and may sit several hours, supported by a bed-chair, or the like, which will greatly conduce to his refreshment. But care must be taken in raising him up, and laying him down, that he make no exertions himself; otherwise the action of the muscles may be sufficient to displace the bone. It is likewise of great importance to keep the patient dry and clean while in this situation: for if he finds himself uncomfortable, he will be perpetually changing his position for ease.

It has been a customary practice when a bone was broken, to keep the limb for five or six weeks continually upon the stretch. But this posture is both uneasy to the patient, and unfavourable to the cure. It is now admittted, that the best situation is to keep the limb a little bent; which may easily be done, either by laying the patient upon his side, or making the bed in such a manner as to favour this position of the limb.

In the treatment of a fracture, care should be taken to examine whether the bone be not shattered or broken into several pieces. In such a case it will sometimes be necessary to have the limb immediately taken off; otherwise a gangrene or mortification may be the consequence.

When a fracture is attended with a wound, the treatment of the latter is in no respect different from that of a common wound.

It is nature only that conducts the cure of a broken bone; and the utmost efforts of art are of no more avail than to lay it in its proper position, and keep it as much so as possible. All tight bandages are prejudicial. The best method of retention is by two or more splints, made of pasteboard, or strong leather. These, if moistened before they are applied, soon accommodate themselves to the shape of the included member, and are sufficient, by the assistance of a very slight bandage, to retain it in its place. The most proper bandage for the purpose is that made with twelve or eighteen tails; which is much easier applied and removed than rollers, at the same time that it is equally retentive. The splints should always be of the same length with the limb, and be furnished with holes adapted to receive the ancles, when the fracture is in the leg.

In fractures of the ribs, instead of a bandage, it may be preferable to apply a broad leather belt pretty tight, and continue it for some weeks.

In all cases of fractured bones, the most proper external application is *oxycrate*, or a mixture of vinegar and water, with which the bandages should be wet at every dressing.

## *Strains.*

Strains, from being generally neglected, are often attended with worse consequences than broken bones. Under the latter circumstance, the patient is incapable of using the injured member; but, in the former, finding a possibility of motion, he endeavours to exercise it, and thereby increases the complaint.

It is a common practice among country people to immerse a strained limb in cold water; and this is a very proper remedy, provided it be done immediately, and not continued too long. But if a swelling comes on before recourse is had to the immersion, this expedient is, then, extremely improper; and, if it be continued too long, instead of bracing, it greatly increases the relaxation.

Many external applications are recommended for strains, some of which are beneficial, some hardly of any effect, and others hurtful. The most safe and useful are the following, viz. warm vinegar, mindererus's ſpirit, volatile liniment, and a poultice of oatmeal, vinegar, and oil. But nothing is more effectual than *eaſe*, continued for a due length of time.

## *Ruptures.*

This diſorder depending generally upon a laxity of the conſtitution, is moſt incident to children and old people, in whom it may be excited by various occaſional cauſes; in the former claſs by crying, coughing, vomiting, or the like; and in the latter by blows, violent exertions of ſtrength, and ſtrains, &c. It has been obſerved that they are moſt frequent among the inhabitants of thoſe countries where oil is much uſed as an article of diet.

Ruptures are extremely various in point of ſituation; and likewiſe in the bowels which produce them. The parts in which they uſually appear are the groin, ſcrotum, labia pudendi, the upper and fore part of the thigh; the umbilicus, or navel; and different points between the interſtices of the abdominal muſcles. Inſtances have occurred of the ſtomach, womb, liver, ſpleen, and bladder, being found to form their contents. But a part of the inteſtinal canal, or a portion of the omentum, or cawl, are known from experience to be the moſt frequent cauſe of their formation.

On the firſt appearance of this diſorder it is commonly of no very conſiderable ſize; ſuch tumors ſeldom acquiring any great bulk at once: but, by repeated deſcents of the bowels it is gradually increaſed, till, in ſome inſtances, it becomes at laſt of great magnitude, and occaſions much diſtreſs to the patient. This ariſes either from an obſtruction to the paſſage of the fæces when the inteſtinal canal forms the tumor, or from a ſtoppage of circulation, occaſioned by ſtricture on the prolapſed parts; ſo that the diſorder will be always more or leſs hazardous, according to the nature of the part ſo protruded.

A rupture being generally inconſiderable at its commencement, ſometimes proves fatal before it is known to be formed. On this account, whenever ſickneſs, vomiting, and obſtinate coſtiveneſs give reaſon to ſuſpect an obſtruction of the bowels, all thoſe places where ruptures uſually happen ought to be carefully examined: for, by neglecting this inquiry, many perſons have been cut off by ruptures who were not ſuſpected to have any ſuch diſorder till after they were dead.

On the firſt appearance of a rupture in an infant, it ought to be laid upon its back, with its head very low. If, in this poſture the gut does not return of itſelf, it may eaſily be put up by gentle preſſure: after which a piece of ſticking-plaſter may be applied over the part, and a proper truſs, or bandage, muſt be conſtantly worn for a confiderable time. The child muft be kept as much as poffible from crying, and from all violent exertions, till the rupture is quite healed.

In adult perfons, when the gut has been forced down with great violence, or happens from any caufe to be inflamed, the cure of a rupture is far more difficult, and fometimes impracticable, by the ufual means of reduction. In fuch a cafe, however, the following method may be purfued:

The patient, having been bled, muft be laid upon his back, with his head very low, and his breech raifed high with pillows. In this fituation, flannel cloths wrung out of a decoction of mallows and chamomile flowers; or, in want of thefe, warm water, muft be applied for a confiderable time, to relax the ftricture upon the gut. A clyfter made of the fame decoction, with a large fpoonful of butter, and an ounce or two of falt, or of water, with a little Caftile foap, may be afterwards thrown up. If thefe fhould not prove fuccefsful, recourfe muft be had to preffure. If the tumor be very hard, confiderable force will be neceffary; but dexterity chiefly is requifite. The operator, at the fame time that he makes a preffure with the palms of his hands, muft, with his finger, artfully introduce the gut by the fame aperture through which it had efcaped. Should thefe endeavours prove ineffectual, it will be proper to make trial of clyfters of the fmoke of tobacco, which have often produced good effects where no other remedy has availed.

The laft refource in an obftinate *hernia* is an operation with the knife; but this is fo nice and difficult, that before it be adopted every other method fhould be tried. After the gut has been returned, the patient muft wear a fteel bandage, or trufs, for a long time.

Thofe who have a rupture ought carefully to avoid all violent exertions of the body, as well as flatulent or windy food, coftivenefs, and catching cold.

## CHAP. XLVI.

### *Cafualties.*

IT is not uncommon for every appearance of life to be fufpended by a fudden and violent accident, at the fame time that there ftill remains a poffibility of reftoring the vital motions by affiduous and well directed efforts. The truth of this obfervation is confirmed by innumerable inftances, which it would be fuperfluous to produce; and it ought to excite in the public a general diſapprobation of that inconſiderate and criminal remiſſneſs which permits the flame of life, when only obſcured, to be irrecoverably extinguiſhed through a total neglect of the means of reſuſcitation. In caſes ſuch as have been mentioned, nothing leſs than a certainty that death has taken place ſhould ever preclude the moſt active exertions to prevent it; but, however ſuſpicion may prevail, and probability favour its ſuggeſtions, there can exiſt no certainty relative to the ſubject until careful inquiry ſhall have clearly aſcertained that the organs eſſential and neceſſary to life are irreparably deſtroyed.

Ignorance and ſuperſtition have both contributed to ſupport the inhuman cuſtom which is at preſent the object of our cenſure. It is a traditional interdiction, derived from the times of rude antiquity, that the body of a perſon killed by accident ſhould not be laid in a houſe that is inhabited. But a more enlightened æra has exploded ſuch barbarous doctrine; and it is now juſtly regarded, not only as a duty, but a highly meritorious office, both to receive into an inhabited houſe the body of a perſon apparently dead from ſome accident, and to exert every effort for reſtoring, if poſſible, the powers of ſuſpended animation.

When a perſon, of a ſudden, ſeems to be deprived of life, the object of immediate inquiry is to examine into the cauſe. If ſuffocation by foul air ſhould appear to have produced the accident, the body ſhould be withdrawn, without the ſmalleſt delay, from the ſpot where it lies, and a free ventilation be procured. If there be no reaſon to ſuſpect ſuch a cauſe, it will then be proper to examine whether reſpiration has been ſtopped by any thing that may have got into the wind-pipe; or whether any dangerous intruſive ſubſtance has made its way into the gullet.

If the vital motions be ſuddenly ſtopped, from any cauſe whatever, except mere weakneſs, the patient ought to be bled. Should the blood not flow, upon opening a vein, the body may be rubbed with warm cloths, ſalt, &c. or it may be immerſed in warm water, or covered with warm grains, aſhes, ſand, or the like, to reſtore the circulation.

## *Subſtances ſtopt in the Gullet.*

One of the moſt common accidents, attended with great danger, is the inadvertently ſwallowing of ſubſtances which are likely to ſtick in the paſſage between the mouth and the ſtomach, and from which ſituation it may be impoſſible, by any contrivance, to bring them up, or to forward their deſcent without hazarding the life of the perſon. This effect may be produced by a lump of food too large for the diameter of the gullet; or by ſharp-pointed ſubſtances, ſuch as pins, nails, and the like; which people often imprudently hold in their mouth, and afterwards, without reflection, ſuffer them to eſcape the palate.

When any ſubſtance is detained in the gullet, there are two ways by which we may endeavour to remove it; and theſe are, either by extracting it, or puſhing it down. The former is by far the ſafeſt way, but not always the eaſieſt. When, therefore, the obſtructing body is of ſuch a nature that no danger can ariſe from its reception into the ſtomach, the expedient moſt adviſable in ſuch an emergency is to puſh it down. The ſubſtances which may be thus protruded with ſafety are, bread, fleſh, fruits, and other aliments. But all indigeſtible ſubſtances, ſuch as cork, wood, bone, &c. ought, if poſſible, to be extracted, eſpecially if theſe bodies be ſharp-pointed, as pins, needles, fiſh-bones, and the like.

When thoſe ſubſtances have not advanced in their paſſage beyond the reach of the hand, we ſhould endeavour to extract them with our fingers; and this method often ſucceeds; when they have proceeded farther, it will be proper to make uſe of nippers, or a ſmall pair of forceps, an inſtrument employed by ſurgeons. If the fingers and nippers fail, or cannot be duly applied, recourſe ſhould be had to the kind of hooks called crotchets. Theſe may be readily made by bending a piece of iron wire at one end. For conducting ſuch an inſtrument with greater ſafety, there ſhould likewiſe be a curvature, or bending, at the other end; which may be tied with a ſtring to ſecure it from ſlipping out of the hand of the operator. The crotchet having paſſed below the ſubſtance which obſtructs the paſſage, and being drawn up again, hooks up with it the offending body. The crotchet may alſo be employed when a ſubſtance ſomewhat flexible, as a pin, or fiſh-bone, ſticks acroſs the gullet; the hook, in ſuch caſes, ſeizing them about their middle part, bends them in ſuch a manner as to facilitate their extraction; or, if they are very brittle ſubſtances, ſerves to break them.

When the obſtructing bodies are ſmall, and only ſtop up a part of the paſſage, and which may either eaſily elude the hook, or, by their reſiſtance, unbend the curvature, a kind of ring may be uſed. For this purpoſe, a piece of fine wire, of a proper length, may be bent into a circle, about the middle, of about an inch diameter, and the long unbent ſides brought parallel, and near each other: theſe are to be held in the hand, while the circular part, or ring, is introduced into the gullet, in order to incloſe the obſtructing body, and ſo to extract it. More flexible rings may be made of thread, ſilk, and ſmall pack-thread; which, for their greater ſtrength, may be waxed. One of theſe is to be tied faſt to a handle of iron wire, whalebone, or any kind of flexible wood, and by this means introduced in order to ſurround the obſtructing ſubſtances, and extract it. To lay hold of the obſtructing body with more certainty, it may ſometimes be proper to paſs ſeveral of theſe rings through one another; thus providing for ſucceſſive chances of action, if one or more rings ſhould fail of the deſired effect. Theſe rings have this advantage, that when the ſubſtance to be extracted is once laid hold of, it may then, by turning the handle, be retained ſo ſtrongly in the ring, thus twiſted, as to admit of being moved every way, and thereby facilitate the extraction.

Another expedient employed on theſe unhappy occaſions is the ſponge; the utility of which is chiefly owing to its property of ſwelling on being wet. If any ſubſtance be ſtopped in the gullet, but without filling up the whole paſſage, a bit of ſponge may be introduced through the vacuity; where, having ſwelled by the moiſture of the ſurrounding parts, or, more ſpeedily, by making the patient ſwallow a few drops of water, it is afterwards drawn back by the handle to which it is faſtened; and, being now too large to return through the narrow paſſage by which it had deſcended, it meets with a reſiſtance from the obſtructing body, and puſhes it upwards.

When all theſe methods fail of extracting the offenſive ſubſtance, there remains one reſource more, which is to make the patient vomit. But this expedient only can be of any ſervice where the obſtructing body is not ſtuck into the ſides of the gullet; as, otherwiſe, vomiting, inſtead of giving relief, might occaſion farther miſchief. If the patient can ſwallow, vomiting may be excited by taking half a drachm of the powder of ipecacuanha made into a draught. If he be not able to ſwallow, an attempt may be made to excite vomiting, by the common practice of tickling his throat with a feather; and if that ſhould not ſucceed, a clyſter of tobacco may be adminiſtered, which has often proved effectual in exciting a motion to vomit, when other attempts for that purpoſe have failed. It is made by boiling an ounce of tobacco in a ſufficient quantity of water.

When the obſtructing body is of ſuch a nature that it may with ſafety be puſhed downwards, this may be attempted by means of a wax candle oiled, and a little heated, ſo as to render it flexible. For the ſame purpoſe may be employed a piece of whalebone, wire, or flexible cane, with a ſponge faſtened to one end. If every effort ſhould prove abortive to extract even thoſe bodies which it is dangerous to admit into the ſtomach, we cannot heſitate a moment with regard to the propriety of puſhing them down into that organ, ſince a precarious alternative is preferable to the certainty which muſt otherwiſe exiſt of the patient's dying in a few minutes; and ſuch a reſolution is more juſtifiable in being ſupported by many inſtances where a ſimilar conduct has been followed with the happieſt effects.

When it is found to be impracticable either to extract or puſh down the obſtructing ſubſtance, it will be proper to deſiſt from any further efforts for that purpoſe; becauſe the inflammation which would enſue from the continuance of them might prove no leſs dangerous to the patient than the obſtruction itſelf.

During the uſe of the above-mentioned means for removing the obſtructing ſubſtance, the patient ſhould frequently ſwallow ſome emollient liquor, ſuch as warm milk and water, or a decoction of mallows; or, if he cannot ſwallow, theſe applications ſhould be introduced into the gullet by injection. They not only ſoften and ſooth the irritated parts, but, when injected with force, prove often more effectual in removing the obſtruction than any other expedient that can be employed.

When, in ſpite of all our endeavours to diſlodge the obſtruction, it ſtill remains immovable, the patient muſt be treated conformably to a ſtate of inflammation. He ought to be bled, kept upon a low diet, and emollient poultices applied round his whole neck; and the ſame treatment will be neceſſary if there be any reaſon to ſuſpect an inflammation of the gullet, though the obſtructing body ſhould be removed.

Inſtances have occurred where the obſtructing body has been diſlodged by a proper degree of agitation. Even a blow on the back has often forced up a ſubſtance which ſtuck in the gullet. But this expedient is yet more efficacious when the ſubſtance gets into the wind-pipe. In this caſe it is likewiſe of advantage to excite vomiting and ſneezing. Pins, which ſtuck in the gullet, have often been diſcharged by riding on horſeback, or in a carriage.

When any indigeſtible ſubſtance, as a coin, has been forced down into the ſtomach, the patient ought to uſe a very mild and ſmooth diet, ſuch as broths, puddings, boiled or roaſted apples, &c. avoiding all heating and irritating food and drink; the latter of which ſhould be milk and water, barley-water, or whey.

When the gullet is ſo completely obſtructed that the patient can receive no nouriſhment by the month, it will be neceſſary to ſupport him by clyſters of broth, ſoup, milk, jelly, and the like.

In caſes where reſpiration is ſo much impeded by an obſtruction in the wind-pipe that there is danger of immediate ſuffocation, the only expedient for protracting the life of the patient is by making a temporary aperture into that paſſage. But this operation, which is termed *bronchotomy*, ſhould be performed by the hand of a ſurgeon.

*Persons apparently Drowned.*

As soon as the body is discovered it ought to be conveyed in a blanket with all expedition to some house, where the process should immediately commence. If the body be that of a child, there is a possibility of its recovering by being laid naked in a bed between two persons stripped to the shirt, who should benevolently contribute their assistance on such an occasion. But if it be the body of a youth, or grown up person, it ought to be laid upon a bed or couch gently sloping, and with the head a little raised. If in winter, the place should be heated with a fire; but if in summer, and the sun shines, the body may be exposed to the warmth of its beams. After being wiped dry with warm cloths it ought to be diligently rubbed with flannel, lightly sprinkled with brandy, rum, or any spirituous liquor. Bottles or bladders, filled with hot water; or heated tiles or bricks, should also be procured, and wrapped up in flannel, be applied to the hands and feet. The warming-pans might likewise be lightly moved along the spine or back bone.

An effort should next be made to inflate the lungs, or fill them with air. For this purpose a person should, with his hand, stop the mouth and one of the nostrils, while another blows gently with a bellows into the open nostril. If a bellows should not be at hand, some benevolent assistant might compensate the deficiency by applying his mouth to that of the object, and breathing forcibly into it. After which the breast ought to be slightly pressed downward to expel the air again, and thus imitate the act of respiration.

If the means hitherto mentioned should not prove effectual, a clyster of mulled wine or some other powerful stimulant, such as warm brandy and water, should be given, and repeated three times in an hour.

The agitation of the body, by moving it in various directions, ought also to be practised. If these various means, though continued during an hour, should still not succeed, the next expedient should be to procure the means of warmth.

Electricity, where there happens to be an apparatus for that purpose, ought also to be tried.

Should any kind of movement, such as twitchings, contractions, &c. be perceptible, there is great reason to expect a happy termination of the process. Every effort should now be exerted with redoubled assiduity. A spoonful or two of tepid or lukewarm water should, if possible, be passed down the throat; and even a little wine, brandy, rum, or whatever of the kind may be at hand. If spirituous liquors be used, they may be diluted with two-thirds of water. The perſon ſhould then be laid in a bed, and kept perfectly quiet in order to enjoy ſome repoſe, by which the reſtoration will be completed.

Such is the method recommended by the Society for conducting the proceſs, the particulars of which are calculated to revive the powers of nature, and excite into freſh action the vital functions of reſpiration and the motion of the heart.

I ſhall only ſubjoin to theſe directions, that the chief means of promoting reſuſcitation is to excite a general warmth. The body ſhould be immediately ſtripped, and every effort made as ſpeedily as poſſible to produce that effect. The beſt thing for the purpoſe is the tepid bath; but if this cannot be procured, the perſon may be covered with warm ſand, aſhes, or thick blankets, in a bed; and heated bricks or ſtones, or bottles with hot water, ſhould be applied to various parts of the body. For it is much better to warm thoroughly perſons apparently dead, than to uſe friction, clyſters, &c. and at the ſame time to ſuffer them to become ſtiff with cold.

After blowing air into the lungs, it would be proper to apply volatile ſalts or ſpirits to the noſtrils.

The time requiſite for effecting theſe purpoſes muſt vary in different perſons, according to the degree of irritability with which the body is endowed. In moſt caſes the end is obtained in about the ſpace of an hour; but there are inſtances of its being retarded to the expiration of four hours. It is therefore adviſible to continue the employment of the means at leaſt to the termination of that period. And if gratitude can ever be due for any benefit received, it muſt be to thoſe who contribute their aſſiſtance in an emergency ſo preſſing and deciſive of the fate of a fellow creature.

The means above recommended are likewiſe applicable in the caſe of ſuſpenſion by the cord. But in this circumſtance a few ounces of blood may be taken from the jugular vein; cupping-glaſſes be applied to the head and neck, and leeches to the temples.

## *Noxious Vapours.*

Air may be rendered unfit for reſpiration either from a defect of the vital principle, or its being impregnated with noxious exhalations, of which there are various kinds.

As both fire and candles conſume a great deal of vital air, it is hurtful to ſit in a ſmall cloſe room where they both are uſed, eſpecially where the air is contaminated by exhalations from the lungs of ſeveral perſons or animals. In ſuch an apartment, the vapours of coal, and other fuel, with the ſmell of candles, or lamps, when the flame is extinguiſhed, are all extremely prejudicial, and have often even proved fatal.

The vapour which exhales from any fermented liquor, while in the ſtate of fermentation in a cloſe veſſel, if imprudently received by any perſon into the lungs, may occaſion inſtantaneous death. On this account it is dangerous to venture into cellars where a large quantity of ſuch liquors are in a ſtate of fermentation, eſpecially if they have been cloſe ſhut up for ſome time.

The ſame effects abovementioned are produced on opening ſubterraneous caves which have been long ſhut up, or on cleaning deep wells which have not been emptied for ſeveral years. No perſon therefore ought to venture into any ſuch place, where dampneſs and a long ſtagnation of the air have produced unwholeſome and mephitic vapours, until theſe have been ſufficiently corrected by the fumes of gunpowder exploded or ſhavings burnt. The common means is by letting down a lighted candle, or throwing in burning fuel. If theſe continue to burn, it is a proof that the air is not corrupted; but if they be ſuddenly extinguiſhed, immediate death would be the conſequence of entering thoſe places, until the air has been purified by the deflagration of gunpowder.

It is common for perſons of a delicate conſtitution to find their breathing oppreſſed in a cloſe apartment, where the air is corrupted by a number of candles, and the reſpiration of a crowded aſſembly. In ſuch circumſtances they ought to withdraw from the ſcene as ſoon as they find themſelves begin to be incommoded. If, after getting into the open air, they continue to feel any uneaſineſs, it will be abated by drinking a little hot lemonade, or water and vinegar of the ſame temperature.

If a perſon has been ſo much affected by the corrupted atmoſphere as to be rendered inſenſible, he ſhould be expoſed to the freſh and open air; and volatile ſalts, or other ſtimulating ſubſtances, held to his noſe. It will next be proper to bleed him in the arm; or, that not ſucceeding, in the neck. His legs ſhould be put into warm water, and afterwards well rubbed with a dry cloth. As ſoon as he can ſwallow, ſome lemonade, or water and vinegar, as before directed, may be given him. It will likewiſe be of advantage to adminiſter active clyſters, which, in defect of more ſtimulating ingredients, may conſiſt of the common clyſter ſharpened with two or three large ſpoonfuls of common ſalt.

A reſpectable practitioner relates the caſe of a man ſuffocated by the ſteam of burning coal, whom he recovered by blowing his breath into the patient's mouth, bleeding him in the arm, and cauſing him to be well rubbed.

And another of the faculty mentions the caſe of a young man who was ſtupefied by the ſmoke of ſea-coal, but was recovered by being plunged into cold water and afterwards laid in a warm bed.

It would ſeem that the practice of plunging perſons ſuffocated by noxious vapours in cold water is conformable to a phyſical principle in the animal œconomy, which can only be aſcertained by obſervation: for it coincides with the common experiment of ſuffocating dogs in the *grotto del cani*, and afterwards recovering them by throwing them into the neighbouring lake.

## *Effects of extreme Cold.*

Extreme cold acts upon the ſurface of the body, particularly the extremities, by conſtricting the veſſels; on which account the circulation is obſtructed, and too great a quantity of blood is forced towards the brain, whence enſues a drowſineſs which terminates in an apoplexy. But ſuch violent effects of cold are ſeldom experienced in this country.

It frequently happens, however, that the hands or feet of travellers are ſo benumbed or frozen, as to be in danger of mortification, if proper means be not immediately uſed to prevent it; and this danger is generally increaſed by the uſual practice of people in ſuch a ſituation. When the hands or feet are pinched with cold, nothing is more common than to hold them to the fire; but nothing at the ſame time is more pernicious, in ſuch circumſtances, than the application of heat. When thoſe parts are greatly benumbed with cold, they ought either to be immerſed in cold water or rubbed with ſnow until they recover their natural warmth and ſenſibility. The perſon afterwards may be removed into an apartment a little warmer, but ſtill be careful not to approach immediately to a fire.

When a perſon has been ſo long expoſed to the cold that every ſymptom of life has diſappeared, he ought to be rubbed all over with ſnow or cold water; or, what may be more immediately efficacious if it can be procured, he may be immerſed in a bath of the coldeſt water. If to this be added two or three handfuls of common ſalt, it will operate ſtill more powerfully. Should one plunge not prove effectual, the patient ſhould be rubbed all over with cloths and again immerſed in the bath. Nor ought we ſoon to deſiſt from the diligent uſe of ſuch means: for there are inſtances of perſons, who, after remaining in the ſnow, or being expoſed to the freezing air during five or ſix ſucceſſive days, and who diſcovered no ſigns of life for ſeveral hours, have, nevertheleſs, been revived by perſevering aſſiduity in ſuch efforts.

## *Effects of extreme Heat.*

In the temperate climate of this country, extreme heat ſeldom operates to the immediate extinction of life; but ſuch incidents are not uncommon in thoſe regions of the globe which lie much nearer to the equator. People exhauſted with heat and fatigue frequently drop down apparently dead in the ſtreets. In ſuch a caſe ſome warm cordial ſhould be poured into the mouth, if practicable; but if this cannot be done, the remedy may be adminiſtered in the form of a clyſter. Volatile ſpirits, and other things of a ſtimulating nature, may be applied to the ſkin, which ſhould alſo be well rubbed with coarſe cloths. Every kind of excitement applied to the ſurface of the body is here of advantage: ſuch as whipping with nettles, or beating with rods; by which means ſome of the ancient phyſicians are ſaid to have revived perſons apparently dead.

---

## CHAP. XLVII.

*Of Fainting-Fits, and other Caſes which require immediate Aſſiſtance.*

STRONG and healthy perſons, of a full habit of body, are often liable to fainting-fits after violent exerciſe, expoſure to great heat, drinking freely of warm or ſtrong liquors, intenſe application to ſtudy, or great agitation of mind.

In caſes of this kind, vinegar ſhould be held to the patient's noſtrils. The ſame remedy, mixed with an equal quantity of warm water, ſhould be applied to his temples, forehead, and wriſts; and two or three ſpoonfuls of vinegar, with four or five times as much water, may, if he can ſwallow, be poured into his mouth.

If the fit proves obſtinate, or degenerates into what is called a *ſyncope*, that is, an abolition of feeling and underſtanding, the patient muſt be bled; after which, a clyſter ſhould be adminiſtered. In the mean time, he ought to be kept perfectly quiet and eaſy; only giving him every half-hour a cup or two of an infuſion of mint, balm, ſage, or any mild herb, with the addition of a little ſugar and vinegar.

When ſwoonings, ariſing from a ſuper-abundance of blood, happen frequently to the ſame perſon, he ſhould, by way of prevention, confine himſelf to a light diet, conſiſting chiefly of bread, fruits, and other vegetables; and uſing, for drink, either ſmall-beer or water. He ſhould likewiſe take a good deal of exerciſe, and be moderate in the indulgence of ſleep.

Fainting-fits, however, are much more frequently occaſioned by a defect than an exceſs of blood; on which account they moſt commonly occur after great evacuations of any kind, obſtinate watching, long faſting, and the like. In thoſe caſes, the treatment muſt be almoſt directly the reverſe of what has been above recommended.

The patient ſhould be immediately laid in bed, with his head low; and, being covered, his legs, thighs, arms, and his whole body be ſtrongly rubbed with hot flannels. Volatile ſalts or ſpirits, Hungary-water, or ſtrong ſmelling herbs, ſuch as rue, mint, or roſemary, may be held to his noſe. His mouth may be wet with a little rum or brandy; and, if he can ſwallow, ſome hot wine, mixed with ſugar and cinnamon, may be poured into his mouth. A piece of flannel, folded two or three times, and dipped in hot wine or brandy, ought to be applied to the pit of the ſtomach, and warm bricks, or bottles filled with hot water, laid to his feet.

By theſe means the patient will probably ſoon begin to recover; and, to promote his reſtoration, he ought now to take a little bread or biſcuit, ſoaked in hot ſpiced wine, or, if ſuch a thing be ready, ſome ſtrong ſoup or broth: continuing to take often, but in ſmall quantities, ſome light ſtrengthening nouriſhment, ſuch as jellies, light roaſt meat, ſoup, and the like, to prevent a return of the fit.

To this claſs belong thoſe fainting-fits which are occaſioned by accidental bleeding, or the violent operation of purgative medicines. Such as are the conſequence of blood-letting ſeldom prove dangerous, and generally terminate on the patient's being laid in a horizontal poſture; in which ſituation perſons who are ſubject to this accident ſhould always be bled. On this occaſion, however, ſhould the fainting not immediately ceaſe, volatile ſpirits may be held to the noſe, and rubbed on the temples.

When fainting proceeds from too ſtrong or acrid purges or vomits, the patient muſt be treated in all reſpects as if he had taken poiſon. He ought to drink plentifully of ſuch liquors as are adapted to blunt the violence of thoſe ſubſtances, and defend the ſtomach and inteſtines from the force of their irritation. This purpoſe will be anſwered by milk, oil, barley-water, warm water, and the like. It will alſo be proper to uſe the ſame materials in the form of clyſters. The patient's ſtrength ſhould afterwards be recruited by generous cordials; with which ſome opiate, as the opiate confection, ſhould be given.

Faintings are ſometimes occaſioned by the quantity or quality of the food. When they proceed from the former, the cure muſt be effected by vomiting, which may be promoted by drinking an infuſion of chamomile flowers. If the nature of the food be the cauſe, ſtimulating applications to the noſtrils and temples muſt be uſed, in the ſame manner as in the caſe of weakneſs. Afterwards, as ſoon as poſſible, he ſhould be made to ſwallow a large quantity of light warm fluid, which may dilute the acrimony of the offending matter, and either promote the difcharge of it by vomiting, or carry it down into the inteftines.

In very delicate conftitutions, fwoonings are fometimes occafioned by difagreable fmells. Upon fuch an emergency the difagreeable object fhould be removed, and the patient carried into the open air, where volatile falts, or other ftimulating things, fhould be held to his nofe.

Fainting-fits often happen in the progrefs of difeafes, particularly fevers. When they happen at the beginning of malignant fevers, they indicate great danger. In all fuch cafes as thefe now mentioned, the heft remedy during the paroxyfm is vinegar, both externally and internally ufed; and after it is over, the free ufe of lemon juice and water, brandy and water, &c. Swoonings which happen in difeafes accompanied with great evacuations, muft be treated as thofe which proceed from weaknefs; reftraining at the fame time the evacuations. When they occur towards the end of a violent fit of an intermitting fever, or at that of the exacerbation of a continual fever, the patient muft be fupported by fmall draughts of wine and water.

Delicate and hyfteric women are very liable to fwooning or fainting-fits after delivery. Thefe are to be cured by generous cordials, and the admiffion of frefh air; by which they might likewife be often prevented. When they proceed from exceffive flooding, the difcharge ought by all means to be reftrained.

In all cafes of fainting, frefh air is of the greateft importance to the patient; of which, however, he is too often deprived by the officious affiduity of his friends, who by crowding around him, perhaps in a fmall apartment, counteract the very means which are the moft proper to reftore him.

Perfons, fubject to fainting-fits fhould do all in their power both to avoid the occafions which excite them, and overcome the conftitutional weaknefs in which they are founded. Every fit of the kind is more or lefs injurious to the future permanency of health, not only by the increafed debility which it occafions, but by the various diforders which may arife from a temporary ftagnation of the blood. Difturbed fecretions, obftructions of veffels, and coagulations of the fluids, are the natural confequences of every fhock which affects fo much the circulation.

## *Intoxication.*

Intoxication is not only extremely pernicious to health, but an excefs of a kind the moft degrading to human nature; and when produced by ardent fpirits, it frequently occafions inftantaneous death. The effects of this *Circean* poison are similar in many respects to those of opium; producing a confusion in the head, a temporary derangement of the understanding, a partial or total abolition of all the senses, and a diminution of the nervous energy. Other kinds of intoxicating liquors, as well as ardent spirits, may prove destructive of life; but being taken in greater quantity, they are more liable to be discharged from the stomach, and thereby prevented from occasioning fatal effects. This is both the readiest and most effectual way in which nature can be relieved from her oppressive load, and vomiting ought always to be excited when the stomach is thus overcharged.

Of those unhappy persons who die in a state of intoxication, the greater part lose their lives from an inability to conduct themselves. Rendered incapable of walking, they tumble down, and, if not immediately destroyed by the accident, lie in some awkward posture, which obstructs the circulation or breathing, till at length they often expire.

A person intoxicated with liquor should never be left to himself till his clothes have been loosened, and himself laid in such a posture as is most favorable for continuing the vital motions, and discharging the contents of the stomach. The best posture for facilitating the latter, is to lay him upon his belly. When asleep he may be laid on his side, with his head a little raised; and particular care should be taken that his neck be no way distorted, or have any thing about it too tight.

The thirst occasioned by drinking strong liquors is most safely allayed by water with a toast, tea, or infusions of common herbs, such as balm, sage, and the like. To excite vomiting, the fittest beverage is an infusion of chamomile-flowers; and, indeed, this is the object which ought always to be promoted in the state of intoxication.

## *Getting Wet.*

Though the accident here mentioned has no title to be comprehended in the list of diseases, yet as it may, if neglected, give rise to many such, and those too of the most dangerous kind, it deserves to be noticed for the purpose of preventing its effects.

This accident is at all times less frequent in towns than in the country, especially since the use of the umbrella has been introduced; but there is no person, however strong his constitution, who may not be affected by it. Indeed, in certain circumstances, a vigorous and athletic man may suffer more violently from it than even the weak and delicate. To both it may prove fatal: and this consideration is a sufficient apology, if any were necessary, for pointing out the method which ought to be pursued on such an occasion by those who would pay due attention to the preservation of health.

When a person is wet he ought never to stand, but to continue in motion till he arrives at a place where he may be suitably accommodated. Here he should strip off his wet clothes, to be changed for such as are dry, and have those parts of his body which have been wet well rubbed with a dry cloth. They should then be washed with brandy, or some other spirituous liquor, and afterwards dry clothes be put on. The legs, shoulders, and arms, are generally the parts most exposed to wet: they should, therefore, be particularly attended to; but, if the whole body has more or less suffered from the accident, the whole should be rubbed and embrocated in the manner already mentioned. It is almost incredible how many diseases may be prevented by adopting this course. Catarrhs, inflammations, rheumatisms, diarrhœa, fevers and consumptions, are the foremost among the train which frequently follow an accident of this kind.

## CHAP. XLVIII.

### *Cosmetics—Warts, and Corns.*

VARIOUS artifices have in all ages been practised for improving the complexion, and removing blemishes, especially those of the face. In ancient times, the expedient was not uncommon among women, of attempting to stain with a black colour the interior part of the eyes; and similar efforts have been made in later periods to change the colour of the eye-brows. But the practice of the cosmetic art, in modern times, is chiefly restricted to that of painting the face; a practice which, however much cultivated by the rudest nations, is not only repugnant to nature, but in the highest degree injurious to the genuine complexion, which it affects to improve. It is likewise, in many cases, no less prejudicial to health; and when the painting is extended over the surface of the breasts, it has, in some instances, been found to prove even fatal.

Nor is it surprising that pernicious effects should ensue from painting the skin, when we consider the nature of the materials generally used for this purpose. They consist, for the most part, of a preparation of lead in disguise, combined with oil, and either scented, or not, with some perfume. When this factitious pigment is applied to the body its effects are to ſhut the pores, to conſtrict the ſmall cutaneous veſſels, and to harden the ſkin; the conſequence of which is, that perſpiration is obſtructed, whence ariſe tooth-achs, and rheumatic pains of the adjacent parts; and the ſkin being thickened as well as hardened, it aſſumes a pallid, coarſe, and haggard, appearance, which, admitting afterwards of no remedy, can only be concealed hy the application of a freſh coat of paint. Thus the practice is perpetuated, and what was at firſt adopted from a chimerical and fantaſtic idea of improving the beauty of the countenance, terminates in the fatal neceſſity of hiding its deformity.

A clearneſs and bloom of the complexion can be improved in no other way than by the preſervation, and, where it is poſſible, the improvement of health. How this may be beſt ſecured has already been ſhown in the chapters on air, exerciſe, &c.

To ſet off the complexion with all the advantage it can attain, nothing more is requiſite than to waſh the face with pure water; or, if any thing farther be occaſionally neceſſary, it is only the addition of a little ſoap, which, however, ſhould be afterwards waſhed off.

An object more ſubſervient to health, and which merits due attention, is the preſervation of the teeth; the care of which, conſidering their importance in preparing the food for digeſtion, is, in general, far from being ſufficiently cultivated. I believe that very few perſons, comparatively, waſh their mouth in the morning; which ought always to be done. Indeed, though the operation ſeems not the moſt delicate to ſpectators at the table, this ought to be practiſed at the concluſion of every meal where either animal food or vegetables are eaten: for the former is apt to leave behind it a rancid acrimony, and the latter an acidity, both of them hurtful to the teeth. Waſhing the mouth frequently with cold water is not only ſerviceable in keeping the teeth clean, but in ſtrengthening the gums, the firm adheſion of which to the teeth is of great importance in preſerving them ſound and ſecure.

Picking teeth properly is alſo greatly conducive to their preſervation; but the uſual manner of doing this is by no means favourable to the purpoſe. A pick-tooth, with moſt people, is uſed in the manner of a tobacco-pipe, or rather as a plug of tobacco, twiſted round and ſqueezed by the lips, in a kind of aukward maſtication; and when it is wielded in the hand of the poſſeſſor, it is more as a weapon of hoſtility than defence to the teeth. When it is neceſſary to pick the teeth, the operation ought to be performed with due care, ſo as not to hurt the gums; but the ſafeſt and beſt way of doing it is always before a looking-glaſs.

Many perſons, while laudably attentive to preſerve their teeth, do them hurt by too much officiousness. They daily apply to them some dentifrice powder, which they rub so hard as not only to injure the enamel by excessive friction, but to hurt the gums even more than by the abuse of the pick-tooth. The quality of some of the dentifrice powders advertised in news-papers is extremely suspicious; and there is reason to think that they are not altogether free of a corrosive ingredient. One of the safest and best compositions for the purpose is a mixture of two parts of scuttle-fish bone, and one of the Peruvian bark, both finely powdered; which is calculated not only to clean the teeth without hurting them, but to preserve the firmness of the gums.

Besides the advantage of sound teeth, from their use in mastication, a proper attention to their treatment conduces not a little to the sweetness of the breath. This is indeed, often affected by other causes existing in the lungs, the stomach, and sometimes even in the bowels; but a rotten state of the teeth, both from the putrid smell emitted by carious bones and the impurities lodged in their cavities, never fails of aggravating an unpleasant breath wherever there is a tendency of that kind.

The smallest eruption on the face is apt to disfigure the countenance, and therefore merits some attention. The most frequent of this kind is pimples, which proceed from an acrimony of the humours, and chiefly infest those who are addicted to the drinking of strong and heating liquors. It is common to wash them with a little Hungary-water, or brandy; but what is better adapted to the purpose, is Goulard's vegeto-mineral water. Topical applications, however, are of advantage only when the pimples arise from a local cause: for when they proceed from a vitiated state of the fluids the eruption cannot be prevented in any other way than by correcting the cause which produces them. In such constitutions the diet ought to be light and cooling, and the body kept gently open.

But a more permanent blemish of the face is the kind of excrescence called a *wart*. This proceeds from no general affection of the system, and is merely a local effect. When warts do not prove troublesome, nothing should be done to them, as they generally either fall off or waste gradually away; but when from their size or situation they require to be removed, there are different methods of treating them. If they be pendulous or have narrow necks, a silk thread waxed may be tied tight round them at the base, and kept in that situation until they fall off.

When their bases are broad, escharotic applications are commonly made use of; but they ought to be of the milder kind. Of these, one of the best is crude sal ammoniac: it should first be moistened in water, and then well rubbed upon the wart two or three times a day. Liquid salt of tartar, and sometimes spirits of hartshorn, have answered the same purpose. Some recommend also the juice of onions, and others that of celandine; but the most effectual application is the tincture of muriated iron, applied every day.

The most troublesome excrescences, however, are corns. These are small hard tubercles, commonly situated on the toes or other parts of the feet, and sometimes on the hands. They are always the effect of pressure; and when seated on the toes or feet, generally arise from tight shoes. When corns are situated on parts much exposed to pressure, they sometimes occasion great pain. Various remedies are recommended for the cure or removal of these tubercles. One is to bathe the part about half an hour in warm water, then to pare as much off them as possible without giving pain, and to apply over them a little wax ointment. If this treatment be frequently repeated, while pressure from the shoes is prevented, they generally fall off. Another method is to allow them to grow to some length through a piece of perforated leather, properly secured by plaster, or by any other means, and afterwards to pick them out, or to cut round their root, by which they may for the most part be easily turned out.

## CHAP. XLIX.

### *Of the Health of Soldiers and Seamen.*

THESE two classes of men, considered in a political view, form a valuable part of the nation; and of so great importance are they to the security of the government, the liberties and interests of the public, that the preservation of their health is an object which merits particular attention. Not more than half a century has elapsed since this branch of medical science began to be cultivated with any degree of success, or indeed even of industry; but within that time it has been constantly prosecuted in many judicious publications.

In respect of the army, it is observed by the learned Sir John Pringle, that the preservatives from diseases are not to depend on medicines, nor on any thing which a soldier can have in his power to neglect. Innumerable instances confirm the justness of this remark; and it is an unquestionable fact, that the preservation of the health of troops depends as much on the observance of due regulations respecting diet, &c. in camp or in quarters as the success of their military exertions does on their discipline and subordination in the field. It is not at present our design to enter into a minute detail of the means for preserving the health of soldiers: all that we propose is to point out the most important objects of consideration relative to the subject.

In all classes of men, the use of proper diet is indispensable for the preservation of health. The food of a soldier may be coarse, but it should be wholesome and abundant, such as is common among the labourers of the country; and the present pay of a British soldier, if properly laid out, can well afford even better.

The men ought to be divided into small messes, and proper stoppages made from their pay to provide food. It should be the business of an officer to see that the meals be regular, sufficient comfortably cooked, and that the men behave at them with due decorum. Great care ought to be taken to prevent the introduction of corrupted flesh, mouldy, or half baked bread, spoiled corn, mixed flour, or other nutritious substances of bad quality.

One meal of animal food is sufficient for a healthy man in twenty-four hours; and it would be a good regulation were that meal taken some hours later than is at present the custom in camp. Digestion is best performed while the body remains at rest. Military exercises should therefore be avoided as much as possible immediately after eating; and those men whose duty calls them to watch during the night, would be better supported by a full than an empty stomach.

Nothing is so agreeable, and at the same time so wholesome to a soldier, after a fatiguing and perhaps a wet march, as some warm soup. To boil the meat is therefore the mode of cooking which ought to be most generally used in the army. Every effort should be made to procure vegetables, to boil with the meat; but it is not necessary to be very delicate in what are selected for this purpose. If the various kinds of cabbage, carrots, parsnips, onions, and potatoes, which are universally approved of, cannot be procured, the wild or water cresses, the brooklime, the scurvy-grass, the wild sorrel, and lettuce, which are to be found in every field, make wholesome as well as agreeable additions to soup. When in a fixed camp, soldiers should be encouraged to cultivate various kinds of culinary vegetables, and especially potatoes. It would conduce much also to the salubrity as well as the nutritious qualities of these soups, were every mess to have a certain quantity of barley, or, what affords more substantial nourishment, decorticated oats, cut groats, dried peas, or rice, to add to their broth. Fresh animal food should always be provided if possible. When circumstances, however, render it necessary to subsist on salted provisions, their injurious consequences may be considerably mitigated, by paying proper attention to their goodness, as well as to the mode of dressing them.

Ripe fruits, in moderate quantity, are wholesome; and contrary to the vulgar prejudice, tend rather to prevent than to induce complaints of the bowels. Unripe fruit of all kinds, especially stone-fruits, are well known to be injurious, and should never be eaten raw.

To prevent an army from being seized with the scurvy, during a season when fresh meat and vegetables are likely to become scarce, it would be prudent to have a large quantity of potatoes, onions, garlic, mustard-seed, leeks, sourcrout, pickled cabbage, &c. and sub-acid fruits laid in store beforehand. These might be sold in moderate quantities, at a low rate, during winter; and all means should at the same time be used to oblige the men to form themselves into messes, and buy a little fresh meat daily. Fermented malt-liquor, cyder, and acescent drinks, are at no time more useful, than when the scurvy is beginning to make its appearance. On such occasions the Russian quass-loaves would be particularly wholesome, and convenient for making small beer. These are composed of oat or rye meal, mixed with ground malt; and, when made into cakes with plain water, are baked and kept for use. They make a pleasant acidulous liquour by being infused twenty-four or thirty hours in boiling water, with a little dried mint or other aromatic herb.

During the prevalence of bloody fluxes, the men ought to be allowed plenty of farinaceous vegetables, such as groats, barley, rice, potatoes, and dried peas; but they should refrain entirely from pot-herbs and green fruits. No objection is made, however, to the free use of ripe fruit. On these occasions they should also use fat and mucilaginous broths; or sago, and a little astringent wine, if it can be procured good; but meagre wines and fermented liquors would be pernicious to their bowels.

It has been observed, that the custom of taking a light but warm breakfast, such as tea or coffee, renders men delicate and susceptible of taking cold. So much were the leaders of the French impressed with the truth of this remark, that warm breakfasts were strictly prohibited in one of their northern armies. Upon the authority of a gentleman who was himself an eye-witness of the fact, every man was allowed half a pint of good wine, which he took with his bread. Few of these men were unfit for duty, though the weather was extremely severe. It may be laid down as a maxim that a soldier will be able to bear fatigue and hardship with vigour and alacrity, in proportion as he lives well. In this country, a pint of good porter, or sound ale, might be substituted for wine. The men should not be allowed to purchase this at pleasure; but it should be regularly issued, and the expense stopped from their pay.

Cheap, excellent, and nourishing puddings may be composed of boiled barley, molasses, and ginger.

Bread, emphatically termed the staff of life, is what the soldier chiefly depends upon for support. While an army is in motion, it is difficult to furnish this article in abundance, and with regularity. It is the settled, but perhaps erroneous custom, to furnish armies with bread fermented and baked into the form of loaves. Biscuits would, on many occasions, be preferable: a loaf sometimes becomes mouldy, and uneatable in a few days; biscuits will keep in perfection for months. Bread baked amidst the hurry and confusion of an army in motion, is apt to be improperly prepared; and in this state it is very unwholesome; but the quality of biscuit made at a distance, and with regularity, may always be depended upon. The hardness of biscuit is removed by soaking it in warm water; and the rawness or doughiness of bread is in some measure corrected by toasting it.

It would be well were the promiscuous sale of distilled spirits to soldiers, wholly prohibited. In hot weather they are peculiarly injurious. The mortality of our troops in the West-Indies has been attributed, by every medical writer, as much to the intemperate use of spirits as to the effects of the climate. It is not denied that in some situations they may be necessary; but that necessity is to be judged of by the physician or commanding officer. In cold damp weather, when a little spirit might be allowable and useful, soldiers would find a tolerable substitute in a draught of hot water with a tea-spoonful of fresh grated ginger in it. This in common cases, would be of equal utility with spirituous liquors, and does not possess the power of intoxicating.

Another article of importance with regard to soldiers is clothing; which is, in general, far from being well adapted to a military life. The stiff bandage that surrounds the neck, and the tight ligatures which constrain the articulations of the loins and the knees, should if possible be avoided. Freedom of respiration is no doubt also impeded by the pressure of the belts crossing upon the chest. In an active campaign, much often depends on rapidity of movement, and promptitude of exertion: but if a certain portion of the strength of each individual be exhausted in counteracting the pressure on his muscles, or in sustaining perhaps an unnecessary burden, the sum of the whole, which might otherwise be employed in supporting unavoidable fatigue, must be considerably diminished.

Many remarks might be made on the other parts of the military dress; but to prosecute the subject with any degree of precision would swell the present chapter to too great a length. Suffice it therefore to obſerve, that prudence, humanity, and ſound policy conſpired to recommend the uſe of woollen clothing for Britiſh ſoldiers, at leaſt during an encampment. Dr. Donald Monro, a judicious and experienced phyſician in the diſeaſes of the army, obſerves, that a woollen ſtock or neck-cloth, with a flannel waiſtcoat and worſted gloves, may be purchaſed for about half a crown per man, and would contribute to preſerve the lives of many: whereas the expence of medicines and recruiting will greatly exceed the price of theſe articles.

Perſonal cleanlineſs is likewiſe an object of great importance in an army; for it is obſerved that thoſe men who are moſt negligent in this reſpect, are the firſt who are infected by diſeaſes. Hence the contagion is frequently ſpread through a whole army, among whom it often proves more fatal than the ſword. The ſtricteſt attention, therefore, is neceſſary to enforce the obſervance of this practice.

---

The method of preſerving the health of ſeamen is in many reſpects the ſame with that which relates to the army. Cleanlineſs and wholeſome diet, in particular, are eſſential in both claſſes. On board ſhips, the practice of frequent ſcraping, ſweeping, and waſhing the decks daily, ſhould never be omitted. In cold weather, if due attention be paid to cleanlineſs, by means of ſcraping and ſweeping well, perhaps it will be ſufficient to waſh the deck once in eight or ten days, as dampneſs, when joined to cold, is a powerful cauſe in producing the ſcurvy and other diſeaſes. Moiſture, when joined to heat and ſtagnant air, is alſo highly prejudicial, and frequently gives riſe to putrid and malignant fevers. The utmoſt attention ſhould therefore be paid to keep between decks as dry as poſſible, by means of ſtoves properly fitted; by frequent ſwabbing; by keeping up a free circulation of air, and every other means of prevention.

Care ſhould be taken not to let any thing acid, or that is apt to ferment and turn acid, remain in the cook's coppers, or other culinary utenſils; as a green ruſt or verdigreaſe may thence be produced, which is well known to be a poiſon of the moſt active and virulent kind.

All the hammocks ſhould be waſhed, cleared, and well dried at ſtated periods, at leaſt once a month, and the clothes and bedding frequently ſpread in rotation, in fine weather, on the booms, or hung up forward for airing.

Seaman likewiſe in hot climates, ſhould have frequent recourſe to bathing in the ſea. This practice not only braces and ſtrengthens the ſyſtem in general, but powerfully aſſiſts the organs of digeſtion, and enables those who use it to bear more fatigue. In a ship, it may be done by having buckets full of salt water thrown over the body, especially during the time that the vessel is within the tropics. But though the practice here recommended is in general highly serviceable, the cold-bath is not to be used when there is much of the prickly heat on the skin, immediately after a full meal, soon after being much heated, nor in the heat of the day.

A due supply of fresh air is indispensable for the preservation of health, as well as life itself. Every attention, therefore, should be paid to its free and constant circulation, and every care taken to keep it in as pure and healthy a state as possible between decks. Wind-sails should be in constant use to ventilate between decks in warm climates. But the most powerful and effectual agent for destroying noxious or putrid air is fire, and the best and safest way of communicating it is by stoves.

The precautions above mentioned are necessary at all times; but in bad weather more particular attention should be paid to dryness and cleanliness, and to the state of the air on the lower decks: for it is in such weather that sickness is most apt to break out.

The diet of seamen is in general less wholesome than that of the army. When the usual allowance of salt beef and pork can be diminished, and other articles, such as peas, potatoes, flour, fruit puddings, &c. be increased, it ought in every instance to be done. There should always be a plentiful supply of vinegar and mustard, as these articles tend greatly to counteract the bad effects of salted or putrid meat. The capsicum or Guinea pepper is an article of daily use amongst the natives of hot countries in wet and sickly seasons; when it seems to fortify the stomach and the whole body against the attack of fever. It is recommended to be infused in vinegar, and regularly served to the ship's company, to use with their meat; and in wet and sickly seasons a quantity of it might be put into the people's peas or soup, in a palatable proportion.

When a ship touches at any port, great caution should be observed with respect to the quantity of fresh meat and vegetables at first allowed; as the usual allowance in a warm climate is by far too much; and most probably gives rise to fluxes, fevers, and a variety of billious disorders. The use of vegetables and fresh meat, therefore, should at first be cautiously moderate, and chiefly used in the form of well prepared soup; increasing the quantity by degrees to the full allowance. The same observation may be made with respect to the article of fruit, of which whatever is used should be perfectly ripe, of the best kind, and served out in proportions. The utility of good fruit, however, as well as all acids, and fermented liquors, in preserving seamen from the ravages of the scurvy, is now generally known.

Water is univerſally an eſſential article in the ſupport of life, and among ſeamen is frequently bad or deficient. Spring water, where it can be had, is always to be preferred; next to that, clear running water, which ſhould be taken from as near the ſource as poſſible. In ſituations where none but unwholeſome water can be procured, the proceſs of boiling will tend much to correct its bad qualities; and where there is reaſon to ſuſpect the eggs of inſects or animalcules in water, this precaution ſhould never be neglected.

If water be hard, the addition of a little pearl-aſh, or ſalt of tartar, will give it the properties of ſoft water. If muddy, the addition of a few grains of alum will cauſe the impurities to ſubſide: or it may be filtrated by forcing a piece of ſponge, or double flannel, tight into any funnel-ſhaped veſſel, and letting the water ſtrain through it; or by paſſing through a barrel of clear ſand, or a filtering ſtone.

To preſerve water from putrefaction, great care ſhould be taken to keep the caſks perfectly clean. The ſmalleſt quantity of corrupted matter being left in them acts as a real ferment, and very quickly diſpoſes the freſh water, with which theſe veſſels are filled, to become putrid in the ſame manner. It is ſaid, that the ſimple proceſs of firing the caſks, in putting the ſtaves together, till a charry coat is formed over the whole ſurface, is a certain means of preſerving water pure and ſweet for any length of time.

To purify a quantity of corrupted water, the method is to add ſix or eight pounds of powdered charcoal to each caſk. It is better to put too much than too little of the powder, and as much diluted vitriolic acid as is ſufficient to communicate to the water a degree of acidity juſt perceptible to the taſte. To prevent the charcoal from ſettling at the bottom of the caſk, in the form of a paſte, it will be proper to ſtir the whole together with a ſtick, at leaſt twice a week.

Before uſing the water ſo preſerved, it ſhould be tried by paſſing a ſmall quantity of it through a ſtrainer, in the form of a jelly-bag, filled with powdered charcoal. If the water thus filtered ſtill have a turbid appearance, a freſh quantity of powdered charcoal muſt be added, till it is become perfectly clear. The whole of the water may then be paſſed through a filtering bag, the ſize of which ſhould be proportioned to the quantity of water.

The habit of daily ſwallowing a quantity of ſpirituous liquor, in its raw ſtate, ſhould be moſt ſcrupulouſly abſtained from; and drams ought never to be given, unleſs after great fatigue, long expoſure to cold, or on getting thoroughly wet. On other occaſions, the ſubſtitute of hot water, with a tea-ſpoonful of grated ginger, above mentioned, may be advantageouſly uſed.

At the end of a long, cold, wet watch, rubbing the body dry, a change of comfortable, dry clothing, and a glaſs of unadulterated ſpirits, would in numberleſs inſtances, prevent many an able ſeaman from appearing next day in the ſick liſt, and eventually, perhaps, be the means of ſaving his life.

The only mode in which liquor can be daily allowed to ſeamen with advantage, is in the form of punch, made either with lime, lemon, or orange juice. The acid, ſugar, and a large proportion of water, tend greatly to correct the bad qualities of the ſpirit, and counteract the bad effects of a ſea-diet, particularly with regard to the ſcurvy.

Sometimes ſailors are unavoidably wet with rain for many days ſucceſſively. In this ſituation the advice of Captain Bligh ſhould be followed; viz. to dip their clothes in the ſalt water and wring them out as often as they become filled with rain. To him, and his unfortunate companions, it felt more like a change of dry clothes than can well be imagined.

In cold, wet weather, much benefit would be derived from the uſe of flannel ſhirts, due attention being paid to cleanlineſs; and ſometimes they would be equally beneficial in warm climates by preventing a check to perſpiration, ſo frequent and dangerous in thoſe parts.

Many economical improvements might yet be made with reſpect both to ſoldiers and ſeamen; but ſuch innovations are commonly gradual, and the work of a conſiderable time.

## CHAP. L.

### *Cold-Bathing, Mineral Waters, and Sea-Water.*

SOME obſervations have already been made on cold-bathing in a preceding chapter;* but the ſubject is of ſo great importance, that it merits more particular attention, were it only to enforce the neceſſity of caution in the uſe of ſo powerful a medicine.

Cold-bathing is promiſcuouſly reſorted to by the votaries both of pleaſure and health; by thoſe whoſe fibres are rigid, and thoſe in whom they are lax; equally by perſons who abound in blood, and perſons deficient in the quantity of the vital fluid. It would, therefore, be repugnant to common ſenſe to ſuppoſe that a thing which operates ſo powerfully upon the body, could poſſibly produce the ſame effects in conſtitutions not only diſſimilar, but di-

* See Chap. X. Book I.

rectly oppoſite to each other. The practice, however, is now become very general for people of all deſcriptions to have recourſe to ſea-bathing in the ſummer, for the purpoſe either of the preſervation or the recovery of health. That, when properly uſed, it contributes in the higheſt degree to both, is a fact which admits of no doubt: but when on the other hand it is greatly miſapplied, the effect is ſo extremely dangerous as often to prove fatal. The truth of this remark will more clearly appear, if we take a view of the obvious effects of cold-bathing.

Cold water, when applied to the body by immerſion, acts both by its gravity and temperature. By ſuddenly conſtricting the veſſels of the ſkin, it forcibly drives the blood to the interior parts of the body, whence ariſes an inſtantaneous oppreſſion of the vital organs. If the blood be in too great quantity, there is danger leſt ſome of the veſſels burſt by the violent diſtention which they ſuffer; and if the vital powers are not ſtrong enough to re-act with force ſufficient to propel the blood outwards, an immediate ſtagnation, with its fatal conſequences, muſt enſue.

Such, therefore, are the effects of cold-bathing when improperly uſed: but when employed in favourable circumſtances it is highly conducive to health. It accelerates the motion of the blood, promotes the different ſecretions, diſſipates incipient obſtructions, and gives permanent vigour to the ſolids.

From what has already been ſaid, ſome idea may be formed of the conſtitutions and caſes in which a recourſe may ſafely be had to cold bathing. It is well adapted to people of a relaxed habit of body, whether this be the effect of conſtitutional or adventitious cauſes, provided that the *viſcera* or various bowels be ſound. Perſons, likewiſe, ſubject to ſlow but habitual diſcharges, ariſing from a laxity of particular parts, are much benefited by it; and in nervous conſtitutions, where the temperature of it is properly adjuſted to the ſenſibility of the patient, it is the moſt powerful remedy.

The adjuſtment of the temperature of the water is a very important conſideration in the practice of bathing; and, on this account, where extreme cold freſh water might prove hurtful, bathing in ſalt water may be uſed both with ſafety and advantage. It is not only more uniform in temperature, but, by its ſtimulating effects on the ſkin, conduces to excite that re-action of the vital powers which is neceſſary to render bathing of any advantage to the health.

The temperature of the ſea, though varying conſiderably in different ſeaſons, is, on the whole, much more uniform than that of any inland water that is ever expoſed to the atmoſphere, and which is not a thermal ſpring, poſſeſſing in itſelf a ſource of heat. The vaſt body of water in the ſea, and the perpetual agitation to which it is expoſed, render it leſs liable to be affected by external changes of temperature, particularly at a conſiderable depth below the ſurface. At its upper part, however, which alone is employed for bathing or drinking, it undergoes great variations of temperature in different times of the year. On the ſhores of England, the ſurface of the ſea is ſeldom, in the ſevereſt weather, lower in temperature than 40°, or higher in the hotteſt ſummer than 65°; whereas the heat of rivers, eſpecially when ſhallow, and their current ſlow, riſes higher, and ſinks lower than each of theſe points.

During the earlieſt period of infancy, waſhing or bathing ought to be practiſed every day. No other expedient tends in a greater degree to ſtrengthen the conſtitution, to ſuppreſs or diminiſh the ſuſceptibility of infection, and to prevent diſeaſes. Bathing is one of the moſt powerful means of purifying the ſkin, of reſtoring free perſpiration, and of preſerving the ſurface of the body from eruptions and other troubleſome diſorders. Children accuſtomed to the bath will more eaſily overcome diſeaſes incident to infancy, particularly the meaſles and ſmall-pox.

Daily bathing in cold water, however is certainly not the proper means of ſtrengthening infants, or improving their health. The contracting power of cold produces rigidity of the fibres, obſtructs the capillary veſſels of the ſurface, and renders the whole ſkin too parched and dry for ſo tender an age.

From the birth of a child to the ſecond year of his age the *tepid* bath only ought to be employed; and after that period the *cool* bath; the conſtitution of infants requiring this gradual change of temperature. During the firſt year of life, they are evidently in want of a moderate degree of warmth, nearly reſembling that to which they were accuſtomed in the womb. New-born babes, or even thoſe under a twelve month old, cannot endure a very cold air, and ought therefore to be treated with additional precaution in bathing.

The luke warm bath is moſt ſuitable to the firſt ſtage of infancy. The Ruſſians, we know, plunge their children in the waters of frozen rivers, and the ſame was the practice of the ancient Germans; but this trial of vital ſtrength is too ſevere to be generally adopted, and coſts the lives of numerous innocents. The ſudden effect of cold is too violent a ſtimulus for the frame of a tender infant, in whoſe mind it perhaps produces all the terrors of inſtant death.

During the firſt three months of its life an infant ought to be daily bathed in moderately warm water; in the next nine months the water ſhould be only lukewarm; after the firſt year its temperature may be ſtill more reduced; and after the ſecond the bath ſhould be cool.

From the third year of its age a child may be bathed in cold water; but it is not here meant in water as cold as ice. It is proper to make a diſtinction between moderately warm, lukewarm, warm, tepid, cool, and cold. By the expreſſion moderately warm, is underſtood that degree of heat when the hand, or, if this be not ſufficiently ſenſible, the foot, may remain in it for ſome time without experiencing the leaſt diſagreeable ſenſation: the lukewarm bath is about the ſame temperature as new milk. The cool bath ſignifies a temperature equal to that of water which has been kept in a room for a conſiderable time, ſo that its chillneſs is taken off: and the cold-bath ought to correſpond with the river water in the height of ſummer.

But it will be proper to elucidate the different temperatures with ſome more preciſion. Immedialy after the birth of a child the water in which it is bathed ought never to exceed the 98th degree of Fahrenheit's thermometer; by progreſſively reducing the warmth of the bath one degree every month, it will ſtand at 86° when the child is one year old; which will produce the ſenſation of what is called lukewarm. If this temperature be ſtill farther reduced in the next twelve months, ſo that the mercury in the glaſs falls to 74°, when the child has completed the ſecond year of its life, it may then with propriety be termed a cool bath.

With reſpect to the manner of uſing the cold bath, few obſervations are neceſſary. It is more ſuitable in ſummer than in winter, eſpecially to thoſe not accuſtomed to it; and the moſt proper time is the morning, or at leaſt before dinner. One ſhould never enter it chilly, but always in a temperate ſtate, inclining rather to warm. A quick immerſion with the head foremoſt is the beſt mode of bathing. When this is not practiſed the head ſhould always be firſt wetted; and there needs no ſtay in the water after the ſhock is received. When an agreeable glow is immediately diffuſed over the body, it is a ſign that the bath has proved ſalutary; but if it be ſucceeded by chillneſs, head-ach, or any internal pain, and this likewiſe repeatedly, there is reaſon to deſiſt from the uſe of it.

But the external uſe of water is not the only way in which the body may be affected by this uſeful and medicinal element. Mineral waters, or thoſe impregnated by nature with peculiar qualities, exert a powerful influence on the animal œconomy when internally uſed; ſome by ſtrengthening the conſtitution, ſome by purging, and others by increaſing the diſcharges of urine, perſpiration, or both. Waters of this kind are to be found in almoſt every country, and in this iſland they are numerous. For the convenience of the reader we ſhall mention ſome of the principal, with the diſeaſes in which they are chiefly celebrated; but without ſpecifying the various ingredients which enter into their compoſition.

## *Malvern Water.*

The extenſive and lofty range of the Malvern hills occupies a great part of the ſouth-weſt of the county of Worceſter, forming a diſtant boundary to the rich vale of the Severn lying to the eaſt, and ſtanding as a frontier between this county and that of Hereford. The village of Great Malvern, ſituated about half way between Ledbury and the city of Worceſter, has long been celebrated for a ſpring of remarkable purity, which, from the reputed ſanctity of its waters, has acquired the name of Holy Well. The water of this well is chiefly uſed externally, in painful and deep ſeated ulcerations, the conſequence of a ſcrophulous habit, and in ſome cutaneous diſorders; but it is alſo uſed with ſome advantage in a few internal diſeaſes. The moſt important of theſe are painful affections of the kidneys and bladder, attended with the diſcharge of bloody, purulent, or fœtid urine; the hectic fever produced by ſcrophulous ulcerations of the lungs; or very extenſive and irritating ſores on the ſurface of the body; and alſo fiſtulas of long ſtanding, which have been neglected, and become conſtant and troubleſome ſores.

The internal uſe of this water is ſometimes attended at firſt with a ſlight nauſea, and not unfrequently, for the firſt day or two, it occaſions ſome degree of drowſineſs, vertigo, or ſlight pain of the head, which comes on a few minutes after drinking it. But this effect is aſcribed to a temporary fulneſs of the head, occaſioned by the great eaſe and rapidity with which the water is abſorbed; and theſe ſymptoms go off ſpontaneouſly after a few days, or may readily be removed by a mild purgative. The effects of this water upon the bowels are by no means uniform: very often it purges briſkly for a few days; at other times the body is rendered coſtive by its uſe, eſpecially in thoſe who are accuſtomed to the uſe of malt-liquors. In all caſes it increaſes the diſcharge of urine, and improves the general health of the patient.

## *Briſtol Water.*

Briſtol Hot Well is ſituated about a mile below the city of Briſtol, and within four miles of the Britiſh channel. The water of this ſpring, from its extraordinary quality of keeping untainted for a great length of time in hot climates, forms a moſt valuable proviſion for long voyages, and is accordingly exported in great quantities to diſtant parts.

The ſenſible effects produced by this water, when freſh from the ſpring, are, at firſt a gentle glow in the ſtomach, ſucceeded ſometimes by a ſlight degree of head-ach and giddineſs, but which ſoon go off. In its effects on the kidneys it nearly reſembles the Malvern water, as it does likewiſe in its operation on the bowels; though on the whole a tendency to coſtiveneſs is the more general conſequence of a continued uſe of Briſtol water; and therefore the uſe of a mild laxative is often neceſſary.

With reſpect to the manner of employing this water medicinally, the time recommended for the firſt doſe is before breakfaſt, as early in the morning as the patient chooſes to riſe, when it is uſual to take two glaſſes; interpoſing between them half an hour ſpent in gentle exerciſe. Two more glaſſes, with the ſame interval, are generally given about the middle period between breakfaſt and dinner; and the water is ſeldom afterwards repeated in the courſe of the day. The ſize of the glaſs varies from a quarter to half a pint, which laſt is reckoned a full doſe: but it never ought to be taken in ſuch a quantity as to cauſe any oppreſſion or ſenſe of weight in the ſtomach.

This water is regarded as beneficial in ſeveral diſorders of the alimentary canal; in the ſymptoms of indigeſtion which often afflict Europeans who have reſided many years in hot climates; in bilious diarrhœas likewiſe, and in ſlight dyſenteries. It has alſo acquired reputation in the cure of the diabetes, or at leaſt in affording conſiderable relief in this malady. But it has, above all, been celebrated in the cure of the conſumption of the lungs; though on this ſubject there is a difference of opinion among medical writers. The ſeaſon for the Hot Wells is generally from the middle of May to October.

## *Matlock Water.*

This water iſſues from a ſpring in a mountainous part of Derbyſhire, where the village of that name is ſituated on the brow of a lime-ſtone hill, at the foot of which flows the rapid ſtream of the Derwent. The cold and tepid ſprings are ſingularly ſituated in this hill. All the tepid waters ariſe from fifteen to thirty yards above the level of the Derwent, whilſt thoſe both above and below are cold; and even the ſources of the latter intermix with thoſe of a higher temperature.

Matlock water is chiefly uſed as a tepid bath, or at leaſt one which comes to the extreme limits of a cold bath. On this account, it produces but little ſhock on immerſion; and is therefore well fitted for thoſe in whom the re-action is too weak to overcome the effects of the ordinary cold bath.

## *Buxton Water.*

Buxton water takes its riſe at the village of Buxton, on the weſtern ſide of the county of Derby. The waters of this place appear to have maintained confiderable reputation in the cure of various difeafes for a longer period, without interruption, than almoft any mineral water in the kingdom. The fprings here are very numerous, and the quantity of water abundant. It is employed largely both in external and internal ufe; and one of thefe modes is often applicable in cafes where the other would be prejudicial. The great recommendation of the Buxton baths is the copious fupply of a very pure water of the high temperature of 82°. As this temperature is feveral degrees below that of the human body, a flight fhock of cold is felt on the firft immerfion into this bath; but this is almoft immediately fucceeded by an agreeable glow over the whole body. The cafes moft relieved by Buxton water, ufed externally, are thofe in which a lofs of action, and fometimes even of perfect fenfation, has affected the limbs, occafioned by long or violent inflammation, or external injury. Thus, the chronic rheumatifm in all its forms, fucceeding to the acute, and where the inflammation has been chiefly feated in moving parts, is often wonderfully relieved by this bath; and the perfon is fo much recovered as to be enabled to ufe the more powerful remedy of fea-bathing, or the common cold bath. The lofs of motion, however, produced by the true palfy will feldom admit of much relief from thefe waters.

With regard to the internal ufe of Buxton water, it is found of confiderable fervice in cafes of weak digeftion, the confequence of luxurious indulgence. Another clafs of diforders much relieved by thefe waters is the painful complaints of the ftone and gravel. The manner of ufing this water is the fame as has been mentioned with refpect to that of Malvern.

## *Bath Waters.*

The city of Bath has long been celebrated for its numerous hot fprings, which are of a higher temperature than any other in this kingdom, and indeed are the only natural waters which we poffefs, that are at all hot to the touch; all the other thermal waters being of a heat below the animal temperature, and only exceeding the general average of the heat of common fprings. There are three principal fources of thefe waters, namely, the king's bath, the crofs bath, and the hot bath, which all arife within a fhort diftance from each other. The fupply of water is fo copious, that all the large refervoirs ufed for bathing are filled every evening with water frefh from their refpective fountains.

Befides the other ingredients in the compofition of this celebrated water, it holds diffolved in it a portion of iron, in a quantity, however, fo extremely fmall, as to be nearly the leaft that is poffible to be detected by chemical tefts. This water, when drunk fresh from the spring, has in most persons the effect of raising and rather accelerating the pulse, increasing the heat, and promoting the secretions. These effects generally appear very soon after drinking the waters, and, in some constitutions, will last for a considerable time. It is, however, particularly in invalids that any such symptoms are observed. This water has also a considerable disposition to pass off by urine, even when taken in a moderate quantity: and this may be regarded as one of its most salutary operations. Its effects on the bowels, like that of all waters which do not contain any purgative salt, is extremely various; but, in general, the use of this water renders the body costive, not so much from any astringency with which it is endowed, as from the want of an active stimulus to the intestines, and probably also from the determination which it occasions to the skin: for, if perspiration be suddenly checked, during the use of Bath water, a purging sometimes ensues.

The stimulating properties of these waters appear to be chiefly exerted in the stomach. When they are likely to prove beneficial, they excite, on being first taken, a pleasing glow in this organ; which is soon succeeded by an increase of appetite and spirits, and a quick determination to the kidneys. On the other hand, when they sit heavy on the stomach, and produce sickness, when they occasion head-ach, thirst and dryness of the tongue, and do not pass off by urine or perspiration, their operation is unfavourable, and the farther use of them is not to be recommended.

One of the most important uses of the Bath water, however, is its external application; and, employed in this way, its effects seem to differ in no respect from those of common water, heated to the same temperature, and similarly applied.

The cases to which this water is peculiarly adapted are mostly of the chronic kind; and by a steady perseverance in this remedy, some very obstinate disorders have given way. The diseases in which it is chiefly beneficial are the *chlorosis* or green sickness, rheumatism, gout, and some kinds of palsy.

## *Tunbridge Water.*

This is the most noted of the simple chalybeates in our island, especially in this part of the kingdom. Tunbridge-Wells is a populous village in the county of Kent, about thirty-six miles south of London. Here are many chalybeate springs, all of which resemble each other very much in chemical properties; but two of these are chiefly used. The effects of this water are evidently of the stimulant kind. Soon after taking a moderate dose, the pulse rises in strength, and the patient, if previously chilly and pale, feels a degree of glow occasioned by the increased circulation. Both the appetite, likewiſe, and the general ſpirits, are improved; though theſe effects are much more ſtriking in ſome than in others, eſpecially in perſons of an irritable and ſanguine habit. It is, however, not uncommon, on beginning the uſe of theſe waters, for the patient to be affected with nauſea, vomiting, and pain about the region of the ſtomach; or elſe a heavineſs of the head, ſlight vertigo, and ſenſe of fulneſs over the whole body. Sometimes theſe ſymptoms are ſo conſtant as to ſuggeſt the propriety of renouncing the uſe of the waters; but in general they are tranſient, and diſappear in a few days, eſpecially when there enſues a permanent increaſe in any of the natural excretions. When the bowels are foul, and loaded with bilious impurities, the water often purges pretty briſkly at firſt, but this effect ceaſes as ſoon as the inteſtines are cleared. All the preparations of iron, and theſe waters among the reſt, are known to tinge the fæces black, a circumſtance in itſelf of no importance, but of which the patient ſhould be appriſed to prevent him from being affected with any groundleſs apprehenſion. The ſecretion which theſe waters moſt commonly excite is that of urine, and is generally in the greateſt quantity where they agree beſt with the conſtitution of the patient. Sometimes they likewiſe induce a more perſpirable ſtate of the body, eſpecially when the uſe of them is accompanied with a good deal of exerciſe.

On the whole, the general operation of theſe chalybeates is to increaſe the various ſecretions in a gradual uniform manner, and at the ſame time to impart to the body a perceptible increaſe of vigour and nervous energy. It is, therefore, chiefly in chronic diſorders, ariſing from ſlow beginnings, and attended with laxity and debility of the ſolids, but without much affection of any of the bowels, that theſe waters are found to be peculiarly uſeful. They are of eminent ſervice in caſes of impaired appetite, ſlow digeſtion, flatulent diſtenſions of the belly, difficult reſpiration ariſing from ſympathy with the ſtomach, and occaſional vomiting of phlegm.

On beginning a courſe of theſe waters, it is a general practice to premiſe ſome evacuation, either a gentle emetic, where the ſtomach is foul, or, what is better, ſome opening medicines. It is likewiſe uſual, where the water is not of itſelf purgative, to intermit its uſe for a day or two after it has been regularly taken for a week or ten days; and to clear the bowels during that interval by ſome proper laxative, or elſe to add a ſmall quantity of vitriolated ſoda or magneſia to the water every two or three days. To perſons of a weak irritable ſtomach, and eſpecially females, the freſh drawn water is apt to prove too cold to the ſtomach, and to occaſion a nauſea or ſickneſs, which always fruſtrates the general intention of the water. To prevent ſuch an effect, it is proper to take the chill off the water; the beſt way of doing which, without prejudice to the water, is to put it into a bottle cloſely corked, and immerſe it in hot water.

In drinking the Tunbridge water, the whole of the quantity daily uſed is taken at two or three intervals, beginning at about eight o'clock in the morning, and finiſhing about noon. The doſe at each time varies from about one to three quarters of a pint, according to the age, ſex, and general conſtitution of the patient, and eſpecially the duration of the courſe: for it is found that theſe waters loſe much of their effect by long habit.

## *Cheltenham Water.*

The ſpring of this denomination has its ſource at Cheltenham, a ſmall town in Glouceſterſhire. The water is decidedly ſaline, and contains much more ſalt than moſt of the waters hitherto mentioned. By far the greater part of the ſalts which it contains are of the purgative kind, and therefore an action on the bowels is a conſtant effect produced, by this medicinal ſpring. Cheltenham water is likewiſe a chalybeate, and if the analyſis given of it be accurate, it is one of the ſtrongeſt that we are acquainted with. It has beſides a ſlight impregnation of ſulphur, but ſo little as to be ſcarcely appreciable, except by very delicate chemical teſts.

The ſenſible effects produced by this water are generally, on firſt taking it, a degree of drowſineſs, and ſometimes head-ach, but which ſoon goes off ſpontaneouſly, even previous to the operation on the bowels. A moderate doſe acts powerfully and ſpeedily as a purgative, but without occaſioning griping, or producing that faintneſs and languor which often ſucceed the operation of the rougher kind of purges. For this and ſome other reaſons, Cheltenham water may be in moſt caſes perſevered in for a conſiderable length of time without producing any inconvenience to the patient; and during its uſe the appetite will be improved, the digeſtive organs ſtrengthened, and the whole conſtitution invigorated.

This medicinal ſpring has been found of eſſential ſervice in the cure of glandular obſtructions, eſpecially thoſe that affect the liver, and the other organs connected with the functions of the alimentary canal; and it has alſo great effect in ſome cutaneous complaints, uſually termed ſcorbutic eruptions.

The ſeaſon of drinking the Cheltenham water is during the whole of the ſummer months. The water ſhould, if poſſible, be always drunk at the fountain head, and never kept long expoſed to the air. The doſe muſt vary conſiderably, both from the great difference of the action of purgatives in different habits, and from the intention with which the water is given. Half a pint of the, water is ſufficient for a ſingle doſe; and this quantity, repeated three or four times during the day at proper intervals, is generally enough to produce the deſired effect on the bowels.

### *Scarborough Water.*

The town where this water iſſues is ſituated at the foot of a very high cliff on the Yorkſhire coaſt, overlooking a ſpacious bay, ſurrounded by lofty rocks. There are here two ſpecies of chalybeate waters, and they differ conſiderably in their compoſition, though riſing nearly contiguous to each other. One of them is a ſimple carbonated chalybeate, ſimilar to the Tunbridge water; the other which is better known, and more frequented, as well as more particularly diſtinguiſhed for its qualities, has, in conjunction with the iron, a conſiderable mixture of purging ſalt, which adds much to its value.

Scarborough water, from its compoſition, may be ranked among the purging chalybeat waters, though the quantity of the purgative ſalt is too ſmall to operate with activity, except an unuſual and often inconvenient doſe be taken. Its general effect, however, even when taken in moderation, is to determine gently to the bowels, rather than to the kidneys, which is the ordinary way in which the ſimple waters paſs off.

With regard to the diſeaſes for which this water may be uſed with advantage, they are in general the ſame as were mentioned in the account of the Cheltenham ſpring. But, in many caſes, it would be adviſable to increaſe the purgative effect of this water by adding ſimilar ſalts, becauſe few ſtomachs could bear ſo many pints of this water as would be requiſite to produce a full evacuation from the bowels. On this account, it is chiefly as an alterative that the Scarborough water can be employed in its natural ſtate.

### *Hartfell Water.*

This chalybeate water iſſues from the baſe of a very high mountain of the ſame name, about five miles from Moffat in Scotland. It is endowed with no inconſiderable ſhare of medicinal virtue in the cure of ſeveral very dangerous diſeaſes. Its firſt effects upon the patient are ſometimes giddineſs and ſickneſs, eſpecially when a large doſe has been taken. Its operation on the bowels is not uniform: ſometimes it produces gripes, and, on firſt uſing it, a diarrhœa not unfrequently follows: but it much oftener occaſions coſtiveneſs, which may be regarded as its moſt natural effect.

This water has been found of great ſervice in diſorders of the ſtomach and bowels, bloody flux, bloody urine, immoderate flow of the *menſes*, or their ſuppreſſion, *fluor albus*, gleet, &c. In general, it may be ſaid to promiſe advantage in all caſes where there is a relaxation of the ſolids. Much benefit has likewiſe been derived from it, employed both internally and externally, in old and languid ulcers, where the texture of the diſeaſed parts is very lax, and the diſcharge profuſe and ill-conditioned.

The doſe of this chalybeate is more limited than that of moſt of the mineral ſprings. The patient, eſpecially if he be of a delicate and irritable habit, ought to begin with a very ſmall quantity: for an over-doſe is apt to be very ſoon rejected by the ſtomach, or to occaſion griping and diſturbance in the inteſtinal canal. Few patients will bear more than an Engliſh pint in the courſe of the day; but this quantity may be long continued in. It is often of advantage to warm the water for delicate ſtomachs; and this may be done without much injuring its properties.

## *Harrowgate Water.*

The villages of High and Low Harrowgate are ſituated in an agreeable country, in the centre of the county of York, adjoining to the town of Knareſborough. The whole of the contiguous diſtrict abounds with mineral ſprings of various qualities, but chiefly ſulphureous and chalybeate. Harrowgate in particular has long been known for its valuable ſprings of both theſe kinds. Some years ago the chalybeate was the only one uſed internally, whilſt the ſulphureous water was confined to external uſe; but at preſent the latter is employed largely as an internal medicine.

The ſulphureous ſprings of Harrowgate conſiſt of four, and they all appear to take their riſe from a large bog at a ſhort diſtance from the wells. They reſemble each other cloſely in all their qualities; but one of them being much more ſtrongly impregnated with the ſulphureous principle than the reſt, it is the only one uſed for drinking, whilſt the three others are devoted to the ſupply of the baths.

The ſenſible effects produced by this water are often a head-ach or giddineſs on beginning to uſe it; with a purgative operation, which is mild, ſpeedy, and ſeldom attended with pain or griping.

Harrowgate water, like that of all the other ſaline ſprings, is uſed in many diſorders of the ſtomach and inteſtines, as well as in the derangements of the biliary ſecretion, which ſo often produce theſe complaints. It is likewiſe of great benefit in the ſcrofula, and in various viſceral obſtructions; but that for which it is moſt celebrated is its efficacy in curing a number of cutaneous diſorders. It is alſo of advantage in the piles, and in ſymptoms produced by ſeveral ſpecies of worms.

This water is generally taken in ſuch doſes as to produce a ſenſible effect on the bowels; for which purpoſe it is found neceſſary to take in the morning three or four glaſſes, of rather more than half a pint each, at moderate intervals.

To correct the nauseous taste with which it is accompanied, it is not unusual to take some aromatic seeds, sugar comfits, and the like; but Dr. Garnett recommends a small quantity of sea-biscuit or coarse bread, which will remove the taste very speedily, and not cloy the stomach. The water should be taken fresh from the spring, and cold, where the stomach can bear it, especially in those cases where the sulphureous ingredient is particularly wanted.

The duration of a course of Harrowgate water varies more than that of most other medicinal springs, on account of the great diversity of the diseases in which it is used. Cutaneous complaints of a bad kind are what require the greatest perseverance; and in these the patient ought to drink the water several months at intervals, especially if he perceives any benefit from the use of it during a few weeks.

## *Moffat Water.*

The village of Moffat is situated at the head of a valley on the banks of the Annan, about fifty-six miles south-west of Edinburgh. It is surrounded by hills, some of which are lofty; and of these the Hartfell mountain has been already noticed for the chalybeate water which springs from its basis. This sulphureous water, the Harrowgate of North Britian, issues from a rock a little below a bog, whence it probably derives its sulphureous ingredient. Almost the only sensible effect which it produces, is that of increasing the discharge of urine. It sometimes indeed purges; but this seems to proceed more from taking it in an excessive quantity, than from any purgative virtue it possesses.

Moffat water has acquired great celebrity for the cure of cutaneous eruptions of every kind. The scrofula is another disorder, in which it has proved of great benefit; but chiefly in the earlier stages and slighter symptoms of this formidable malady. It often, however, disperses glandular tumours without suppuration, or any bad consequence. This water is also employed in many bilious complaints; in cases of weak digestion, and general want of action in ihe alimentary canal, as well as in troublesome symptoms of the gravel and stone.

In drinking it, the quantity usually prescribed is from one to three bottles every morning; but this allowance is much too large for persons of a delicate stomach. It should, however, be used pretty freely in such doses and intervals as the patient can bear*.

* The common people frequently take, in one morning, from three to five Scots pints (or from six to ten English quarts); and an instance is mentioned by Mr. Milligin of a man who in eight hours swallowed the enormous quantity of thirty-two English quarts, and without feeling any other inconvenience than a slight giddiness and head-ach.

*Sea-Water.*

This, if we except ſome brine-ſprings and ſalt-lakes, is by far the ſtrongeſt in ſaline matter of all the natural waters which are medicinally employed. The water of the ſea, as it waſhes the ſhores of our iſland, is a very heterogenous compound, containing a conſiderable quantity of ſaline ſubſtances, and holding ſuſpended an infinite number of minute animal and vegetable particles, compoſed of all the variety of marine productions that abound in this element.

It is fully aſcertained by experiments, that the proportion of ſalt in ſea-water varies conſiderably at different depths, and in different latitudes. In general, the water at the tropics is ſalter than at the poles, and the ſurface leſs ſalt than at a conſiderable depth. The water of our own coaſts contains, at an average, about $\frac{1}{30}$ of its weight of ſalt.

The diſorders for which ſea-water may be uſed internally are, in general, the ſame for which all the ſimple ſaline waters may be employed, and have been already enumerated. The internal employment of ſea-water, however, is chiefly made an auxiliary to its external application, which is now ſo generally uſed. It is chiefly recommended in ſcrofulous affections, and hard indolent tumors in certain glands, particularly thoſe of the neck. In all ſuch caſes, however, the uſe of it is almoſt entirely confined to thoſe periods of the diſeaſe when there is no tendency to a hectic fever.

Sea-water ſhould be taken in ſuch doſes as to prove moderately purgative; the increaſe of this evacuation being the peculiar object for which it is employed. About a pint is generally ſufficient for the purpoſe; and this ſhould be taken in the morning at two doſes, with an interval of about half an hour between each. It is ſeldom neceſſary to repeat the doſe at any other time of the day. But it is often neceſſary to perſevere for a long time in the uſe of the ſea-water; and, happily, this perſeverance is ſeldom productive of any bad conſequences to general health. Dr. Ruſſel mentions caſes where a pint of this water has been taken daily for 200 mornings, without any interruption, which produced a continued courſe of moderate purging; yet the appetite continued all this time perfectly good, and the health improved.

## CHAP. LI.

### *Of Empirics.*

AFTER a long attention to the cure of diseases, it is mortifying to reflect how much this arduous province is infested by a race of ignorant and shameless empirics, who are daily tampering with the public credulity, to the destruction of numbers of lives. It may safely be affirmed, that a very considerable part of the annual deaths in the capital and its vicinity, exclusive of those in other parts, are occasioned by the profligate temerity of these unprincipled impostors. There is hardly a news-paper that does not teem with the audacious falsehoods, and pompous pretensions, of this imposing class of mercenary, and yet (I use not too harsh an expression) tolerated murderers. What man who is conversant with physic can peruse without indignation the public advertisements of these quacks; in which every one arrogates to himself the possession of superlative knowledge, and ascribes to his respective nostrum such contradictory and inconsistent qualities as were never yet united in any one medicine in the world?

To the disgrace, however, of the public credulity, not a few of these impostors attain to a degree of opulence that is seldom acquired even in the scientific and legitimate prosecution of medical practice. The artifices which they employ to delude the multitude are well known to many. Having picked up the name of some extremely active medicine, the bold and indiscriminate use of which must therefore be proportionably dangerous, they immediately resolve on converting it into a nostrum, and endeavour to disseminate its unrivalled praises either by advertisements or hand-bills. But being themselves totally illiterate, they have, for this purpose, recourse to some other person, whom they engage for a stipulated reward to fabricate the pernicious illusion. A hyperbolical panegyric on the wonderful remedy is accordingly vamped up, and preparations are made for commencing a lucrative trade with the public. Should the channel of communication be the public papers, it is a settled point, that if daily or frequent advertisements can be supported for the space of some months, the fame of the medicine, whatever be its real character, is established. The better to promote this purpose, innumerable authorities in favour of the nostrum are asserted in general terms; venality is again exerted to furnish specific testimonials in its support; and if, among the number of unfortunate purchasers or patients, there exists any person who has not only taken it with impunity, but even with some advantage, (and what extremely powerful medicine may not ſometimes by chance have good effects?) the fortuitous incident is immediately blazoned with all the oſtentation of intereſted zeal and affected popularity; and a reference to uncorrupted teſtimony reſounded through every channel of information. By a ſtrange aſſociation, truth now is confidently adduced in ſupport of falſehood; and the recovery of one or two perſons is rendered the unhappy means of draining the purſe, undermining the health, and deſtroying the lives of thouſands.

Such, in fact, is the general progreſs of empiriciſm. Were the taſk not invidious, and the objects too deſpicable for any other than juridical cognizance, which they merit in a ſuperlative degree, the repreſentat ion here given might be ſupported by unqueſtionable authority. It is hoped, however, that enough has been ſaid to influence the minds of the judicious with reſpect to this iniquitous practice, which becomes every day more alarming, and threatens the more credulous part of the community with the moſt fatal effects.

This country, through the bleſſing of Providence, has been for many ages exempted from the horrors of the famine, the peſtilence, and the ſword; but the infatuation of a numerous body of the people has ſubjected it to the ravages of another public calamity, which, though generally more ſlow in its operation than any of the former, is equally deſtructive in the end. Humanity ſhudders at the horrible depredations committed on the human conſtitution by this empirical tribe, who ſubſiſt by public deluſion, and riot, where they can, in the irreparable ruin of thoſe whom they entice into their ſnares. What conſumptive viſages, what enfeebled frames, what mutilated bodies, and what palſied limbs, are the miſerable monuments of that ignorance and criminal temerity by which they are actuated!

In certain diſeaſes, it is doubtleſs an object of importance to the unfortunate patients, that their cure ſhould be conducted with ſecrecy, and likewiſe to many, at the ſmalleſt poſſible expenſe; but they do not conſider that, while they are economical in this article, they are fatally prodigal of health. They ſneak, under night, to the manſion with the gilded lamps, or enter it perhaps by a private door in the day time; not reflecting that the ſame deluſion and folly which occaſioned their diſeaſe, now leads them to complete their deſtruction. They graſp with eagerneſs the pill box or the phial, which they are aſſured contains the elixir of ſpeedy and effectual convaleſcence; but, alas! the flattering hope proves of ſhort duration. They may feel perhaps, for a little, a ſuppreſſion of the ſymptoms of their diſeaſe; but the deſtructive embers are ſmothered, not extinguiſhed; and, while preying upon the vitals, are acquiring a malignity which will again break forth with redoubled violence.

It is not, however, in one diſeaſe only, nor in the lower claſs of the people, that this infatuated credulity operates; we find it prevail even amongſt thoſe from whoſe ſuperior ſituations in life more diſcernment might be expected; but who have nevertheleſs become voluntary dupes to the meaneſt artifices of empiriciſm. Witneſs the ſucceſsful impoſture practiſed with regard to the inſpection of urine; the viſionary notion of charms, and the whimſies of animal magnetiſm!

But it is time that ſuch chimerical doctrines ſhould be conſigned to the regions of barbariſm, and flouriſh no longer in a ſoil where almoſt every other phyſical prejudice has been rooted up and exploded by the progreſs of ſcience. To effect this ſalutary purpoſe, nothing can have a more powerful tendency than the view which has been given, in the preceding pages, of the cauſes and cure of diſeaſes. By removing the myſterious veil which for a long time concealed this uſeful branch of knowledge from the eyes of the public, it ought, on one hand, to preclude for ever all recourſes to empirical impoſtors, and, on the other, to ſhow in what caſes it will be proper to call in the aſſiſtance of a phyſician. Within the bounds preſcribed by this limitation any perſon of an ordinary capacity may act in conformity to the rules which have been delivered. By this means a prudent economy will be conſulted, unhappy patients will no longer be ſhipwrecked on the dangerous rocks of empiriciſm, with all their deceitful allurements, but will be conducted through the ſafeſt and moſt direct road to the recovery of health, when that deſirable object is practicable.

Ah! in what perils is vain life engag'd!
What slight neglects, what trivial faults destroy
The hardiest frame! Of indolence, of toil,
We die; of want, of superfluity:
The all-surrounding heaven, the vital air,
Is big with death. And though the putrid south
Be shut; tho' no convulsive agony
Shake, from the deep foundations of the world,
Th' imprison'd plaugues; a secret venom oft
Corrupts the air, the water, and the land.
What livid deaths has sad Byzantium seen!
How oft has Cairo, with a mother's woe,
Wept o'er her slaughter'd sons and lonely streets!
Even Albion, girt with less malignant skies,
Albion the poison of the Gods has drunk,
And felt the sting of monsters all her own.

ARMSTRONG.

THE END.

# APPENDIX:

CONTAINING

## AN ALPHABETICAL ACCOUNT

OF THE

*Substances most commonly employed in Medicine,*

WITH THE

## VIRTUES AND USES OF EACH,

*AS CONFIRMED BY EXPERIENCE AND OBSERVATION:*

ALSO

*The Method of Preparing and Compounding ſuch Medicines as are recommended in the preceding Work, with the Addition of ſeveral others which may be uſeful:*

*An Account of Acids, Abſorbents, Alkaline and Neutral Salts:*

*A Liſt of the moſt uſeful Simples, and Medicinal Preparations for a Medicine Cheſt:*

*A Table of Doſes for different Ages; with the Denominations of the Apothecary's Weights, and Engliſh Wine-meaſure: and,*

*A Gloſſary, explaining the Medical Terms neceſſarily uſed in the Work.*

# APPENDIX.

*An Alphabetical Account of the Subſtances moſt commonly employed in Medicine; with the Virtues and Uſes of each, as confirmed by Experience and Obſervation.*

### *Aloes, Socoterine.*

THIS ſubſtance is obtained from the aloes plant, which is a native of Africa, and flowers moſt part of the year. A tract of mountains, about fifty miles from the Cape of Good Hope, is wholly covered with the aloes plants where the planting of them therefore is unneceſſary; but in Jamaica and Barbadoes they were firſt brought from Bermuda, and gradually propagated themſelves.

The ſocotorine aloes is ſo named from being formerly brought from the iſland Socotria, or Zocotria, at the mouth of the Red Sea. It comes wrapt in ſkins, and is of a bright ſurface, and in ſome degree pellucid: in the lump, of a yellowiſh red colour, with a purpliſh caſt; when reduced into powder, of a golden colour. It is hard and friable in the winter, ſomewhat flexible in the ſummer, and ſoftens between the fingers. Its bitter taſte is accompanied with an aromatic flavour, but not ſufficient to prevent its being diſagreeable: the ſmell, however, is not very unpleaſant, and ſomewhat reſembles that of myrrh.

All the kinds of aloes conſiſt of a reſin united to a gummy matter, and diſſolve in pure ſpirit, proof ſpirit, and proof ſpirit diluted with half its weight of water; the impurities only being left. They diſſolve alſo, by the aſſiſtance of heat, in water alone; but, as the liquor grows cold, the reſinous parts ſubſide.

Aloes is a well known purgative; a property which it poſſeſſes not only when taken internally, but alſo by external application. This cathartic quality of aloes does not, like moſt of the others of this claſs, reſide in the reſinous part of the drug, but in the gum; for the pure reſin has little or no purgative power. Aloes, taken in large doſes, often produces much heat and irritation, particularly about the rectum, from which it ſometimes occaſions a bloody diſcharge. To thoſe, therefore, who are ſubject to the hæmorrhoids, and to women in a ſtate of pregnancy, the exhibition of it has been productive of conſiderable miſchief: but, on the contrary, by thoſe of a phlegmatic conſtitution, or ſuffering by uterine obſtructions, and in ſome caſes of diſpepſy, palſy, gout, and worms, aloes may be employed as a laxative with peculiar advantage. Its purgative effects are not always in proportion to the quantity taken; and as its principal uſe is rather to obviate coſtiveneſs than to operate ſtrongly, this ought to be no objection to its uſe.

Reſpecting the choice of the different kinds of aloes, it may be obſerved, that the ſocotorine contains more gummy matter than the hepatic, and hence is found to purge with more certainty and greater irritation. It is, therefore, moſt proper where a ſtimulus is required, or for promoting the uterine diſcharge: while the hepatic is better calculated for the purpoſe of a common purgative; and alſo, by containing more reſin, anſwers better for external application, conſidered as a vulnerary.

Small doſes of aloes, frequently repeated, not only cleanſe the ſtomach and bowels, but likewiſe attenuate and diſſolve viſcid juices in the remoter parts, quicken the circulation, warm the habit, and promote the uterine and hæmorrhoidal fluxes. It is particularly ſerviceable to perſons of a phlegmatic temperament and ſedentary life, and where the ſtomach is oppreſſed and weakened; but in dry bilious habits it proves injurious, by immoderately heating the blood and inflaming the bowels.

Aloes is likewiſe, on account of its bitterneſs, ſuppoſed to kill worms, either taken internally, or applied in plaſter to the umbilical region. It is alſo highly ſerviceable for reſtraining external hæmorrhages, and cleanſing and healing wounds and ulcers.

The ancients gave aloes in much larger doſes than is cuſtomary at preſent. Modern practice rarely exceeds a ſcruple, and limits the greateſt doſe to two ſcruples. For the common purpoſes of this medicine, ten or twelve grains are ſufficient: taken in theſe or leſs quantities, it acts as a gently ſtimulating laxative, capable of removing, if duly continued, very obſtinate obſtructions.

Aloes, in doſes of a few grains, is occaſionly mixed into pills, with a third or equal parts of ſome ſaponaceous or reſolvent ſubſtance, ſuch as extract of liquorice or gentian, white ſoap, or the like. It is a ſlow but ſure-working purge, and is generally taken at bed-time, ſeldom operating until the next day. It is ſometimes employed in larger doſes, to produce the bleeding piles, when they have been ſuddenly and injuriouſly ſuppreſſed.

### *Alum.*

This is a salt artificially produced from certain minerals, by calcining and exposing them to the air; after which the alum is elixated by means of water. The largest quantities are prepared in England, Germany, and Italy.

Alum is a powerful astringent, and is reckoned particularly serviceable for restraining hæmorrhages, and immoderate secretions from the blood; but less proper in intestinal fluxes. In violent hæmorrhages, it may be given in doses of fifteen or twenty grains, nay even to half a drachm, and repeated every bour, or half hour, till the bleeding abates. In other cases, smaller doses are most advisable: for, if large, they are apt to nauseate the stomach, and occasion violent constipation of the bowels. It is best administered with draggon's blood, or gum-kino, gum-arabic, spermaceti, or opium. It is used also externally, in astringent and repellent lotions, gargles, and collyria, or eye-waters.

### *Ammoniac, Gum.*

We have no certain account of the plant which produces this juice: it is said, however, to be an exudation from a species of ferula. This gum has a nauseous sweet taste, followed by a bitterness, and a peculiar smell, not very grateful. It is an useful medicine in hysteric disorders, proceeding from a deficiency of the menstrual evacuations, and in obstructions of the abdominal viscera. It likewise proves of considerable service in some kinds of asthma, where the lungs are oppressed by viscid phlegm. Externally it softens and ripens hard tumors: a solution of it in vinegar is recommended by some for resolving even scirrhous swellings.

### *Angustura-Bark.*

This is the bark of a tree growing in the interior parts of Africa. It is a powerful bitter, joined with an aromatic, and, as is supposed, likewise, with a narcotic principle; and has been thought to exceed the Peruvian bark, both as a tonic and antiseptic. This bark is best prepared by infusion. It has been employed for the same intentions as the Peruvian bark. In intermittents it is sometimes inferior; but in low fevers, and those of the putrid kind, it has seemed more efficacious. In head-achs, attended with fever, but proceeding from the stomach; in dysentery and dyspepsy, it has been of great service. From various experiments, the Angustura-bark appears to be a powerful antiseptic.

## *Arabic, Gum.*

This is produced from a plant called mimoſa Nilotica, which grows in great abundance over the vaſt extent of Africa; but gum-arabic is chiefly obtained from thoſe trees which are ſituated near the equatorial regions. It is uſually imported into England from Barbary, in large caſks or hogſheads. Gum-arabic of a pale yellowiſh colour is moſt eſteemed. It does not admit of ſolution by ſpirit or oil, but in twice its quantity of water it diſſolves in a mucilaginous fluid, of the conſiſtence of a thick ſyrup, and in this ſtate anſwers many uſeful purpoſes, by rendering oily, reſinous, and fat ſubſtances miſcible with water.

The glutinous quality of gum-arabic is preferred to moſt other gums and mucilaginous ſubſtances as a demulcent, in coughs, hoarſeneſſes, and other catarrhal affections, in order to obtund irritating acrimonious humours, and to ſupply the loſs of abraded mucus. It is likewiſe very generally employed in heat of urine, and ſtrangury; but to produce any conſiderable effect in theſe complaints, it ought to be taken in the quantity of ſeveral ounces in the day. It is the opinion of Dr. Cullen, "that even this "mucilage, as an internal demulcent, can be of no ſervice beyond "the alimentary canal."

## *Aſafœtida.*

This is the concrete juice of a large umbelliferous plant growing in Perſia. It has a bitter, acrid, pungent taſte, and is well known by its peculiar nauſeous fœtid ſmell, the ſtrength of which is the ſureſt teſt of its goodneſs. This odour is extremely volatile, and of courſe the drug loſes much of its efficacy by keeping.

Aſſafœtida is a medicine of very general uſe, and is certainly a more efficacious remedy than any of the other fœtid gums. It is moſt commonly employed in hyſteric and hypochondriac diſorders, flatulent colics, and in moſt of the diſeaſes termed nervous. But its chief uſe is derived from its antiſpaſmodic effects; and it is thought to be the moſt powerful remedy we poſſeſs for thoſe peculiar convulſive and ſpaſmodic affections which often recur in the firſt of the diſeaſes above mentioned, both taken into the ſtomach and in the way of clyſter. It is alſo recommended in obſtructions of the *menſes*, aſthmatic complaints, againſt worms, and as having a tendency to produce ſleep. Where we wiſh it to act immediately as an antiſpaſmodic, it ſhould be uſed in a fluid form, as that of tincture.

*Balm.*

This plant, when in perfection, has a pleaſant ſmell, ſomewhat of the lemon kind, and a weak, roughiſh, aromatic taſte. Some writers have entertained ſo high an opinion of balm, that they aſcribed to it the virtue of prolonging life beyond the uſual period. Strong infuſions of the herb, drunk as tea, and continued for ſome time, have done ſervice in a weak lax ſtate of the viſcera. Balm is now chiefly uſed as a diluent in febrile diſeaſes; and, when acidulated with juice of lemons, makes a very pleaſant drink.

*Bark, Peruvian.*

This is the bark of a very large tree, a native of Peru. There are ſeveral ſpecies of this bark, differing from each other in colour; but, at preſent, the uſe of the bark is chiefly confined to the pale and red kind; and the nearer the former reſembles the latter, the more it is eſteemed.

The bark firſt acquired its reputation for the cure of intermittent fevers; and in theſe, when properly exhibited, it rarely fails of ſucceſs. In remittent fevers, eſpecially during the times of remiſſion, it may alſo be employed with great ſucceſs. In continued fevers, of the nervous and putrid kind, the bark is very generally uſed, as well ſuited to counteract the debility or putreſcency which marks the progreſs of the diſorder. Of late, the bark has been much employed in acute rheumatiſm, particularly after the violence of the diſeaſe has been in ſome meaſure moderated by antiphlogiſtic treatment, or when evident remiſſions take place. In the confluent ſmall-pox, after the maturation of the puſtules is completed, or where ſymptoms of putreſcency, or a diſſolved ſtate of the blood, ſupervene, the bark cannot be too liberally employed.

The other diſeaſes in which the bark is recommended, are gangrenous ſore throats, and indeed every ſpecies of gangrene: ſcarlatina, dyſentery, all hemorrhages of the paſſive kind; likewiſe other increaſed diſcharges; ſome caſes of dropſy, eſpecially when unattended with any particular local affection; ſcrofula, ill conditioned ulcers, rickets, ſcurvy, ſtates of convaleſcence, or recovery from diſeaſes, certain ſtages of conſumption of the lungs, &c.

*Broom, Common.*

The tops and leaves of broom have a nauſeous taſte, which they impart, by infuſion, both to water and ſpirit. They are commended for their purgative and diuretic qualities, and have therefore been fuccefsfully employed in hydropic cafes. The afhes of broom have alfo been much ufed in dropfies; but the efficacy of this preparation depends entirely upon the alkaline falt, and not in the leaft upon the vegetable from which it is obtained.

### *Buckbean*, or *Water Trefoil.*

This plant is common in every part of England: it grows in marfhes and ponds, producing flowers about the latter end of June. The whole plant is fo extremely bitter, that, in fome countries, it is ufed as a fubftitute for hops in the preparation of malt liquors.

Marfh trefoil has gained great reputation in fcorbutic and fcrofulous diforders, in dropfy, jaundice, afthma, rheumatifm, and worms. Inveterate cutaneous difeafes have been removed by an infufion of the leaves, drunk to the quantity of a pint a day, at proper intervals, and continued fome weeks. From one to two fcruples of the leaves in powder may be given two or three times a day; or perhaps a ftrong infufion is preferable.

### *Burdock.*

This plant is common in wafte grounds and road fides: it flowers in July and Auguft, and is well known by the burs or fcaly heads, which ftick to the clothes. The part chiefly ufed for medical purpofes is the root: it has no fmell, but taftes fweetifh, with a flight aufterity and bitterifhnefs. A decoction of it has of late been ufed in rheumatic, fcorbutic, dropfical, and other diforders. It is made by boiling two ounces of the frefh root in three pints of water to two; which, when intended as a diuretic, fhould be taken in the courfe of two days, or, if poffible, in twenty-four hours.

### *Camphor.*

This is a fubftance extracted from the wood and roots of a tree growing in different parts of the Eaft-Indies. Pure camphor is very white, pellucid, and fomewhat unctuous to the touch; of a bitterifh, aromatic, acrid tafte, yet accompanied with a fenfe of coolnefs; of a very fragrant fmell, fomewhat like that of a rofemary, but much ftronger. It is totally volatile, and inflammable; foluble in vinous fpirits, oils, and the mineral acids; not in water, alkaline liquors, nor the acids of the vegetable kingdom.

Camphor is efteemed one of the moft efficacious diaphoretics; and has long been celebrated in fevers, malignant and epidemical diſtempers. In the delirium of fevers, where opiates fail of procuring ſleep, and often aggravate the ſymptoms, this medicine frequently ſucceeds. In ſpaſmodic and convulſive affections it is alſo of great ſervice, and even in the epilepſy it has been uſeful. The taſte of camphor is beſt corrected by vinegar; which ſeems even to render it leſs diſagreeable to the ſtomach.

*Cardamom.*

Cardamom-ſeeds are very warm, pungent, aromatic, and grateful, frequently employed as ſuch in practice. They are ſaid to have this advantage, that, notwithſtanding their pungency, they do not, like thoſe of the pepper kind, immoderately heat or inflame the bowels. They are conſidered as warm, cordial ſtomachics, and may be taken in powder from five to ten grains or more.

*Caraway.*

The ſeeds of caraway have an aromatic ſmell, and a warm, pungent taſte. They are frequently employed as a ſtomachic and carminative in flatulent colics and the like. They contain a large proportion of oil; and except ſome peculiarity in odour, neither their ſeeds nor their oil differ in their virtues from thoſe of aniſe.

*Caſtor-oil.*

This is obtained from the ſeeds of the plant called ricinus, or Palma Chriſti. It is now come into frequent uſe as a quick but gentle purgative. The common doſe of the oil is a table-ſpoonful, or half an ounce; but many perſons require a double quantity.

*Catechu.*

This ſubſtance, commonly known by the name of terra Japonica, is an inſpiſſated vegetable juice, prepared in the Eaſt-Indies from the fruit, as is ſuppoſed, of a ſpecies of palm-tree. Catechu may be uſefully employed for moſt purpoſes where an aſtringent is indicated, provided the moſt powerful be not required. But it is particularly uſeful in fluxes of the belly; and where theſe require the uſe of aſtringents, we are acquainted with no one equally beneficial. It is alſo employed in uterine diſcharges, in laxity and debility of the viſcera in general, in catarrhal affections, and various other diſeaſes where aſtringents are neceſſary. It is often ſuffered to diſſolve leiſurely in the mouth, as a topical aſtringent for laxities and exulcerations of the gums, for aphthous ulcers in the mouth, and ſimilar affections.

*Centaury.*

Centaury is juſtly eſteemed to be the moſt efficacious bitter of all the medicinal plants indigenous in this country. It has been recommended as a ſubſtitute for gentian, and, by ſeveral, thought to be a more uſeful medicine. Many authors have obſerved that, along with the tonic and ſtomachic qualities of a bitter, centaury frequently proves purgative; but it is probable that this ſeldom happens, unleſs it be taken in very large doſes. The tops of centaury are commonly given in infuſion, but they may alſo be taken in powder, or prepared into an extract.

*Chamomile.*

Both the leaves and flowers of this plant have a ſtrong though not an ungrateful ſmell, and a very bitter nauſeous taſte; but the latter exceed in bitterneſs, and are conſiderably more aromatic. Chamomile flowers give out their virtues both to water and rectified ſpirit: when theſe have been dried, ſo as to be pulverable, the infuſions prove more grateful than when they are freſh, or but moderately dried.

Theſe flowers poſſeſs the tonic and ſtomachic qualities uſually aſcribed to ſimple bitters, having very little aſtringency, but a ſtrong odour of the aromatic and penetrating kind; from which they are alſo judged to be carminative, emmenagouge, and, in ſome meaſure, antiſpaſmodic and anodyne. They have been long ſucceſsfully employed for the cure of intermittents; as well as of fevers of the irregular nervous kind, accompanied with viſceral obſtructions. That chamomile flowers may be effectually ſubſtituted for Peruvian bark in the cure of intermittent fevers, appears from the teſtimony of ſeveral reſpectable phyſicians, among whom is Dr. Cullen. He informs us that he has employed theſe flowers, and agreeable to the method of Hoffman, by giving, ſeveral times during the intermiſſion, from half a drachm to a drachm of the flowers in powder; by which he has cured intermittent fevers. He has found, however, that the flowers were attended with this inconvenience, that, given in a large quantity, they readily run off by ſtool, defeating thereby the purpoſe of preventing the return of the paroxyſms; and he has found, indeed, that, without joining with them an opiate, or an aſtringent, he could not commonly employ them.

Theſe flowers have been found uſeful in hyſterical affections, flatulent or ſpaſmodic colics, and dyſentery; but, from their laxative quality, Dr. Cullen tells us, that he has found them hurtful in diarrhœas. A ſimple watery infuſion of them is frequently taken, in a tepid ſtate, for the purpoſe of exciting vomiting, or for promoting the operation of emetics. Externally the flowers are uſed in diſcutient fomentations.

### *Cinnamon.*

The true cinnamon-tree is a native of Ceylon, where it grows common in the woods and hedges, and is uſed by the Ceylonese for fuel and other domeſtic purpoſes. The ſpice ſo well known to us by the name of cinnamon, is the inner bark of the tree. It is one of the moſt grateful of the aromatics; of a very fragrant ſmell, and a moderately pungent, glowing, but not fiery taſte, accompanied with conſiderable ſweetneſs, and ſome degree of aſtringency. Its aromatic qualities are extracted by water in infuſion, but more powerfully by it in diſtillation, and in both ways alſo by a proof ſpirit applied. Cinnamon is a very elegant and uſeful aromatic, more grateful both to the palate and ſtomach than moſt other ſubſtances of this claſs: by its aſtringent quality it likewiſe ſtrengthens the viſcera, and proves of great ſervice in ſeveral kinds of alvine fluxes, as well as immoderate diſcharges from the uterus. The eſſential oil of cinnamon, in doſes of a drop or two diluted by means of ſugar, mucilages, &c. is one of the moſt immediate cordials and reſtoratives in langours and all debilities.

### *Coltsfoot.*

This plant, otherwiſe called tuſſilago, has a rough mucilaginous taſte, but no remarkable ſmell. The leaves have always been of great fame, as poſſeſſing demulcent and pectoral virtues; whence it is eſteemed uſeful in pulmonary conſumptions, coughs, aſthmas, and in various catarrhal ſymptoms. Fuller recommends coltsfoot as a valuable medicine in ſcrofula; and Dr. Cullen, who does not allow it any powers as a demulcent and expectorant, found it ſerviceable in ſome ſtrumous affections. It may be uſed as tea, or given in the way of infuſion, to which liquorice or honey may be a uſeful addition.

### *Columbo-root.*

This is a root brought from Columbo, a town in the iſland of Ceylon, whence it takes its name; but we know not as yet to what ſpecies of plant it belongs. The ſmell of the root is weakly aromatic, not diſagreeable; the taſte bitter and ſomewhat acrid; when chewed, it almoſt diſſolves in the mouth. By keeping, it is very apt to be worm-eaten, and its bitteriſhneſs diminiſhed.

The columbo-root has long been a medicine of great repute among the natives of Ceylon, in diforders of the ftomach and bowels; and by the experiments of Dr. Percival and others, it is found to be of great efficacy in various difeafes depending on the ftate of the bile; fuch as the bilious colic, bilious fevers, habitual vomitings, dyfentery, &c. It has befides been employed with great advantage in weaknefs of digeftion. Water is not fo complete a menftruum as fpirits, but to their united action it yields a flavoured extract in very confiderable quantity. The dofe of the powder ufually given is from one fcruple to two.

*Contrayerva.*

The root of this plant has a peculiar kind of aromatic fmell, with a light aftringent warm bitterifh tafte, and on being long chewed it difcovers fomewhat of a fweetifh fharpnefs. The anti-poifonous virtues formerly afcribed to this root have been long very juftly exploded as entirely chimerical, fo that it is now employed merely as a diaphoretic of a moderately ftimulating kind; being poffeffed of lefs pungency than any other of thofe medicines ufually denominated alexipharmic. Putrid and nervous fevers are the difeafes in which contrayerva is chiefly ufed.

*Cowhage.*

This plant, otherwife called cow-itch, is a native of the Eaft and Weft-Indies. It bears pods thickly covered with fharp hairs, which penetrate the fkin, and occafion a moft troublefome itching. It is efteemed an efficacious remedy againft worms. The manner in which it is employed is, to mix the hairy matter fcraped off from the pods, with fyrup or molaffes, into a thin electuary; of which a tea-fpoonful is given to a child two or three years old, and double the quantity to an adult. The dofe is adminiftered in the morning, fafting, for three fucceffive days, after which a dofe of rhubarb is given. Its effects are reprefented as remarkably powerful and certain, without the leaft dangerous confequence.—The manner in which thefe hairy fpiculæ act as a vermifuge feems to be purely mechanical; for neither the tincture nor the decoction is endowed with any quality deftructive of worms.

*Dandelion.*

This herb is fo very common, that a plot of ground can fcarcely be feen where it does not prefent its yellow flowers. The expreffed juice is bitter and fomewhat acrid, but not equal in bitternefs to the root, which poſſeſſes a greater medicinal power than any other part of the plant. It is much commended in obſtructions of the viſcera, particularly of the liver. The leaves, roots, flower-ſtalks, and juice of dandelion have all been ſeparately employed for medicinal purpoſes, and ſeem to differ rather in degree of ſtrength than in any eſſential property. The expreſſed juice, therefore, or a ſtrong decoction of the roots, have moſt commonly been preſcribed, from one ounce to four, two or three times a day. The plant ſhould be always uſed freſh: even extracts prepared from it appear to loſe much of their power by keeping.

*Elecampane.*

This plant is ſeldom to be met with in a wild ſtate, but it is commonly cultivated in gardens, whence the ſhops are ſupplied with the root, which is the part directed for medicinal uſe. This root, in its recent ſtate, has a weaker and leſs grateful ſmell than when thoroughly dried and kept for a length of time, by which it is greatly improved. Its taſte, on firſt being chewed, is glutinous and ſomewhat rancid, quickly ſucceeded by an aromatic bitterneſs and pungency. An extract made with water poſſeſſes the bitterneſs and pungency of the root, but in a leſs degree than that made with ſpirit.

The ancients entertained a high opinion of elecampane, which is recommended for promoting expectoration in humoural aſthmas and coughs: liberally taken, it is ſaid to excite urine, and looſen the belly. In ſome parts of Germany, large quantities of this root are candied, and uſed as a ſtomachic, for ſtrengthening the tone of the viſcera in general, and for attenuating viſcid humours.

*Elm.*

This tree is frequent in various parts of Great-Britain. The inner tough bark, which is directed for uſe by the diſpenſatories, has no remarkable ſmell, but has a bitteriſh taſte, and abounds with a ſlimy juice, recommended in nephritic caſes, and externally as a uſeful application to burns. The external bark is brittle, contains but little mucilage, and is wholly deſtitute both of ſmell and taſte. The internal bark of the branches is more bitter than that of the trunk, and therefore more efficacious.

The complaints for which the elm-bark is chiefly recommended are thoſe of the cutaneous kind allied to herpes and lepra. Dr. Lyſons mentions five caſes of inveterate eruptions, both dry and humid, or thoſe forming incruſtations, which were ſucceſsfully treated by a decoction of this bark, prepared from four ounces of it taken freſh, and boiled in two quarts of water to one: of this the patients were uſually directed to drink half a pint twice a day.

But as he added nitre to the decoction, and also frequently had recourse to purgatives, it may be doubted whether these cures ought to be wholly ascribed to the elm-bark. Other authorities, however, confirm its utility in cutaneous diseases. In very obstinate cases it is necessary to persevere in the use of the decoction for some months.

### *Fern, Male.*

This is a native of Great-Britain, and grows about the borders of woods near rivulets, and in stony rocky places. The root of it has lately been greatly celebrated for its effects upon the tape-worm, or tænia lata of Linnæus; and this vermifuge power of fern-root seems to have been known to the ancients, after whom it has been recommended by several practical writers. The use of it, however, was very generally neglected till some years ago. Madame Nonfer, a surgeon's widow in Switzerland, acquired great celebrity by employing a secret remedy as a specific in the cure of the tape-worm. This secret was thought of such importance by some of the principal physicians in Paris, who were deputed to make a complete trial of its efficacy, that it was purchased by the French king, and afterwards published by his order. The method of cure has been stated as follows: After the patient has been prepared by an emollient clyster, and a supper of panada, with butter and salt, he is directed to take in the morning, while in bed, a dose of two or three drachms of the powdered root of male fern (the dose for infants is one drachm.) The powder must be washed down with a draught of water, and two hours after a strong purge, composed of calomel and scammony, is to be given, proportioned to the strength of the patient. If this should not operate in due time, it is to be followed by a dose of purging salt; and if the worm be not expelled in a few hours, this process is to be repeated at proper intervals. Of the success of this, or a similar mode of treatment, in cases of tænia, there can be no doubt, as many proofs of it in this country afford sufficient testimony; but whether the fern-root or the strong cathartic be the principal agent in the destruction of the worm, may admit of a question; and the latter opinion, we believe, is the more generally adopted by physicians. It appears, however, from some experiments made in Germany, that the tænia has in several instances been expelled by the repeated exhibition of the root, without the assistance of any purgative.

### *Fox-Glove.*

This plant is known in botany by the name of digitalis purpurea. Its leaves have a bitter nauseous taste, but no remarkable ſmell: they have been long uſed externally to ſores and ſcrofulous tumours with conſiderable advantage. Reſpecting the internal uſe of this plant, we are told of its good effects in epilepſy, ſcrofula, and phthiſis; but the incautious manner in which it was employed rendered it a dangerous remedy. Yet while digitalis was generally known to poſſeſs ſuch medicinal activity, its diuretic effects, for which it is now deſervedly eſteemed, were wholly overlooked. It has at length been diſcovered to be an excellent remedy in dropſical diſorders; but the management of it with ſucceſs, or even with ſafety, requires a degree of ſkill and obſervation, which can only be expected in thoſe who are converſant in the practice of phyſic.

*Fumitory.*

The leaves of fumitory, which are the part of the plant directed for medicinal uſe by the Edinburgh college, are extremely ſucculent, and have no remarkable ſmell, but a bitter and ſomewhat ſaline taſte. Fumitory has been ſuppoſed by ſeveral phyſicians of great authority, both ancient and modern, to be very efficacious in opening obſtructions and infractions of the viſcera, particularly thoſe of the hepatic ſyſtem. It is alſo highly commended for its power of correcting a ſcorbutic and acrimonious ſtate of the fluids; and has therefore been employed in different cutaneous diſeaſes. When taken in pretty large doſes, it proves diuretic and laxative, eſpecially the juice, which may be mixed with whey, and uſed as a common drink. Dr. Cullen claſſes this plant among the tonics. He ſays, "I have found it uſeful in many caſes in which bitters are preſcribed; but its remarkable virtues are thoſe of clearing the ſkin of many diſorders. For this it has been much commended; and I have myſelf experienced its good effects in many inſtances of cutaneous affections, which I would call lepra. I have commonly uſed it by expreſſing the juice, and giving that to two ounces twice a day: but I find the virtues remain in the dried plant, ſo that they may be extracted by infuſion or decoction in water; and the foreign diſpenſatories have prepared an extract of it, to which they aſcribe all the virtues of the freſh plant."

*Garlic.*

These roots are of the bulbous kind, of an irregularly roundiſh ſhape, with ſeveral fibres at the bottom: each root is compoſed of a number of ſmaller bulbs, called cloves of garlic, incloſed in one common membranous coat, and eaſily ſeparable from one another. All the parts of this plant, but particularly the roots, have a ſtrong offenſive ſmell, and an acrimonious, almoſt caustic taste. The root applied to the skin inflames, and often exulcerates the part. Its smell is extremely penetrating and diffusive. When the root is applied to the feet, its scent may soon be perceived in the breath; and when taken internally, its smell is communicated to the urine, or the matter of an issue, and perspires through the pores of the skin.

This root, from its pungency, warms and stimulates the solids, and attenuates tenacious juices. Hence, in cold phlegmatic habits, it proves a powerful expectorant, diuretic, and emmenagogue; and, if the patient be kept warm, a sudorific.

In humoural asthmas, and catarrhous disorders of the breast, in some scurvies, flatulent colics, hysterical and other diseases proceeding from laxity of the solids, and cold sluggish indisposition of the fluids, it has generally good effects; and has likewise been found serviceable in some hydropic cases.

Too free an use of garlic is apt to occasion head-achs, flatulencies, thirst, febrile heats, inflammatory distempers, and sometimes discharges of blood from the hæmorrhoidal vessels. In hot bilious constitutions, where there is already a degree of irritation, where the juices are too thin and acrimonious, or the viscera unsound, this stimulating medicine is obviously improper, and never fails to aggravate the distemper.

The most commodious form for the taking of garlic is that of a bolus or pill, infusions of it being so acrimonious as to render it unfit for general use.

Garlic made into an ointment with oils, &c. and applied externally, is said to resolve and discuss cold tumors, and has been by some greatly esteemed in cutaneous diseases.

## *Gentian.*

This plant is a native of the Alps, and according to the Hortus Kewensis was first cultivated in Britain in the time of Gerard, towards the close of the sixteenth century. But the gentian with which our shops are supplied is imported from the mountainous parts of Switzerland, Germany, &c.

The root, which is the only medicinal part of the plant, has little or no smell, but to the taste it manifests great bitterness—a quality which is extracted by aqueous, spirituous, and vinous menstrua, though not in so great a degree by water as by spirit; and the extract of this root, prepared from the watery infusion, is less bitter than that made from the spirituous tincture.

Gentian is the principal bitter now employed by physicians; and as the intense bitters are generally admitted to be not only tonic and stomachic, but also anthelmintic, antiseptic, emmenagogue, anti-arthritic, and febrifuge, this root has a better claim to the poſſeſſion of theſe powers than moſt of this kind.

Many dyſpeptic complaints, though ariſing from debility of the ſtomach, are more effectually relieved by bitters than by Peruvian bark; and hence may be inferred their ſuperior tonic power on the organs of digeſtion. And the gentian, joined with equal parts of tormentil or galls, we are told by Dr. Cullen, conſtantly ſucceeded in curing intermittents, if given in ſufficient quantity.

As a ſimple bitter, the gentian is rendered more grateful to the ſtomach by the addition of an aromatic; and for this purpoſe orange peel is commonly employed.

### *Ginger.*

The ginger plant is a native of the Eaſt-Indies, and is ſaid to grow in the greateſt perfection on the coaſt of Malabar and Bengal; but it is now plentifully cultivated in the warmer parts of America and in the Weſt-India iſlands, whence chiefly it is imported into Europe. In 1731 it was firſt introduced into this country by Mr. P. Miller, and is ſtill cultivated in the dry ſtoves of the curious. The flowers have a ſweet fragrant ſmell, and the leaves and ſtalks, eſpecially when bruiſed, alſo emit a faint ſpicy odour; but the hot acrid aromatic taſte is entirely confined to the root.

Ginger gives out its virtues perfectly to rectified ſpirit, and in a great meaſure to *water*. According to Lewis, its active principles are of a remarkably fixed nature; for, a watery infuſion of this root being boiled down to a thick conſiſtence, diſſolved afreſh in a large quantity of water, and ſtrongly boiled down again, the heat and pungency of the root ſtill remained, though with little or nothing of its ſmell. Ginger is generally conſidered as an aromatic, leſs pungent and heating to the ſyſtem than might be expected from its effects upon the organs of taſte. Dr. Cullen thinks, however, that there is no real foundation for this remark. It is uſed as an antiſpaſmodic and carminative. The caſes in which it is more immediately ſerviceable are flatulent colics, debility and laxity of the ſtomach and inteſtines, and in torpid and phlegmatic conſtitutions to excite briſker vaſcular action. It is ſeldom given but in combination with other medicines.

### *Ground-Ivy.*

This plant has a peculiar ſtrong ſmell, and its taſte is bitteriſh, and ſomewhat aromatic. It was formerly in conſiderable eſtimation, and ſuppoſed to poſſeſs great medicinal powers, but which later experience has been unable to diſcover. The qualities of this plant have been defcribed, by different authors, as pectoral, detergent, apperient, diuretic, vulnerary, corroborant, errhine, &c. and it has been varioufly recommended for the cure of thofe difeafes to which thefe powers feemed moft adapted, but chiefly in pulmonary and nephritic complaints. In obftinate coughs it is a favourite remedy with the common people, who probably experience its good effects by ftill perfevering in its ufe. Ray, Mead, and fome others, fpeak of its being ufefully joined with fermenting ale; but Dr. Cullen obferves, "It appears to me frivololous. In fhort, in many cafes where I have feen it employed, I have had no evidence either of its diuretic or of its pectoral effects. In common with many other of the verticillatæ, it may be employed as an errhine, and in that way cure a head-ach, but no otherwife by any fpecific quality." It is ufually taken in the way of infufion, or drunk as tea.

### *Guaiacum.*

This tree is a native of the Weft-India iflands, and the warmer parts of America. The wood, gum, bark, fruit, and even the flowers of this tree have been found to poffefs medicinal qualities. The general virtues of this plant are thofe of a warm ftimulating medicine. It ftrengthens the ftomach and other vifcera, and remarkably promotes the cuticular and urinary difcharges. Hence, in cutaneous diforders, and others proceeding from obftructions of the excretory glands, and where fluggifh ferous humours abound, it is eminently ufeful. In rheumatic and other pains it is adminiftered with fuccefs; but in thin emaciated habits, and an acrimonions ftate of the fluids, it often does harm. Conjoined with mercury and foap, and in fome cafes with bark or fteel, it has been found remarkably ufeful as an alterative. The gum-refin of guaiac is generally given from fix grains to twenty at a dofe; but the latter will be apt to purge brifkly. It may either be adminiftered by itfelf, or in a fluid form, by means of mucilage, or the yolk of egg.

### *Hellebore, black.*

This plant is a native of Auftria and Italy, and was unknown to the gardens in this country till cultivated by Gerard in 1596. If the weather be fufficiently mild, it flowers in January, and hence has obtained the name of Chriftmas flower.

The tafte of the frefh root is bitterifh, and fomewhat acrid. It alfo emits a naufeous acrid fmell; but being long kept, both its fenfible qualities and medicinal activity fuffer very confiderable diminution.

It ſeems to have been principally from its purgative quality that the ancients eſteemed this root ſuch a powerful remedy in maniacal diſorders, with a view to evacuate the *atra bilis*, from which theſe mental diſeaſes were ſuppoſed to be produced: but though evacuations be often found neceſſary in various caſes of alienations of mind, yet, as they can be procured with more certainty and ſafety by other medicines, this catholicon of antiquity is now almoſt entirely abandoned. Modern practice regards it chiefly as an alterative; in which light it is frequently employed in ſmall doſes for attenuating viſcid humours, promoting the uterine and urinary diſcharges, and opening inveterate obſtructions of the remoter glands. It often proves a very powerful emmenagogue in plethoric habits, where ſteel is ineffectual, or improper. It is alſo recommended in dropſies, and ſome cutaneous diſeaſes. The watery extract of this root, made after the manner directed in the diſpenſatories, is one of the beſt and ſafeſt preparations of it, when deſigned for a cathartic, as it contains both the purgative and diuretic parts of the hellebore: it may be given in a doſe from ten grains to a ſcruple, or more. A tincture of this drug is alſo ordered in the diſpenſatories, which is preferred for the purpoſes of an alterative and deobſtruent. Of this a tea-ſpoonful, twice a day, may be conſidered a common doſe.

### *Hemlock.*

This plant is commonly found about the ſides of fields, under hedges, and in moiſt ſhady places, and flowers in June and July. It has a peculiar fœtid ſmell, and a ſlightly aromatic, herbaceous, and ſomewhat nauſeous taſte.

With regard to its virtue when taken internally, it has been generally accounted poiſonous; which it doubtleſs is, in a high degree, when uſed in any conſiderable quantity. The ſymptoms produced by hemlock, when taken in immoderate doſes, are related by various authors, the principal of which has been collected by Haller and others, and ſtated in the following terms: "Internally taken, it occaſions anxiety, heartburn, vomiting, proſtration of appetite, convulſions, blindneſs, vertigo, madneſs, and death itſelf."

Baron Stoerck was the firſt phyſician who brought hemlock into repute as a medicine of extraordinary efficacy. He found that in certain ſmall doſes it may be taken with great ſafety; and that, without in the leaſt diſordering the conſtitution, or even producing any ſenſible operation, it ſometimes proves a powerful reſolvent in many obſtinate diſorders. Though we have not in this country any direct facts, like thoſe mentioned by Stoerck, proving that inveterate ſcirrhuſes, cancers, ulcers, and many other diſeaſes hitherto deemed irremediable, were completely cured by the cicuta; we have, however, the teſtimonies of ſeveral eminent phyſicians, ſhowing that ſome complaints, which had reſiſted other powerful medicines, yielded to hemlock; and that even ſome diſorders, which, if not really cancerous, were at leaſt ſuſpected to be of that tendency, were greatly benefited by this remedy. In glandular ſwellings, chronic rheumatiſms, in various fixed and periodical pains, the cicuta is now very generally employed, and from daily experience it appears in ſuch caſes to be a very efficacious remedy. It has alſo been found of great advantage in the hooping-cough. Externally the leaves of hemlock have been applied with good effect to ulcers, indurated tumours, and gangrenes.

*Honey.*

This is entirely a vegetable juice: for though depoſited by the bees, which extract and carry it into their cells, it never enters their body, nor receives any tincture from their fluids. Honey is obtained from the honey-comb, either by ſeparating the combs, and laying them flat upon a ſieve, through which it ſpontaneouſly percolates; or by including the comb in canvas bags, and forcing out its contents by a preſs. The former ſort is the purer; the latter containing a good deal of wax, and other impurities. There is another ſort ſtill inferior to the two foregoing, obtained by heating the combs before they are put into the preſs. The beſt kind of honey is thick, of a whitiſh colour, an agreeable ſmell, and a very pleaſant taſte. Both the colour and flavour differ according to the plants from which the bees collect it; the ſweet herbs, ſuch as roſemary, marjoram, and thyme, affording the moſt delicate juices.

Honey, conſidered as a medicine, is a very uſeful detergent and aperient, powerfully diſſolving viſcid juices, and promoting the expectoration of tough phlegm. Hence it has proved of great benefit to perſons afflicted with aſthmatic complaints; but for this purpoſe it muſt be taken in conſiderable quantity, as an article of diet. In ſome conſtitutions it diſagrees with the bowels, and is apt to occaſion griping or purging; but this inconvenience, it is ſaid, is in ſome meaſure obviated by previouſly boiling the honey.

*Horehound.*

The leaves of horehound have a moderately ſtrong ſmell, of the aromatic kind, but not agreeable, which by drying is improved, and by keeping for ſome months is in great meaſure diſſipated. Their taſte is very bitter, penetrating, diffuſive, and durable in the mouth. This plant was greatly extolled by the ancients for its efficacy in removing obſtructions of the lungs and other viſcera. It has chiefly been employed in humoural aſthmas, obſtinate coughs, and pulmonary conſumptions. Inſtances are alſo mentioned of its ſucceſsful uſe in ſcirrhous affections of the liver, jaundice, cachexies, and menſtrual ſuppreſſions.

That horehound poſſeſſes ſome ſhare of medicinal power may be inferred from its ſenſible qualities, but its virtues do not appear to be clearly aſcertained; and the character it had formerly acquired is ſo far depreciated, that it is rarely preſcribed by phyſicians. A drachm of the dry leaves in powder, or two or three ounces of the expreſſed juice, or an infuſion of half a handful of the freſh leaves, have been directed for a doſe. This laſt mode is uſually practiſed by the common people, with whom it is ſtill a favourite remedy in coughs and aſthmas.

## *Horſe-Cheſnut.*

The fruit of this tree is eaten by ſheep, goats, deer, oxen, and horſes. It contains much farinaceous matter, which, by undergoing a proper proceſs, ſo as to diveſt it of its bitterneſs and acrimony, probably might afford a kind of bread. Starch has been made of it, and found to be very good. It appears alſo to be endowed with a ſaponaceous quality, as it is uſed particularly in France and Switzerland, for the purpoſe of cleaning woollens, and in waſhing and bleaching linens.

With a view to its errhine power, the Edinburgh college has introduced it into the Materia Medica. As a ſmall portion of the powder, ſnuffed up the noſtrils, readily excites ſneezing; even the infuſion or decoction of the fruit produces this effect; it has therefore been recommended for the purpoſe of producing a diſcharge from the noſe, which, in ſome complaints of the head and eyes, is found to be of conſiderable benefit.

On the continent the bark of the horſe-cheſnut tree is held in great eſtimation as a febrifuge, and, upon the credit of ſeveral reſpectable authors, appears to be a medicine of great efficacy; and that it may be ſubſtituted for the Peruvian bark in every caſe in which the latter is indicated, with equal, if not ſuperior, advantage.

## *Horſe-Radiſh.*

The root of this plant, which has long been received into the Materia Medica, is alſo well known at our tables. It affects the organs both of taſte and ſmell with a quick penetrating pungency:

but contains neverthelefs, in certain veffels, a fweet juice, which fometimes exudes in little drops upon the furface. Its pungent matter is of a very volatile kind, being totally diffipated in drying, and carried off in evaporation or diftillation by water and rectified fpirit. As the pungency exhales, the fweet matter of the root becomes more fenfible, though this alfo is in a great meafure diffipated or deftroyed. It impregnates both water and fpirit, by infufion or by diftillation, very richly with its active matter. In diftillation with water, it yields a fmall quantity of effential oil, exceedingly penetrating and pungent.

With refpect to the medical virtues of horfe-radifh, we fhall infert the opinion of Dr. Cullen. "The root of this only is employed, and it affords one of the moft acrid fubftances of this order (filiquofa) and therefore proves a powerful ftimulant, whether externally or internally employed. Externally, it readily inflames the fkin, and proves a rubifacient that may be employed with advantage in palfy and rheumatifm; and if its application be long continued, it produces blifters. Taken internally, I have faid in what manner its ftimulant power in the fauces may be managed for the cure of hoarfenefs*. Received into the ftomach, it ftimulates this, and promotes digeftion; on which account it is properly employed as a condiment with our animal food. If it be infufed in water, and a portion of this infufion be taken with a large draught of warm water, it readily proves emetic, and may either be employed by itfelf to excite vomiting, or to affift the operation of other emetics. Infufed in water, and taken into the ftomach, it proves ftimulant to the nervous fyftem, and is thereby ufed in palfy; and if employed in large quantity it proves heating to the whole body: and hereby it proves often ufeful in chronic rheumatifm, whether arifing from fcurvy or other caufes. Bergius has given us a particular method of exhibiting this root, which is by cutting it down, without bruifing, into very fmall pieces; and thefe, if fwallowed without chewing, may be taken down in large quantity,

* The doctor here refers to the article Erysimum, the juice of which, mixed with an equal part of honey or sugar, is strongly recommended for the cure of hoarseness which proceeds from an interrupted secretion of mucus, and which stimulants of the acrid kind are found most efficacious in restoring. When the erysimum was not at hand, the doctor substituted a syrup of horse-radish. He says, "I have found that one drachm of the root, fresh, scraped down, was enough for four ounces of water, to be infused in a close vessel for two hours, and made into a syrup, with double its weight of sugar. A tea-spoonful or two of this syrup swallowed leisurely, or at least repeated two or three times, we have found often very suddenly effectual in relieving hoarseness." Mat. Med, vol. ii. p. 167.

to that of a table-ſpoonful: and the author alleges, that, in this way, taken every morning for a month together, this root has been extremely uſeful in arthritic caſes; which, however, I ſuppoſe to have been of the rheumatic kind. It would ſeem that in this manner employed, analogous to the uſe of unbruised muſtard-ſeed, it gives out in the ſtomach its ſubtile volatile parts, that ſtimulate conſiderably without inflaming. The matter of horſe-radiſh; like the ſame matter of the other ſiliquoſe plants, carried into the blood-veſſels, paſſes readily into the kidneys, and proves a powerful diuretic, and is therefore uſeful in dropſy; and we need not ſay, that in this manner, by promoting both urine and perſpiration, it has been long known as one of the moſt powerful antiſcorbutics.

## *Hyſſop.*

This plant, ſuppoſed to be different from the hyſſop mentioned in the Old Teſtament, is a native of Siberia, and the mountainous parts of Auſtria, and flowers from june till September. The leaves have an aromatic ſmell, and a bitteriſh, moderately warm taſte. They give out their active matter both to water and to rectified ſpirit; but to the latter moſt perfectly. Dr. Cullen claſſes this and all the verticillated plants as ſtimulants; and this quality is to be aſcribed to the quantity of eſſential oil which they contain. The hyſſop, therefore, may be eſteemed aromatic and ſtimulant; and, with a view to theſe effects, Bergius recommends it as an emmenagogue and anti-hyſteric: but it is chiefly employed as a pectoral, and has been long thought an uſeful medicine in humoural aſthmas, coughs, and catarrhal affections. For this purpoſe an infuſion of the leaves, ſweetened with honey or ſugar and drunk as tea, is recommended by Lewis. The external application of hyſſop is ſaid to be particularly efficacious in the way of fomentation and poultice, in contuſions, and for removing the blackneſs occaſioned by the extravaſated fluids.

## *Jalap.*

This is the root of an American convolvulus, brought to us in thin tranſverſe ſlices from Xelapa, a province of New Spain. It has ſcarcely any ſmell, and very little taſte; but, to the tongue and to the throat, manifeſts a ſlight degree of pungency. The medicinal activity of jalap reſides principally, if not wholy, in the reſin, which, though given in ſmall doſes, occaſions violent griping. The gummy part bears an inconſiderable proportion to the reſinous, and is found to have little or no cathartic power; but, as a diuretic, it is extremely active.

That jalap is an efficacious and ſafe purgative, daily experience muſt evince; but, according as the root contains more or leſs reſin, its effects muſt of courſe vary. Hoffman thought it particularly improper and unſafe to adminiſter this medicine to children; but Dr. Cullen obſerves, that if jalap "be well triturated, before exhibition, with a hard powder, and the cryſtals of tartar are the fitteſt for the purpoſe, it will operate in leſſer doſes than when taken by itſelf, and, at the ſame time, very moderately, and without griping. Except when given in very large doſes, I have not found it to be heating to the ſyſtem; and if it be triturated with hard ſugar, it becomes, in moderate doſes, a ſafe medicine for children; which in this form they will readily receive, as the jalap itſelf has very little taſte."

Jalap, in large doſes, or when joined with calomel, is recommended as an anthelmintic and a hydragogue. The doſe of the ſimple powder is commonly from one ſcruple to two.

*Ipecacuanha.*

This root is divided into two ſorts, Peruvian and Brazilian: but the eye diſtinguiſhes three kinds, viz. the aſh-coloured or grey, brown, and white; of which the aſh-coloured is that uſually preferred in the ſhops. It was firſt introduced into this country with the character of an almoſt infallible remedy in dyſenteries and other inveterate fluxes, and alſo in diſorders proceeding from obſtructions of long ſtanding; nor has it loſt much of its reputation by time. The uſe of ipecacuanha in fluxes is thought to depend upon its reſtoring perſpiration; for in theſe caſes, eſpecially in dyſentery and diarrhoea, the ſkin is dry and tenſe; and while the common diaphoretics uſually paſs off by ſtool, ſmall doſes of this root have been adminiſtered with the beſt effects, proving both laxative and diaphoretic. In the ſpaſmodic aſthma, Dr. Akenſide remarks, that where nothing contraindicates repeated vomiting, he knows no medicine ſo effectual as ipecacuan. In violent paroxyſms a ſcruple procures immediate relief. Where the complaint is habitual, from three to five grains every morning, or from five to ten every other morning, may be given for a month or ſix weeks.

This medicine has alſo been ſucceſsfully uſed in hæmorrhages. Several caſes of uterine diſcharges are mentioned by Dahlberg, in which one third or half a grain was given every four hours till it effected a cure. Theſe ſmall doſes are likewiſe found of great uſe in catarrhal and even conſumptive caſes, as well as in various ſtates of fever. Ipecacuanha, particularly in the ſtate of powder, is now advantageouſly employed in almoſt every diſeaſe in which vomiting is indicated; and when combined with opium, under the form of ſudorific powder, it furniſhes us with the moſt uſeful and active ſweating medicine which we poſſeſs. It is alſo given with advantage in very ſmall doſes, even when it produces no ſenſible operation. The full doſe of ipecacuanha in ſubſtance is a ſcruple, though leſs doſes will frequently produce an equal effect.

## *Juniper.*

Both the tops and berries of this plant are directed for medicinal uſe, but the latter are uſually preferred, and are brought to us chiefly from Holland and Italy. They have a moderately ſtrong, not diſagreeable, ſmell, and a warm, pungent, ſweetiſh taſte, which, if they are long chewed, or previouſly well bruiſed, is followed by a conſiderable bitterneſs. The ſweetneſs appears to reſide in the juice or ſoft pulpy part of the berry; the bitterneſs, in the ſeeds; and the aromatic flavour, in oily veſicles, ſpread throughout the ſubſtance both of the pulp and the ſeeds, and diſtinguiſhable even by the eye. The freſh berries yield, on expreſſion, a rich, ſweet, honey-like, aromatic juice; if previouſly powdered, ſo as to thoroughly break the ſeeds, which is not done without great difficulty, the juice proves tart and bitter. The ſame differences are obſervable alſo in tinctures and infuſions made from the dry berries, according as the berry is taken entire or thoroughly bruiſed. They give out nearly all their virtue both to water and rectified ſpirit.

Theſe berries are chiefly uſed for their diuretic effects: they are alſo conſidered as ſtomachic, carminative, and diaphoretic.—Of the efficacy of juniper berries in many hydropical affections, we have various relations by phyſicians of great authority. Theſe, however, ſeem not to be perfectly agreed which preparation of the juniper is moſt efficacious. But, as it is now ſeldom, if ever, relied upon for the cure of dropſies, and only called to the aid of more powerful remedies, perhaps one of the beſt forms under which the berries can be uſed is that of a ſimple infuſion. This, either by itſelf, or with the addition of a little gin, is a very uſeful drink for hydropic patients. The juniper has alſo been recommended in nephritic caſes, uterine obſtructions, ſcorbutic affections, and ſome cutaneous diſeaſes; and in the two laſt mentioned complaints the wood and tops of the plant are ſaid to have been employed with more advantage than the berries.

## *Kino.*

This is a red aſtringent gum from Gambia, ſuppoſed to exude from inciſions made in the trunks of certain trees called *pan de ſangue*, growing in the interior parts of Africa. It is very friable, ſo as to be crumbled in pieces by the hands; of an opake, dark reddiſh colour, inclining to black; when reduced to powder, of a deep brick red. It has a reſemblance to catechu, but is more red and aſtringent.

This gum has been found uſeful in ſome uterine hæmorrhages, particularly after child-bearing. One part of kino united with three parts of alum, Dr. Cullen ſays, has proved one of the moſt powerful aſtringents with which he was ever acquainted. This compoſition may be given from five to fifteen grains or more, every four hours, in uterine and pulmonary hæmorrhage. Forty grains of gum-arabic added to one drachm of kino, and a proper quantity of ſyrup of white poppy, forms an agreeable aſtringent linctus or lambative; of which a tea-ſpoonful may be taken occaſionally.

### *Lavender.*

The fragrant ſmell of the flowers of this plant is well known, and to moſt people agreeable: to the taſte they are bitteriſh, warm, and ſomewhat pungent; the leaves are weaker and leſs grateful. Lavender has been an officinal plant for a conſiderable time. Its medicinal virtue reſides in the eſſential oil, which is ſuppoſed to be a gentle corroborant and ſtimulant of the aromatic kind, and is recommended in nervous debilities, and various affections proceeding from a want of energy in the animal functions.

### *Liquorice.*

This is a native of the ſouth of Europe, but has been long cultivated in Britain, particularly at Pontefract in Yorkſhire, Workſop in Notinghamſhire, and Godalming in Surry. But it is now planted by many gardeners in the vicinity of London, by whom the metropolis is ſupplied with the roots, which after three years growth, are dug up for uſe, and are found to be in no reſpect inferior for medical purpoſes to thoſe produced in their native climate.

Liquorice root, lightly boiled in a little water, gives out nearly all its ſweetneſs: the decoction, preſſed through a ſtrainer, and inſpiſſated with a gentle heat, till it will no longer ſtick to the fingers, affords a better extract than that brought from abroad, and its quantity amounts to near half the weight of the root.

This root contains a great quantity of ſaccharine matter, joined with ſome proportion of mucilage; and hence has a viſcid, ſweet taſte. From the time of Theophraſtus it has been a received opinion that it very powerfully extinguiſhes thirſt; which, if true, is more remarkable, as ſweet ſubſtances, in general, have a contrary effect. It is in common uſe as a pectoral or emollient in catarrhal defluxions on the breaſt, coughs, hoarſeneſs, &c. Infuſions or extracts made from it afford likewiſe very commodious vehicles for the exhibition of other medicines; the liquorice-taſte concealing that of unpalatable drugs more effectually than ſyrups, or any other ſubſtance of the ſaccharine kind.

*Maidenhair.*

The leaves of this plant have a mucilaginous, ſweetiſh, ſubaſtringent taſte, without any particular flavour. They are eſteemed uſeful in diſorders of the breaſt, proceeding from a thickneſs and acrimony of the juices; and are likewiſe ſuppoſed to promote the expectoration of tough phlegm, and to open obſtructions of the viſcera. They are uſually directed in infuſion or decoction, with the addition of a little liquorice. A ſyrup prepared from them, though it has now no place in our diſpenſatories, is frequently to be met with in the ſhops, both as prepared at home and imported from abroad. A little of theſe ſyrups mixed with water makes a very pleaſant draught. The ſyrup brought from abroad has an admixture of orange flower-water.

*Manna.*

This is the juice of certain trees of the aſh-kind growing in Italy and Sicily, either naturally concreted on the plants, or exſiccated and purified by art. From inciſions made in the trees, the manna ſometimes flows in ſuch abundance, that it runs upon the ground, by which it becomes mixed with various impurities, unleſs carefully prevented by thoſe who are employed in obtaining it.

Manna is well known as a gentle purgative, ſo mild in its operation, that it may be given with ſafety to children and pregnant women. In ſome conſtitutions, however, it produces troubleſome flatulencies, and therefore requires the addition of a ſuitable aromatic, eſpecially when given to an adult, where a large doſe is neceſſary: it is therefore uſually aſſiſted by ſome other purgative of a more powerful kind.

*Marjoram, Wild.*

This plant grows in many parts of Britain, eſpecially on dry chalky hills, or gravelly ſoils, and produces its flowers in July and Auguſt. It has an agreeable aromatic ſmell, approaching to that of ſweet marjoram, and a pungent taſte much reſembling thyme, to which it is likewiſe thought to be more nearly allied in its medicinal qualities than to any of the other verticillatæ, and therefore deemed to be emmenagogue, tonic, ſtomachic, &c. The dried leaves, uſed inſtead of tea, are ſaid to be exceedingly grateful. They are alſo employed in medicated baths and fomentations.

### *Marjoram, Sweet.*

This plant is thought to be the amaracus of the ancients, mentioned by Virgil and Catullus. It has long been cultivated in our gardens, and in frequent uſe for culinary purpoſes. The leaves and tops have a pleaſant ſmell, and a moderately warm, aromatic, bitteriſh taſte. The medicinal qualities of this agree with thoſe of wild marjoram; but, being more fragrant, it is deemed to be better adapted to thoſe complaints known by the name of nervous; and may be therefore employed with the ſame intentions as lavender. In its recent ſtate, we are told that it has been ſucceſsfully applied to ſcirrhous tumours of the breaſt.

### *Marſh-Mallow.*

This plant, under the name of althæa, has long been in general uſe among practitioners in every country where the ſcience of medicine is cultivated. The virtues of it conſiſts in a mucilaginous matter, with which it abounds, and which renders it emollient and demulcent. It therefore proves ſerviceable in a thin acrimonious ſtate of the juices, and where the natural mucus of the membranes is abraded. It is chiefly recommended in ſharp defluxions upon the lungs, hoarſeneſſes, dyſenteries, and likewiſe in nephritic and calculous complaints. It is uſed in decoction or infuſion.

### *Mezereon.*

This plant is extremely acrid, eſpecially when freſh, and if retained in the mouth, excites great and long continued heat and inflammation, particularly of the throat and fauces. The berries alſo have the ſame effects, and, when ſwallowed, prove a powerful corroſive poiſon, not only to man, but to dogs, wolves, foxes, &c. The bark and berries of mezereon, in different forms, have been long externally uſed to obſtinate ulcers and ill-conditioned ſores. In France the former is ſtrongly recommended as an application to the ſkin, which, under certain management, produces a continued ſerous diſcharge, without bliſtering; and is thus rendered uſeful in many chronic diſeaſes of a local nature, anſwering the purpoſe of what has been called a perpetual bliſter, while it occaſions leſs pain and inconvenience.

The bark of the root is the part chiefly in uſe, two drachms of which, with half an ounce of bruiſed liquorice, are boiled in three pints of water till reduced to two: of this from four to eight ounces are taken four times a day. This has been found very efficacious for reſolving venereal nodes, and curing other remains of the venereal diſeaſe, which mercury, taken in large quantities, had failed to effect. Dr. Cullen found a caſe of ulcerations in many different parts of the body, for which mercury had likewiſe been taken without ſucceſs, entirely cured by the uſe of mezereon decoction for two or three weeks.

### *Mugwort.*

This plant grows plentifully in fields, hedges, and waſte places, and flowers in June. The leaves have a light aromatic ſmell, and an herbaceous bitteriſh taſte. They are principally celebrated as uterine and anti-hyſteric. An infuſion of them is ſometimes drunk, either alone or in conjunction with other ſubſtances, in ſuppreſſion of the menſtrual evacuations. In ſome parts of the kingdom, mugwort is in common uſe as a pot-herb.

### *Muſk.*

This is a grumous ſubſtance like clotted blood, found in a little bag ſituated near the umbilical region of a particular kind of animal met with in China, Tartary, and the Eaſt-Indies. Muſk has a bitteriſh ſub-acrid taſte, a fragrant ſmell, agreeable at a diſtance, but, when ſmelt near, ſo ſtrong as to be diſagreeable, unleſs weakened by the admixture of other ſubſtances. It is a medicine of great eſteem in the eaſtern countries; but among us it has been for ſome time very little uſed, even as a perfume, on a ſuppoſition of its occaſioning vapours, &c. in weak females, and perſons of a ſedentary life. It appears, however, from late experience, to be, when properly managed, a remedy of great ſervice, even againſt thoſe diſorders which it has been ſuppoſed to produce. In convulſive and other diſeaſes it has been found to produce extraordinary good effects; and Dr. Cullen conſiders it as the moſt powerful antiſpaſmodic with which we are acquainted. It is moſt effectual when given in ſubſtance, and muſt be adminiſtered in large doſes; from ten to thirty grains. Even when theſe large doſes are found to be effectual, they muſt be repeated at ſhort intervals till the diſeaſe is entirely ſubdued. Dr. Cullen once procured immediate relief to a patient labouring under ſevere head-ach and delirium from the gout, by adminiſtering fifteen grains of genuine muſk at a doſe. He alſo relieved a gentleman afflicted with a ſpaſm of the pharynx, preventing deglutition, and almoſt reſpiration, by muſk, when other remedies had failed; and as the diſeaſe continued to recur, at times, for many years after, it was only obviated or relieved by the uſe of mulk. It has given relief in ſeveral circumſtances of the gout, when retrocedent, affecting the ſtomach, lungs, and particularly the head, when adminiſtered in large doſes, or at leaſt by repeating them after ſhort intervals. In fine, muſk ſeems to be adapted to all caſes of convulſive diſorders for which opium is uſually preſcribed.

## *Muſtard.*

This plant is diſtinguiſhed into two kinds, namely, the black or common, and the white. The ſeeds of the former are directed by the London College, and thoſe of the latter by that of Edinburgh: but they manifeſt no remarkable difference to the taſte, nor in their general effects, and therefore anſwer equally well for the uſes of the table and for the purpoſes of medicine.

Muſtard is conſidered to promote appetite, aſſiſt digeſtion, attenuate viſcid juices, and, by ſtimulating the fibres, to prove a general remedy in paralytic and rheumatic affections. Beſides its ſtimulant qualities, it frequently, if taken in conſiderable quantity, opens the body, and increaſes the urinary diſcharge, whence it has been found uſeful in dropſical complaints. It was alleged by Haller, that the uſe of muſtard diſpoſes the humours to putreſcency; an opinion which he was probably led to entertain from a ſuppoſition that it contained volatile alkali: for it is well known that ſome of the pungent plants, when in a ſtate of putrefaction, give out this alkali by diſtillation, and hence have been termed alkaleſcent plants. But the fermentation of theſe vegetable ſubſtances may be ſo directed as to be of the aceſcent kind, and the alkali obtained from them ſeems not to have exiſted in the vegetable in a ſeparate ſtate. The great pungency of theſe plants, therefore, is not to be aſcribed to the volatile alkali, but to the eſſential oil which they contain.

Bergius informs us, that he found muſtard of great efficacy in curing vernal intermittents; for which purpoſe he directed a ſpoonful of the whole ſeeds to be taken three or four times a day, during the intermiſſion; and, when the diſeaſe was obſtinate, he added flower of muſtard to the bark. Externally theſe ſeeds are frequently uſed as a ſinapiſm, or ſtimulating poultice. Muſtard-ſeed may be moſt conveniently given entire or unbruiſed, and to the quantity of a table ſpoonful or half an ounce for a doſe.

## *Nettle, Stinging.*

The present practice pays very little regard to this plant; yet, if the testimony of many respectable authors is to be credited, it seems to merit more attention. The juice, taken from two to four ounces, is recommended in nephritic complaints, and internal hæmorrhages. The nettle is a common remedy among the people of Brunswick in an incipient consumption. When the juice is not to be obtained, the powder is used, mixed with honey or sugar. Externally it has been employed as a rubifacient; a method of cure which has been called *urtication*, and found efficacious in restoring excitement to paralytic limbs, or in other cases of torpor or lethargy. Withering tells us, that a nettle leaf put upon the tongue, and then pressed against the roof of the mouth, is sometimes efficacious in stopping a bleeding at the nose.

## *Nightshade, Deadly.*

This plant, otherwise named belladonna, or solanum lethale, has been for ages known as a strong poison of the narcotic kind; and the berries, though less powerful than the leaves, furnish us with many instances of their fatal effects, particularly upon children, who are readily tempted to eat this fruit by its alluring appearance and sweet taste. The number of these berries necessary to produce deleterious effects may probably depend upon the state of maturity in which they are eaten: if not more than three or four, according to Haller's account, no bad consequence ensues. But when a greater number of berries are taken into the stomach, scarcely half an hour elapses before violent symptoms supervene, viz. vertigo, delirium, great thirst, painful deglutition, and retching, followed by phrenzy, grinding of the teeth, and convulsions, which usually precede death.

The leaves of the nightshade were first used externally to discuss scirrhous and cancerous tumours, and also as an application to ill-conditioned ulcers. Their good effects in this way at length induced physicians to employ them internally for the same disorders; and a considerable number of well-authenticated facts evince them to be a very serviceable and important remedy. At the same time it must be acknowledged, that many cases of this sort have occurred in which the belladonna has been employed without success. This, however, may be said of every medicine; and though Dr. Cullen repeatedly experienced its inefficacy, yet the facts he adduces in confirmation of this plant are clear and decisive. "I have," says he, "had a cancer of the lip entirely cured by it; a scirrhosity in a woman's breast, of such a kind as frequently proceeds to cancer, I have found entirely difcuffed by the ufe of it; a fore a little below the eye, which had put on a cancerous appearance, was much mended by the internal ufe of the belladonna: but the patient, having learned fomewhat of the poifonous nature of the medicine, refufed to continue the ufe of it; upon which the fore again fpread, and was painful, but, upon a return to the ufe of the belladonna, was again mended to a confiderable degree: when the fame fears again returned, the ufe of it was again laid afide and with the fame confequence of the fore becoming worfe. Of thefe alternate ftates, connected with the alternate ufe of, and abftinence from, the belladonna, there were feveral of thefe alternations which fell under my own obfervation."

The fenfible effects produced by the leaves of this plant taken in medicinal dofes are ufually by the fkin, the urinary paffages, and fometimes by ftool; in larger dofes, troublefome drynefs of the mouth and throat, giddinefs and dimnefs of fight are experienced.

That the advantages derived from the internal ufe of belladonna are only in proportion to the evacuations effected by it, is a conclufion which we cannot admit as fufficiently warranted by the facts adduced upon this point.

As this plant is very uncertain in its operation, the proper dofe is with difficulty afcertained: the moft prudent manner of adminiftering it is by beginning with one grain or lefs; which may be gradually increafed, according to its effects. Six grains are confidered as a very large dofe. The root feems to partake of the fame qualities as the leaves, but is lefs virulent.

## *Nutmeg.*

The feeds or kernels of this denomination are the produce of a tree which is a native of the Eaft-Indies, particularly the Molucca Iflands, and have long been ufed both for culinary and medical purpofes. The medicinal qualities of nutmeg are fuppofed to be aromatic, anodyne, ftomachic, and reftringent; and, with a view to the laft mentioned effects, it has been much ufed in diarrhœas and dyfenteries. To many people the aromatic flavour of nutmeg is very agreeable; they fhould beware, however, of ufing it in too large quantities, as it is apt to affect the head, and even to manifeft a foporific power in fuch a degree as to prove extremely dangerous. Bontius fpeaks of this as a frequent occurrence in India; and Dr. Cullen relates a remarkable inftance of fuch an effect of the nutmeg, which fell under his obfervation; and hence concludes, that in apoplectic and paralytic cafes this fpice may be very improper

## *Nitre.*

Nitre, or ſaltpetre, is a ſalt extracted in Perſia and the Eaſt-Indies from certain earths that lie on the ſides of hills; and artificially produced in ſome parts of Europe from animal and vegetable ſubſtances rotted together (with the addition of lime and aſbes) and expoſed for a length of time to the air, without the acceſs of which nitre is never generated. The ſalt extracted from the earths by means of water is purified by colature and cryſtallization.

Nitre is a medicine of extraordinary uſe in many diſorders. Beſides the aperient quality of neutral ſalts in general, it has a manifeſtly cooling one, by which it quenches thirſt, and abates febrile heats and commotions of the blood. It has one great advantage above the cooling medicines of the acid kind, that it does not coagulate the animal juices. Blood, which is coagulated by all the mineral acids, and milk, &c. by acids of every kind, are by nitre rendered more dilute, and preſerved from coagulation. It nevertheleſs ſomewhat thickens thin, ſerous, acrimonious humours, and occaſions an uniform mixture of them with ſuch as are more thick and viſcid; by which means it prevents the ill conſequences which would otherwiſe enſue from the former.

This medicine for the moſt part promotes urine; ſometimes gently looſens the belly; but, in cold phlegmatic habits, very rarely has this effect, though given in large doſes. Alvine fluxes, proceeding from too great acrimony of the bile, or inflammation of the inteſtines, are ſuppreſſed by it: in choleric and febrile diſorders it generally excites ſweat: but in malignant caſes, where the pulſe is low and the ſtrength much reduced, it retards this ſalutary evacuation and the progreſs of eruptions.

It is given from five to thirty grains, with equal quantities of ſugar or gum-arabic well powdered, and diſſolved in barley-water or thin gruel. It is thus adminiſtered repeatedly as a cooling medicine, in acute fevers, and other inflammatory diſorders; though it may be given with great ſafety, and generally to better advantage, in large quantities: the only inconvenience is its being apt to ſit uneaſy on the ſtomach.

## *Oak.*

The aſtringent effects of the oak were ſufficiently known to the ancients, by whom different parts of the tree were uſed; but it is the bark which is now generally directed for medicinal uſe. Oak-bark manifeſts to the taſte a ſtrong aſtringency, accompanied with a moderate bitterneſs; qualities which are extracted both by water and by rectified ſpirit. Its univerſal uſe and preference in the tanning of leather is a proof of its great aſtringency; and, like other aſtringents, it has been recommended in agues, and for reſtraining hæmorrhages, alvine fluxes, and other immoderate evacuations. A decoction of it has likewiſe been advantageouſly employed as a gargle, and a fomentation or lotion in the bearing down of the rectum and uterus.

To this valuable tree we are indebted for galls, which in the warm climates of the Eaſt are found upon its leaves. They are occaſioned by a ſmall inſect, called cynips, with four wings, which depoſits an egg in the ſubſtance of the leaf, by making a ſmall perforation through the under ſurface. The gall preſently begins to grow, and the egg in the centre of it changes to a worm; this worm again changes to a nymph, and the nymph to the flying inſect above mentioned, which, by eating its paſſage out, leaves a round hole: and thoſe galls which bave no holes are found to have the dead inſect remaining in them.

Galls appear to be the moſt powerful of the vegetable aſtringents; and, as a medicine, they are applicable to the ſame indications as the oak-bark. Reduced to a ſine powder, and made into an ointment, they have been found of great ſervice in hæmorrhoidal affections. Their efficacy in intermittent fevers was tried by Mr. Poupart, by order of the Academy of Sciences; and from his report it appears, that the galls had ſucceeded in many caſes; and alſo that they had failed in many other caſes, which were afterwards cured by the Peruvian-bark.

### *Opium.*

This juice is obtained from the poppy in Egypt, Perſia, and ſome other provinces of Aſia. The opium prepared about Thebes in Egypt, hence named Thebaic opium, has been uſually eſteemed the beſt; but this is not now diſtinguiſhed from that collected in other places.

The general effects of this medicine are, to relax the ſolids, and render them leſs ſenſible of irritation; to cheer the ſpirits, caſe pain, procure ſleep, and to promote perſpiration. When its operation is over, the pain and other ſymptoms which it had for a time abated, return, and generally with greater violence than before, unleſs the cauſe has been removed by the ſweat or relaxation which it occaſioned.

The operation of opium is generally attended with a ſlow but ſtrong and full pulſe, a dryneſs of the mouth, a redneſs and ſlight itching of the ſkin, and followed by a degree of nauſea, a difficulty of reſpiration, lowneſs of the ſpirits, and a weak languid pulſe,

The principal indications of opium are great watchfulneſs, immoderate evacuations, proceeding from acrimony and irritation, cramps or ſpaſmodic contractions of the nerves, and violent pains of almoſt every kind. In theſe caſes, opiates procure at leaſt a temporary relief, and an opportunity for other medicines, properly interpoſed, to take effect.

Opium ſometimes fruſtrates the intention of the phyſician, and, inſtead of procuring reſt, occaſions great anxiety, vomiting, &c. Taken on a full ſtomach, it often proves emetic. Where the patient is exhauſted by exceſſive evacuations, it occaſions generally great lowneſs. It has been obſerved to operate more powerfully in perſons of a lax habit than in the oppoſite circumſtances. While it uſefully reſtrains præternatural diſcharges, proceeding from irritation, it proves injurious in thoſe that ariſe from a contrary cauſe, as in the colliquative diarrhœa attending the hectic fever.

In hæmorrhages excited by irritation, and unattended with inflammation, opium is uſeful. In the dyſentery it may be occaſionally employed to moderate the violence of the ſymptoms, though not conſidered as a remedy. In the latter ſtages of diarrhœa, when the acrimony producing the diſeaſe has been carried off in a great meaſure, opium is an efficacious remedy. In the cholera morbus, and water-braſh, it is chiefly to be relied upon. Joined with laxatives, it is employed in the colic. In different ſpecies of *tetanus* opium is ſucceſsful, and affords relief to various ſpaſmodic and convulſive ſymptoms occurring in ſeveral diſeaſes, as aſthma, epilepſy, &c.

In intermittent fevers, opium has been ſtrongly recommended, as an effectual means of ſtopping the return of the febrile paroxyſms, and has been given before the fit, in the cold ſtage, in the hot fit, and during the interval, with the beſt effects; producing immediate relief, and in a ſhort time curing the patient. But in theſe fevers the beſt practice, perhaps, is to unite opium with the bark, which enables the ſtomach to bear the latter doſes, and adds conſiderably to its efficacy.

With regard to the doſe of opium, one grain is generally ſufficient, and often too large a one. Its doſe, however, varies in different perſons, and in different ſtates of the ſame perſon. A quarter of a grain will in one adult produce effects which ten times the quantity will not do in another; and a doſe that might be fatal in the colic or cholera would not have the ſmalleſt effect in many caſes of tetanus, or mania. Given in the way of clyſter, it has the ſame effects as when taken into the ſtomach; but, to anſwer the purpoſe, double the quantity muſt be employed.

Opium taken into the ſtomach in an immoderate doſe, by thoſe not accuſtomed to the uſe of it, proves a narcotic poiſon producing giddineſs, tremors, convulſions, delirium, ſtupor, and, finally, fatal apoplexy.

Opium applied externally gives eaſe in many pains, but does not, as ſome have ſuppoſed, ſtupefy the part, or render it inſenſible of pain. Uſed immoderately, it is ſaid to produce the ſame ill effects as when taken to exceſs internally.

## *Pennyroyal.*

This plant has a warm pungent flavour, ſimilar to that of mint, of which it is a ſpecies, but more acrid, and leſs agreeable both in ſmell and taſte. Pennyroyal certainly poſſeſſes the general properties of the other mints: it is ſuppoſed, however, to be of leſs efficacy as a ſtomachic, but more uſeful as a carminative and emmenagogue, and is more commonly employed, in hyſterical affections. We are told by Boyle, and others, that it has been ſucceſsfully uſed in the hooping-cough; but the chief purpoſe for which it has long been adminiſtered is promoting the uterine evacuation. With this intention, Haller recommends an infuſion of the herb with ſteel, in white wine, which he never knew to fail of ſucceſs. In the opinion of Dr. Cullen, however, mint is in every reſpect a more effectual remedy than pennyroyal; and "nothing but the neglect of all attempts to eſtabliſh principles could have made phyſicians think of this as a peculiar medicine different from the other ſpecies." Conformably to this remark, it may be obſerved that pennyroyal is leſs frequently uſed now than formerly.

## *Peppermint.*

The ſpontaneous growth of this plant is ſaid to be peculiar to Britain; but as it is commonly preferred to the other ſpecies of mint, its cultivation has long been extended over Europe, and that employed here is commonly raiſed in gardens. This ſpecies has a more penetrating ſmell than any of the other mints, and a much ſtronger and warmer taſte, pungent and glowing like pepper, from which it has obtained its name. Its ſtomachic, antiſpaſmodic, and carminative qualities render it uſeful in flatulent colics, hyſterical affections, retchings, and other ſymptoms of indigeſtion, acting as a cordial, and often producing immediate relief.

## *Plantain, or Way-bread.*

The common great plantain was formerly reckoned amongſt the moſt efficacious of vulnerary herbs; and by the peaſants the leaves are now commonly applied to fresh wounds and cutaneous sores. Inwardly they have been used in phthisical complaints, spitting of blood, and in various fluxes both alvine and hæmorrhagic. The seeds, however, seem better adapted to relieve pulmonary diseases than the leaves, as they are extremely mucilaginous. The roots have also been recommended for the cure of tertian intermittents, and, from the experience of Bergius, not undeservedly. An ounce or two of the expressed juice, or the like quantity of a strong infusion of plantain may be given for a dose: in agues, the dose should be double the quantity, and taken at the commencement of the fit.

### *Poppy White.*

This species is said to have been named white poppy from the whiteness of its seeds: a variety of it however, is well known to produce black seeds: the double-flowered white poppy is also another variety; but for medicinal purposes any of these may be employed indiscriminately, as we cannot discover the least difference in their sensible qualities or effects.

The seeds, according to some authors, possess a narcotic power; but there seems to be no foundation for this opinion: they consist of a simple farinaceous matter, united with bland oil, and in many countries are eaten as food. As a medicine, they have been usually given in the form of emulsion, in catarrhs, stranguries, &c.

The heads or capsules of the poppy, which are directed for use in the dispensatories, like the stalks and leaves, have an unpleasant smell, somewhat like that of opium, and an acrid bitterish taste. Both the smell and taste reside in a milky juice, which abounds chiefly in the cortical part of the capsules. These capsules are powerfully narcotic, or anodyne: boiled in water, they impart to the menstruum their narcotic juice, together with the other juices which they have in common with vegetable substances in general. The liquor, strongly pressed out, suffered to settle, clarified with whites of eggs, and evaporated to a due consistence, yields an extract which possesses the virtues of opium, but requires to be given in double its dose to answer the same intention, which it is said to perform without occasioning a nausea and giddiness, the usual effects of opium. The syrup of white poppies, as directed by both colleges, is a useful anodyne, and often succeeds in procuring sleep where opium fails; it is more especially adapted to children. White poppy heads are also used externally in fomentations, either alone, or more frequently added to the decoction for fomentation, which consists of the leaves of southernwood, the tops of sea worm-wood, chamomile flowers, and bay-berries.

### *Quassia.*

This is a native of South-America, particularly of Surinam, and alſo of ſome of the Weſt-India iſlands. The root, wood and bark, of this tree are all comprehended in the catalogues of the Materia Medica; but as the roots are perfectly ligneous, they may be medically conſidered in the ſame light as the wood, which is now moſt generally employed, and ſeems to differ from the bark in being leſs intenſely bitter; the latter is therefore thought to be a more powerful medicine. Quaſſia has no ſenſible odour; its taſte is that of a pure bitter, more intenſe and durable than that of almoſt any other known ſubſtance. It imparts its virtues more completely to watery than to ſpirituous menſtrua. Quaſſia derived its name from a negro named Quaſſi, who employed it with uncommon ſucceſs, as a ſecret remedy in the malignant epidemic fevers which frequently prevailed at Surinam. In conſequence of a valuable conſideration, this ſecret was diſcloſed to Daniel Rolander a Swede, who brought ſpecimens of the quaſſia-wood to Stockholm in the year 1756; and ſince that time the effects of this drug have been very generally tried in Europe, and numerous teſtimonies of its efficacy publiſhed by many reſpectable authors. Various experiments with quaſſia have likewiſe been made, with a view to aſcertain its antiſeptic powers, from which it appears to have conſiderable influence in retarding the tendency to putrefaction. This effect, profeſſor Murray thinks, cannot be attributed to its ſenſible qualities, as it poſſeſſes no aſtringency whatever; nor can it depend upon its bitterneſs, as gentian is much more bitter, yet leſs antiſeptic. The medicinal virtues aſcribed to quaſſia are thoſe of a tonic, ſtomachic, antiſeptic, and febrifuge. It has been found very effectual in reſtoring the tone of the ſtomach, producing appetite for food, aſſiſting digeſtion, expelling flatulency, and removing habitual coſtiveneſs, occaſioned by debility of the inteſtines, and common to a ſedentary life.

### *Rhubarb.*

Rhubarb is the root of a plant of the dock kind, which grows ſpontaneouſly in China, Turkey, and other parts of the Eaſt; but the propagation of it has lately been introduced into our own country, with a degree of ſucceſs which promiſes in time to ſuperſede the uſe of the foreign root. This excellent purgative operates without violence or irritation, and may be given with ſafety even to pregnant women and children. Beſides its purgative quality, it is celebrated for an aſtringent one, by which it ſtrengthens the tone of the ſtomach and inteſtines, and proves uſeful in fluxes of the belly arifing from a laxity of the fibres. Rhubarb in fubftance operates more powerfully as a purgative than any of the preparations of it; and its qualities are more perfectly extracted by water than by rectified fpirit. The dofe, when intended as a purgative, is from a fcruple to a drachm or more.

*Rofe, Hundred-leaved.*

Moft of the rofes, though much cultivated in our gardens, are far from being diftinctly characterifed. Thofe denominated varieties are extremely numerous, and often permanently uniform; and the fpecific differences, as hitherto pointed out, are in many refpects fo inadequate to the purpofe of fatisfactory difcrimination, that it is difficult to fay which are fpecies, and which are varieties only. The London college, following Gerard and Parkinfon, has ftill retained the name rofa damafcena; but the damafk rofe is another fpecies, widely different from the hundred-leaved, as appears from the defcriptions given of it by Du Roi and Miller.

The petals are directed for medicinal ufe: they are of a pale red colour, and of a very fragrant odour; which to moft people is extremely agreeable, and therefore this and moft of the other rofes are much ufed as nofegays. In fome inftances, however, under certain circumftances, they have produced alarming fymptoms; fuch as inflammations of the eyes, faintings, hyfterical affections, abortion, &c. Perfons confined in a clofe room with a large quantity of rofes have been in danger of immediate extinction of life. From the experiments of Prieftley and Ingenhoufz this effect feems owing to the mephitic air, which thefe and moft other odoriferous flowers exhale.

The petals impart their odoriferous matter to watery liquors, both by infufion and diftillation. On diftilling large quantities, there feparates from the watery fluid a fmall portion of a fragrant butyraceous oil, which liquefies by heat and appears yellow, but concretes in the cold into a white mafs. A hundred pounds of the flowers, according to the experiments of Tachenius and Hoffman, afforded fcarcely half an ounce of oil. The fmell of this oil exactly refembles that of rofes, and is therefore much ufed as a perfume. It poffeffes very little pungency, and has been highly recommended for its cordial and reftorative virtues.

*Rofe, Red.*

This is a native of the South of Europe, and is now common in our gardens, flowering in June and July. The flowers poffefs neither the fragrance nor the laxative power of thofe of the hundred-leaved, but are chiefly valued for their aſtringent qualities, which are moſt conſiderable before the petals expand, and therefore in this ſtate they are choſen for medicinal uſe, and ordered by diſpenſatories in different preparations, ſuch as thoſe of a conſerve, a honey, an infuſion, and a ſyrup. The preparations, eſpecially the firſt and ſecond, have been highly eſteemed in phthiſical caſes, particularly by the Arabian phyſicians. Avicenna and Meſue mention ſome remarkable inſtances of this kind which were cured by the roſes. Riverius alſo cites ſeveral others; and the caſe of Krugar, related in the German Ephemerides, has been thought a ſtill more evident proof of the efficacy of the conſerve of roſes in a conſumption of the lungs: but as the uſe of the conſerve was conſtantly joined with that of milk and farinaceous ſubſtances, together with proper exerciſe in the open air, it has been doubted whether theſe recoveries could be wholly imputed to the roſes, though their mild aſtringent and corroborant virtues certainly contributed much. In ſome of the caſes alluded to, twenty or thirty pounds of the conſerve were taken in the ſpace of a month. The quantity commonly uſed is far too inconſiderable to produce beneficial effects.

The infuſion of roſes is a grateful cooling ſubaſtringent, uſeful in ſpitting of blood, and ſome other hæmorrhagic complaints, as a gargle: its efficacy, however, depends chiefly on the acid. For the latter purpoſe, the honey of roſes is alſo frequently uſed.

### *Roſemary.*

This plant has a fragrant ſmell, and a bitteriſh pungent taſte. The leaves and tops are the ſtrongeſt in their ſenſible qualities. Roſemary gives out its virtues completely to rectified ſpirit, but only partially to water. It is reckoned one of the moſt powerful of thoſe plants which ſtimulate and corroborate the nervous ſyſtem; and has therefore been recommended in various affections, ſuppoſed to proceed from debility, or defective excitement of the nerves; as in certain head-achs, deafneſs, giddineſs, palſy, &c. and in ſome hyſterical and dyſpeptic ſymptoms. Dr. Cullen ſuppoſes the ſtimulant power of roſemary inſufficient to reach the ſanguiferous ſyſtem; it has, however, the character of being an emmenagogue; and the only diſeaſe in which Bergius ſtates it to be uſeful, is the chloroſis or green-ſickneſs. It is a principal ingredient in what is known by the name of Hungary-water.

*Rue.*

This plant is extremely common in our gardens, where it retains its verdure the whole year. It has a ſtrong ungrateful ſmell, and a bitter, hot, penetrating taſte: the leaves are ſo acrid, that by much handling they are ſaid to irritate and inflame the ſkin; and the plant in its natural and uncultivated ſtate is reported to poſſeſs theſe ſenſible qualities ſtill more powerfully. Both water and rectified ſpirit extract its virtues, but the latter more powerfully than the former.

Rue was much uſed by the ancients, who aſcribed to it many virtues. Hippocrates commends it as a reſolvent and diuretic, and attributes to it the power of reſiſting the action of contagion, and other kinds of poiſons; and with this intention it was uſed by Mithridates. But this imaginary quality of the rue is now little credited. It is doubtleſs, however, a powerful ſtimulant, and may be conſidered like other medicines of the foetid kind, to have attenuating, deobſtruent, and antiſpaſmodic powers, and to be more peculiarly adapted to phlegmatic habits or weak and hyſterical conſtitutions, ſuffering from retarded or obſtructed ſecretions. By ſome it is employed in the way of tea.

*Sage.*

This has a fragrant ſtrong ſmell, and a warm, bitteriſh, aromatic taſte, like other plants containing an eſſential oil: it gives out its properties more perfectly to ſpirituous than to aqueous menſtrua. In ancient times ſage was celebrated as a remedy of great efficacy; but at preſent it is conſidered as of little importance in the Materia Medica; and, though frequently employed as a ſudorific, it ſeems to have no advantage over other plants that render the fluids in which they are infuſed more agreeable to the ſtomach. By ſome it has been ſucceſsfully uſed even for the purpoſe of reſtraining inordinate ſweating. As poſſeſſing a ſmall ſhare of aromatic and aſtringent power, it may prove a ſerviceable tonic in ſome caſes of debility of the ſtomach and nervous ſyſtem. The Chineſe, who are ſaid to have experienced the good effects of ſage in this way, eſteem it highly, and prefer it to their own tea. It appears from experiments, that ſage is endowed with the power of reſiſting the putrefaction of animal ſubſtances.

*St. John's Wort.*

This plant was in great eſteem with the ancients, who preſcribed it in the hyſteric and hypochondriac diſeaſes, and in madneſs.

They even imagined that it had the power of curing demoniacs, whence it obtained the name of *fuga dæmonum*. It was alſo recommended internally for wounds, bruiſes, ulcers, ſpitting of blood, bloody urine, gravel, dyſentery, agues, worms, and outwardly as an anodyne, and as a diſcutient and detergent. It is now, however, rarely uſed, and its name is omitted in the Materia Medica of the laſt edition of the Edinburgh Pharmacopœia.

### *Salt Wort, Prickly.*

This plant is a native of Britain, and common on the ſea-ſhore, flowering in July and Auguſt. Salt-wort, as well as various other plants, on being burned, is found to afford the foſſil alkali. A ſpecies of it grows abundantly on that part of the Spaniſh coaſt which is waſhed by the Meditterranean Sea, and ſupplies all the beſt ſoda conſumed in Europe, which by us is called Spaniſh or Alicant ſoda, and by the Spaniſh merchants *barilla de Alicante.*

To detail the peculiar properties of this alkali, would lead us too far, and is properly the province of chemiſtry. It is in common uſe in the manufacture of glaſs and ſoap, and as the latter is an article of the Materia Medica, we ſhall proceed to conſider its medicinal effects.

All the ſoaps, of which there are ſeveral kinds, are compoſed of expreſſed vegetable oils, or animal fats, united with alkaline lixivia. The white Spaniſh ſoap, being made of the finer kinds of olive-oil, is the beſt, and therefore preferred for internal uſe.

The virtues of ſoap, according to Bergius, are detergent, reſolvent, and aperient; and its uſe is recommended in jaundice, gout, calculous complaints, and in obſtructions of the viſcera. The efficacy of ſoap, in the firſt of theſe diſeaſes, was experienced by Sylvius, and ſince recommended very generally by various authors who have written on this complaint; and it has alſo been thought of uſe in ſupplying the place of bile in the inteſtines. The utility of this medicine in the jaundice was inferred chiefly from its ſuppoſed power of diſſolving biliary concretions; but it has loſt much of its reputation in this diſorder, from gall-ſtones being found, in many, after death, who had been daily taking ſoap for ſeveral months, and even years.

Of its good effects in calculous affections of the urinary paſſages, eſpecially when diſſolved in lime-water, by which its efficacy is conſiderably increaſed, we have the teſtimony of ſeveral. With Boerhaave, ſoap was a general medicine; for, as he attributed moſt complaints to a viſcidity of the fluids, he, and moſt of the Boerhaavian ſchool, preſcribed it in conjunction with different reſinous and other ſubſtances, in gout, rheumatiſm, and various viſceral complaints.

Acids ſhould never be uſed with ſoap, becauſe they decompound it, by uniting with the alkaline ſalt, and thus ſeparating it from the oil. In moderate quantity, ſoap ſeldom can enter the circulation in its perfect ſtate; becauſe there being always more or leſs of an acid in the ſtomach, the ſoap muſt be decompounded. It is therefore conſidered as a very good corrector of acidity in the ſtomach and bowels. If any ſervice is to be expected from ſoap as a deobſtruent and detergent, it muſt be given in larger doſes than are commonly preſcribed, or they ſhould be much more frequently repeated. Soap is externally uſed as a reſolvent; and, united with rectified ſpirit, camphor, and eſſential oils, it forms an agreeable application for ſuperficial tumours, or others more deeply ſeated, ſtrains, bruiſes, &c. The ſoft ſoaps are more penetrating and acrimonious than the hard, and are only uſed for ſome external purpoſes.

### *Sarſaparilla.*

This plant is a native of America, and was, more than two hundred years ago introduced into Spain as an undoubted ſpecific in venereal diſorders. It was alſo celebrated as an efficacious medicine in ſome other diſeaſes of the chronic kind. But whether owing to a difference of climate, or other cauſes, European practitioners ſoon found that it by no means anſwered the character which it had acquired in the Spaniſh Weſt-Indies, and therefore it became very much neglected. Many phyſicians, however, ſtill conſider the ſarſaparilla as a medicine of much efficacy; and though they admit that by the uſe of this root alone we are not to expect a cure of the lues venerea, yet they aſſert that when it is given along with mercury, the diſeaſe is much ſooner ſubdued; and that ulcers, nodes, and other ſymptoms of this diſorder, which reſiſted the effects of repeated ſalivations, have afterwards diſappeared by the continued uſe of ſarſaparilla. Notwithſtanding the unfavourable opinion of a great authority reſpecting ſarſaparilla, it is in frequent uſe at moſt of the London hoſpitals, after the uſe of mercury, in venereal complaints. Sarſaparilla is alſo recommended in rheumatic affections, ſcrofula, and cutaneous diſorders, or where an acrimony of the fluids prevails. It may be given in decoction or powder, and ſhould be continued in large doſes for a conſiderable time.

## *Saſſafras.*

The ſaſſafras-tree is a native of North-America, whence the wood is now uſually imported into this country. It has a fragrant ſmell, and a ſweetiſh, aromatic, ſubacrid taſte. The root, wood, and bark, agree in their medicinal qualities; but the bark is the moſt fragrant, and thought to be more efficacious than the woody part.

Saſſafras is uſed as a mild, corroborant, diaphoretic, and ſweetener in ſcorbutic, venereal, cachectic, and catarrhal diſorders. Its ſuppoſed medicinal virtues where formerly held in great eſtimation, but it is now thought to be of very little importance, and ſeldom employed but in conjunction with other medicines of a more powerful nature.

Watery infuſions of ſaſſafras, made both from the cortical and woody part, raſped or ſhaved, are commonly drunk as tea; but the ſpirituous tincture, or extract, which contains both the volatile and fixed parts of the medicine, appears to be preferable.

## *Savin.*

This is a native of the ſouth of Europe and the Levant, but has long been cultivated in our gardens. It is a powerful and active medicine, particularly noted for producing a determination to the uterus, and thereby proving emmenagogue. It heat and ſtimulates the whole ſyſtem very conſiderably, and is ſaid to promote the more fluid ſecretions.

The power which this plant poſſeſſes in opening uterine obſtructions is conſidered to be ſo great, that we are told it has been frequently employed for infamous and unnatural purpoſes. It ſeems probable, however, that its effects in this may have been exaggerated, ſince it is found very frequently to fail as an emmenagogue; though this in ſome meaſure may be aſcribed to the ſmallneſs of the doſe in which it has uſually been adminiſtered. Dr. Cullen obſerves, "that ſavin is a very acrid and heating ſubſtance, and I have been often, upon account of theſe qualities, prevented from employing it in the quantity perhaps neceſſary to render it emmenagogue. I muſt own however, that it ſhows a more powerful determination to the uterus than any other plant I have employed; but I have been frequently diſappointed in this, and its heating qualities always require a great deal of caution." Dr. Home appears to have had very great ſucceſs with this medicine: for in five caſes of obſtructions of the menſes, which occurred at the Royal Infirmary at Edinburgh four were cured by the ſavin, which he gave in powder from a ſcruple to a drachm twice a-day. He ſays it is well ſuited to the debile, but improper in plethoric habits, and therefore orders repeated bleedings before its exhibition. Externally, ſavin is recommended as an eſcharotic to foul ulcers, warts, &c.

### *Saxifrage, Burnet.*

This plant is a native of Britain, and grows in dry meadows and paſtures. The root has a grateful, warm, very pungent taſte, which is entirely extracted by rectified ſpirit. It promiſes, from its ſenſible qualities, to be a medicine of conſiderable efficacy, though little regarded in common practice. Stahl, Hoffman, and other German phyſicians, are extremely fond of it, and recommend it as an excellent ſtomachic, reſolvent, detergent, diuretie, diaphoretic, and alexipharmic. They frequently gave it with ſucceſs in ſcorbutic and cutaneous diſorders, foulneſs of the blood and juices, tumours and obſtructions of the glands, and diſeaſes proceeding from a deficiency of the fluid ſecretions in general. Boerhaave directs the uſe of this medicine in aſthmatic and hydropic caſes where the ſtrongeſt reſolvents are indicated.

By ſeveral writers it is recommended as a ſtomachic, and in all caſes where phlegmatic humours are thought to prevail, not only in aſthmas and dropſies, but alſo in catarrhal coughs, hoarſeneſs, and the ſerous ſore throat. Hoffman conſiders it as an excellent emmenagogue. In the way of gargle it has been employed for diſſolving viſcid mucus, and to ſtimulate the tongue when that organ becomes paralytic. It may be given in doſes of a ſcruple in ſubſtance, and in infuſion to two drachms.

### *Scurvy-graſs.*

This plant has an unpleaſant ſmell, and a warm, acrid, bitter taſte. Its active matter is extracted by maceration both in watery and ſpirituous menſtrua, and accompanies the juice obtained by expreſſion. The moſt conſiderable part of it is of a very volatile kind; the peculiar penetrating pungency totally exhaling in the exſiccation of the herb, and in the evaporation of the liquors. Its principal virtue reſides in an eſſential oil, ſeparable in a very ſmall quantity, by diſtillation with water.

This plant is antiſeptic, attenuant, aperient, and diuretic; and is ſaid to open obſtructions of the viſcera and remoter glands, without heating or irritating the ſyſtem. It has been long conſidered as the moſt efficacious of all the antiſcorbutic plants, and its ſenſible qualities are ſufficiently powerful to confirm this opinion. In what is called the ſcorbutic rheumatiſm, conſiſting of wandering pains of long continuance, this plant, combined with arum and wood-forrel, is highly recommended both by Sydenham and Lewis. As an antifcorbutic, it is beft ufed frefh, in the manner of fallad, or taken in the form of expreffed juice, as directed in the difpenfatories.

*Seneka, or Rattlefnake-root.*

This root difcovers no remarkable fmell, but has a peculiar kind of fubtile, pungent, penetrating tafte. Its virtue is extracted both by water and fpirit, though the powder in fubftance is fuppofed to be more efficacious than either the decoction or tincture. The watery decoction, on firft tafting, feems not unpleafant, but the peculiar pungency of the root quickly difcovers itfelf, fpreading through the fauces, or exciting a copious difcharge of faliva, and frequently a fhort cough.

The rattlefnake-root was firft introduced to the attention of phyficians about feventy years ago, by Dr. John Tennent, whofe intercourfe with the Indian nations led him to difcover that they poffeffed a fpecific medicine againft the poifon of the rattlefnake, which, in confequence of a ftipulated reward, was revealed to him, and found to be the root of this plant, employed by the Indians both internally and externally. Cafes afterwards occurred, under his own obfervation, which fully convinced him of the efficacy of this medicine; and as the Doctor remarked that pleuritic or peripneumonic fymptoms were generally produced by the action of this poifon, he thence inferred that the rattlefnake-root might alfo be an ufeful remedy in difeafes of this kind. It was accordingly tried in pleurifies, not only by Dr. Tennent himfelf, but by feveral of the French academicians and others, who all unite in teftimony of its good effects. In many of thofe cafes, however, recourfe was had to the lancet, and even the warmeft advocates for the feneka admit, that, in the true pleurify, repeated bleeding is at the fame time not to be neglected. The reputation which this root obtained in peripneumonic affections, induced fome to employ it in other inflammatory diforders, in which it proved ferviceable, particularly the rheumatifm. It has alfo been prefcribed with much fuccefs in dropfies. The ufual dofe is from one fcruple to two of the powder, or two or three table-fpoonfuls of a decoction, prepared by boiling an ounce of the root in a pint and a half of water till it is reduced to one pint.

*Senna.*

This plant is a native of Egypt. It alfo grows in fome parts of Arabia, efpecially about Mocha; but as Alexandria has ever been the great mart from which it has been exported into Europe, it has long been diſtinguiſhed by the name of Alexandrian ſenna, or ſena.

The leaves of ſenna have rather a diſagreeable ſmell, and a ſub-acrid, bitteriſh, nauſeous taſte. They give out their virtue both to watery and ſpirituous menſtrua, and have long been employed as a purgative. How bitterneſs aids the operation of ſenna we know not; but it is obſerved by Dr. Cullen, "that when ſenna was infuſed in the infuſum amarum, a leſs quantity of ſenna was neceſſary for a doſe than the ſimple infuſions of it." The ſame author has remarked, "that as ſenna ſeldom operates without much griping, its frequent uſe is a proof how much moſt part of practitioners are guided by imitation and habit." Senna however, when infuſed in a large proportion of water, as a drachm of the leaves to four ounces of water, rarely occaſions much pain of the bowels, and, to thoſe who do not object to the bulkineſs of the doſe, may be found to anſwer all the purpoſes of a commmon purgative. For covering the taſte of ſenua Dr. Cullen recommends coriander ſeeds; but for preventing its griping, he thinks that the warmer aromatics, ſuch as cardamoms or ginger, would be more effectual.

## *Simaruba.*

The ſimaruba kept in the ſhops is the bark of the roots of this tree, which has been many years celebrated for its virtues in the cure of the dyſentery. In the years 1718 and 1723, an epidemic flux prevailed very generally in France, which reſiſted all the medicines uſually employed in ſuch caſes; ſmall doſes of ipecacuanha, mild purgatives, and all aſtringents were found to aggravate, rather than to relieve, the diſeaſe. Under theſe circumſtances recourſe was had to the bark of the ſimaruba, which proved remarkably ſucceſsful, and firſt eſtabliſhed its character in Europe as a valuable medicine. Moſt authors who have written on the ſimaruba agree, that in fluxes it reſtores the loſt tone of the inteſtines, allays their ſpaſmodic motions, promotes the ſecretions by urine and perſpiration, removes that lowneſs of ſpirits attending dyſenteries, and diſpoſes the patient to ſleep: the gripes and teneſmus are taken off, and the ſtools are changed to their natural colour and conſiſtence. In a moderate doſe, it occaſions no diſturbance nor uneaſineſs, but in large doſes it produces ſickneſs at the ſtomach and vomiting.

More recent experience has evinced, that this medicine is only ſucceſsful in the third ſtage of the dyſentery, where there is no fever, where the ſtomach likewiſe is no way hurt, and where the gripes and teneſmus are only continued by the weakneſs of the bowels. In ſuch caſes Dr. Monro gave two or three ounces of the decoction every five or ſix hours, with four or five drops of laudanum, and found it a very effectual remedy. The late Sir John Pringle, Dr. Huck Saunders, and many others, prescribed the simaruba bark in old and obstinate dysenteries and diarrhoeas, especially those brought from warm climates.

Dr. Wright recommends two drachms of the bark to be boiled in twenty-four ounces of water to twelve; the decoction is then to be strained and divided into three equal parts, the whole of which is to be taken in twenty-four hours, and when the stomach is reconciled to this medicine, the quantity of the bark may be increased to three drachms.

It may not be improper here to subjoin what is said of the simaruba by Dr. Cullen. "We can perceive nothing in this bark but that of a simple bitter; the virtues ascribed to it in dysentery have not been confirmed by my experience, or that of the practitioners in this country; and, leaving what others are said to have experienced to be further examined and considered by practitioners, I can only at present say, that my account of the effect of bitters will perhaps explain the virtues ascribed to simaruba. In dysentery I have found an infusion of chamomile flowers a more useful remedy."

### *Sloe-Tree.*

The fruit of the sloe, or, as it is frequently called, black-thorn, is so sharp and austere as not to be eatable till thoroughly mellowed by frosts: its juice is extremely viscid, so that the fruit requires the addition of a little water, in order to admit of expression. The juice obtained from the unripe fruit, and inspissated to dryness by a gentle heat, is the German acacia, and has been usually sold in the shops for the Egyptian acacia, from which it differs in being harder, heavier, darker coloured, of a sharper taste, and more especially in giving out its astringency to rectified spirit.

Sloes have been recommended in diarrhoeas, hæmorrhagic affections, and as gargles in tumefactions of the tonsils and uvula. Dr. Cullen considers the sloe as the most powerful of the austere fruits, and adds that he has often found it an agreeable and useful astringent. Dr. Withering says, "The tender leaves dried are sometimes used as a substitute for tea, and is, I believe, the best substitute that has yet been tried. The fruit bruised, and put into wine, gives it a beautiful red colour, and a pleasant sub-acid roughness. Letters written upon linen or woollen with the juice of this fruit will not wash out.

*Snake-root.*

This is a ſpecies of the ariſtolochia, growing in Virginia, and Carolina. It has an aromatic ſmell, approaching to that of a valerian, but more agreeable, and a warm, bitteriſh, pungent taſte, which is not eaſily concealed or overpowered by a large admixture of other materials.

Snake-root was firſt recommended as a medicine of extraodinary power in counteracting the poiſonous effects of the bites of ſerpents, and it has ſince been much employed in fevers, particularly thoſe of the malignant kind; a practice which ſeems to be founded on a ſuppoſition that the morbific matter of theſe fevers is ſomewhat analogous to the poiſon of the ſerpents, and that its influence upon the human ſyſtem might be obviated by the ſame means Modern phyſicians, however, have exploded the theory of antidotes.

Serpentaria is thought to poſſeſs tonic and antiſeptic virtues, and is generally admitted to be a powerful ſtimulant and diaphoretic; and in ſome fevers where theſe effects are required, both this and contrayerva have been found very uſeful medicines. The doſe of ſnake-root is uſually from ten to thirty grains in ſubſtance, and to a drachm or two in infuſion.

*Soap.* See *Salt-wort.*

*Sorrel-Wood.*

This delicate little plant is totally inodorous, but has a grateful acid taſte, approaching nearly to that of the juice of lemons, or the acid of tartar, which it alſo reſembles in a great meaſure in its medicinal effects, being eſteemed cooling, antiſcorbutic, and diuretic. It is recommended by Bergius in inflammatory, bilious, and putrid fevers. The principal uſe, however, of the acetoſella is to allay inordinate heat, and to quench thirſt; for which purpoſe, a pleaſant whey may be made by boiling the plant in milk. An eſſential ſalt is prepared from this plant, known by the name of eſſential ſalt of lemons, and commonly uſed for taking ink-ſtains out of linen.

*Sorrel, Common.*

The leaves of common ſorrel have an agreeable acid taſte, like that of wood-ſorrel, and are medicinally employed for the ſame purpoſes. Sorrel taken in conſiderable quantity, or uſed variouſly prepared as food, will be found of advantage where a cooling and antiſcorbutic regimen is required.

### *Southernwood.*

This plant is a native of France, Spain, and Italy. It was cultivated here by Gerard, and its odour renders it ſo generally acceptable, that there are few gardens in which it is not to be found. But though it bears very well the cold of our winters, it very rarely is ever known to flower in this country.

The leaves and tops of ſouthernwood have a ſtrong, and, to moſt people, an agreeable ſmell: its taſte is pungent, bitter, and ſomewhat nauſeous. It has been regarded as ſtomachic, carminative, and deobſtruent; and is ſuppoſed to ſtimulate the whole ſyſtem, more particularly that of the uterus. But though it ſtill retains a place both in the London and Edinburgh Pharmacopœias, it is now rarely uſed, unleſs in the way of fomentation.

### *Spear-mint.*

This plant grows wild in many parts of England, but is more rarely met with in this ſtate than the pepper-mint. It is not ſo warm to the taſte as the laſt mentioned, but has a more agreeable flavour, and is therefore preferred for culinary uſes, and more generally cultivated in our gardens.

On drying, the leaves loſe about three-fourths of their weight, without ſuffering much loſs of their ſmell or taſte. Cold water, by maceration for ſix or eight hours on the dried herb, and warm water in a ſhorter time, become richly impregnated with its flavour. By diſtillation, a pound and a half of the dried leaves communicate a ſtrong impregnation to a gallon of water; but the diſtilled water proves more elegant if drawn from the freſh plant in the proportion of ten pints from three pounds.

Spear-mint poſſeſſes the ſame medicinal qualities which have been noticed of pepper-mint; but the different preparations of the former, though more pleaſant, are perhaps leſs efficacious. It contains much eſſential oil, but of an odour ſomewhat leſs agreeable than that of lavender and marjoram. It is therefore leſs employed as a cephalic; but it acts very powerfully on the parts to which it is immediately applied, and therefore conſiderably on the ſtomach, invigorating all its functions. It acts eſpecially as an antiſpaſmodic, and therefore relieves pains and colic depending upon ſpaſm. It will alſo ſtop vomiting proceeding from ſuch a cauſe; but there are many caſes of vomiting in which it is of no ſervice; and in thoſe caſes any wiſe depending upon inflammatory irritation in the ſtomach itſelf, or in other parts of the body, it aggravates the diſeaſe, and increaſes the vomiting. Practitioners are of opinion, that the infuſion of mint in warm water agrees better with the ſtomach than the diſtilled water, which is often ſomewhat empyreumatic.

Lewis obſerves, that it is ſaid by ſome to prevent the coagulation of milk; and hence it has been recommended to be uſed along with milk diets, and even in cataplaſms and fomentations for reſolving coagulated milk in the breaſts. Upon experiment, the curd of milk, digeſted in a ſtrong infuſion of mint, could not be perceived to be any otherwiſe affected than by common water; but milk, in which mint leaves were ſet to macerate, did not coagulate near ſo ſoon as an equal quantity of the ſame milk kept by itſelf.

### *Spermaceti.*

This is an unctuous flaky ſubſtance, of a white colour, and a ſoft butyraceous taſte, without any remarkable ſmell; ſaid to be prepared from the fat of the brain of the whale, by boiling and purifying it with alkaline lixivia. The virtues of this concrete are thoſe of an emollient. It is of conſiderable uſe in pains and eroſions of the inteſtines, in coughs proceeding from thin ſharp defluxions, and, in general, in all caſes where the ſolids require to be relaxed, or acrimonious humours to be ſoftened. For external purpoſes, it readily diſſolves in oils; and, for internal uſe, may be united with watery liquors into the form of an emulſion, by the intervention of almonds, gums, or yolk of an egg. Sugar does not render it perfectly miſcible with water; and alkalies, which change other oils and fats into ſoap, have little effect upon ſpermaceti. This drug ought to be kept very cloſely from the air, otherwiſe its white colour ſoon changes into a yellow, and its mild unctuous taſte into a rancid and offenſive one. After it has ſuffered this diſagreeable alteration, both its colour and quality may be recovered by ſteeping it in alkaline liquors, or in a ſufficient quantity of ſpirit of wine.

### *Squill, or Sea-Onion.*

This plant is a native of Spain, Sicily, and Syria, growing in ſandy ſituations on the ſea-coaſt, and was firſt cultivated in England about a hundred and fifty years ago. The red-rooted variety has been ſuppoſed to be more efficacious than the white, and is therefore ſtill preferred for medicinal uſe. It is very nauſeous to the taſte, intenſely bitter and acrimonious, but without any perceptible ſmell.

The root of the ſquill appears to manifeſt a poiſonous quality to ſeveral animals; in proof of which we have the teſtimonies of

Hillefield, Bergius, Vogel, and others. Its acrimony is ſo great, that even if much handled, it exulcerates the ſkin; and if given in large doſes, and frequently repeated, it not only excites nauſea, gripes, and vomiting, but it has been known to produce ſtrangury, bloody urine, violent purging, heartburn, hæmorrhoids, convulſions, with fatal inflammation and gangrene of the ſtomach and bowels. But as many of the more active ſubſtances of the Materia Medica, by injudicious adminiſtration, become equally deleterious, theſe effects of the ſquill do not derogate from its medicinal virtues. On the contrary, this drug, under proper management, and in certain caſes and conſtitutions, is a medicine of great utility in the cure of many obſtinate diſeaſes. It powerfully ſtimulates the ſolids, and attenuates viſcid juices; by which qualities it promotes expectoration, urine, and (if the patient be kept warm) ſweat. In dropſical caſes, it has long been eſteemed one of the moſt certain and efficacious diuretics with which we are acquainted, and uſually employed in humoral aſthmas as an expectorant. In all pulmonic affections, excepting only thoſe of actual inflammation, ulcer, or ſpaſm, the ſquill has been experienced to be a uſeful medicine.

The preparations of ſquills kept in the ſhops, are, a conſerve, ſyrup, vinegar, oxymel, and pills; but practitioners do not always confine themſelves to theſe. When the root is intended as a diuretic it has moſt commonly been uſed in powder, as being in this ſtate leſs diſpoſed to nauſeate the ſtomach; and to the powder it has been the practice to add neutral ſalts, ſuch as nitre, or cryſtals of tartar, eſpecially if the patient complained of much thirſt: others recommend calomel; and, with a view to render the ſquill leſs offenſive to the ſtomach, it has been uſual to join with it an aromatic. The doſe of dried ſquills is from two to four or ſix grains, once a day, or half this quantity twice a day; afterwards to be regulated according to its effects. The doſe of the other preparation of the ſquill, when freſh, ſhould be four times this weight; for this root loſes, in the proceſs of drying, four-fifths of its original weight; and this loſs is merely a watery exhalation.

## *Tamarind.*

This is the fruit of a tree, which appears, upon various authorities, to be a native of both the Indies, America, Egypt, and Arabia. The pulp of the tamarind, with the ſeeds, connected together by numerous tough ſtrings or fibres, are brought to us freed from the outer ſhell, and commonly preſerved in ſyrup. This fruit contains a large proportion of acid with the ſaccharine matter, and is therefore not only employed as a laxative, but alſo for abating thirst and heat in various inflammatory complaints, and for correcting putrid disorders, especially those of a bilious kind. When intended merely as a laxative, it may be of advantage to join it with manna, or purgatives of a sweet kind, by which its use is rendered safer and more effectual. Three drachms of the pulp are usually sufficient to open the body; but, to prove moderately cathartic, one or two ounces are required.

## *Tansy.*

This plant grows wild by road-sides, and the borders of fields; and is frequently also cultivated in gardens, both for culinary and medicinal uses. According to Bergius, the virtues of tansy are tonic, stomachic, anthelmintic, emmenagogue, and resolvent; qualities usually attributed to bitters of the warm or aromatic kind. Tansy has been much used as a vermifuge; and testimonies of its efficacy are given by many respectable physicians. Not only the leaves but the seeds have been employed with this intention, and substituted for those of santonicum. Some have entertained a high opinion of it in hysteric disorders, particularly those proceeding from a deficiency or suppression of the uterine purgations. This plant is given in the quantity of half a drachm or more for a dose; but it is more commonly taken in infusion, and drunk as tea.

## *Tar.*

This substance is properly an empyreumatic oil of turpentine, and has been much used as a medicine both internally and externally. Tar-water or water impregnated with the more soluble parts of tar, was upwards of half a century ago a very popular remedy in various obstinate disorders, both acute and chronic; especially in the small-pox, scurvy, ulcers, fistulas, rheumatism, asthma, coughs, cutaneous complaints, &c. and though its medicinal efficacy was greatly exaggerated by the publications of Bishop Berkeley, Prior, and others, yet Dr. Cullen acknowledges that he experienced this preparation in several cases to be a valuable medicine, and that it appeared to strengthen the tone of the stomach, to excite appetite, promote digestion, and to cure all symptoms of dyspepsia. At the same time it manifestly promotes the excretions, particularly that of urine. From all these effects, there is reason to conclude, that in many disorders of the system this medicine may be highly useful.

An ointment of tar, which has been chiefly employed in cutaneous disorders, is directed in the dispensatory both of London and Edinburgh. In respect of tar, Dr. Cullen informs us that he had met with an empirical practice of a singular kind. "A leg of mutton is laid to roast; and whilst it continues roasting, a sharp skewer is frequently thrust into the substance of the mutton, to give occasion to the running out of the gravy; and with the mixture of the tar and gravy to be found in the dripping-pan, the body is to be anointed all over for three or four nights successively; whilst for the same time the body-linen is to be worn. This is alleged to be a remedy in several cases of lepra; and I have had one instance of its being employed in a lepra ichthyosis with great success: but for reasons readily to be apprehended, I have not had opportunities of repeating the practice."

## *Tartar.*

This is a substance which is thrown off from wines to the sides and bottom of the cask, and consists of the vegetable alkali supersaturated with acid. When taken from the cask, it is found mixed with an earthy, oily, colouring matter. It is purified by dissolving it in boiling water, and separating the earthy part by filtering the solution. This, while cooling, deposits irregular crystals, containing the colouring matter, which is separated by boiling the mass with white clay. The tartar, thus purified, is called cream of tartar. If this be exposed to a red heat, its acid flies off, and what remains is the vegetable alkali, or salt of tartar.

Crystals of tartar are in common use as a laxative, and mild cathartic. They are also esteemed for their cooling and diuretic qualities, and therefore have been much employed in dropsies, and other cases requiring an antiphlogistic treatment. Dr. Cullen says, "that in large doses they act like a purgative, in exciting the action of the absorbents in every part of the system, and that more powerfully than happens from the operation of any entirely neutral salt." Hence arises their utility in the cure of dropsies. It must, however, be remarked, that they do not readily pass off by the kidneys, unless taken with a large quantity of water; and therefore when intended as a diuretic, they ought to be given in a liquid form, as Dr. Holme has directed. The dose is to be regulated according to the circumstances, from a drachm to two ounces.

## *Thyme, Garden.*

This herb has an agreeable aromatic smell, and a warm pungent taste. Bergius considers thyme as resolvent, emmenagogue, diuretie, tonic, and stomachic; but we find no disease mentioned in which its use is particularly recommended either by him or other writers. As agreeing in common with the natural order of the verticillatæ, its aromatic qualities may be found equally uſeful in ſome of thoſe complaints for which lavender, ſage, roſemary, &c. are uſually employed.

*Tobacco.*

Tobacco was firſt imported into Europe about the middle of the ſixteenth century. The different ſorts of tobacco and ſnuffs now prepared from this plant are to be attributed to the difference of the climate and ſoil in which it is raiſed, and the peculiar mode of manufacture, rather than to any eſſential difference in its natural qualities. The vaſt conſumption of tobacco, in the various ways of uſing it, ſufficiently evinces the importance of an enquiry into its effects upon the body; and this having been treated with much attention by Dr. Cullen, we are perſuaded that no apology will be thought neceſſary for tranſcribing the ſentiments of the learned profeſſor on this intereſting ſubject. "Tobacco (ſays he) is a well known drug, of a narcotic quality, which it diſcovers in all perſons, even in ſmall quantity, when firſt applied to them. I have known a ſmall quantity of it ſnuffed up the noſe produce giddineſs, ſtupor, and vomiting; and when applied in different ways, in larger quantity, there are many inſtances of its more violent effects, even of its proving a mortal poiſon. In all theſe inſtances, it operates in the manner of other narcotics. But along with its narcotic qualities it poſſeſſes alſo a ſtrongly ſtimulant power; perhaps with reſpect to the whole ſyſtem, but eſpecially with reſpect to the ſtomach and inteſtines; ſo as readily, even in no great doſes, to prove emetic and purgative.

"By this combination of qualities, all the effects of tobacco may be explained; but I ſhall begin with conſidering its effects as they appear in the uſe of it as an article of living.

"As ſuch it has been employed by ſnuffing, ſmoking, and chewing; practices which, as having been for two hundred years paſt common to all Europe, need not be deſcribed here. Like other narcotics, the uſe of it may be introduced by degrees; ſo that its peculiar effects, even from large quantities employed, may not, or may hardly at all appear: but this does not at all contradict the account I have given of its quality with reſpect to perſons unaccuſtomed to it: for even in theſe, the power of habit has its limits; ſo that in perſons going but a little beyond the doſe to which they have been accuſtomed, very violent effects are ſometimes produced.

"On this ſubject it is to be remarked, that the power of habit is often unequal; ſo that in perſons accuſtomed to the uſe of tobacco, a leſſer quantity than what they had been accuſtomed to will often have ſtronger effects than had before commonly appeared. I knew a lady who had been for more than twenty years accuſtomed to take ſnuff, and that at every time of the day; but ſhe came at length to obſerve, that ſnuffing a good deal before dinner took away her appetite: and to find, that a ſingle pinch, taken any time before dinner, took away almoſt entirely her appetite for that meal. When, however, ſhe abſtained entirely from ſnuff before dinner, her appetite continued as uſual; and after dinner, for the reſt of the day, ſhe took ſnuff pretty freely without any inconvenience.

"This is an inſtance of the inequality of the power of habit in exerting its effects: but in what caſes this may take place, we cannot determine, and muſt now go on in marking its uſual and ordinary powers. When ſnuff, that is, tobacco in powder, is firſt applied to the noſe, it proves a ſtimulus, and excites ſneezing; but by repetition that effect entirely ceaſes.

"When ſnuff is firſt employed, if it be not both in ſmall quantity and be not thrown out immediately by ſneezing, it occaſions ſome giddineſs and confuſion of the head; but by repetition theſe effects ceaſe to be produced, and no other effect of it appears in the accuſtomed, when not taken beyond the accuſtomed quantity. But even in the accuſtomed, when it is taken beyond the uſual quantity, it produces ſomewhat of the ſame giddineſs and confuſion of head that it did when firſt employed; and in ſeveral caſes, theſe effects in the accuſtomed, depending on a larger doſe, are not only more conſiderable, as they act on the ſenſorium, but as they appear alſo in other parts of the ſyſtem, particularly in the ſtomach, occaſioning a loſs of appetite, and other ſymptoms of a weakened tone in that organ.

"With reſpect to this, it is to be obſerved, that perſons who take a great deal of ſnuff, though they ſeem, from the power of habit, to eſcape its narcotic effects, yet as they are often liable to go to exceſs in the quantity taken, ſo they are ſtill in danger from theſe effects operating in an inſenſible manner; and I have obſerved ſeveral inſtances of their being affected in the ſame manner as perſons are from the long continued uſe of other narcotics, ſuch as wine and opium; that is, by a loſs of memory, by a fatuity, and other ſymptoms of the weakened or ſenile ſtate of the nervous ſyſtem, induced before the uſual period.

"Among other effects of exceſs in ſnuffing, I have found all the ſymptoms of dyſpepſia produced by it, and particularly pains of the ſtomach, occurring every day. The dependance of thoſe upon the uſe of ſnuff became very evident from hence, that upon an accidental interruption of ſnuffing for ſome days, theſe pains did not occur; but upon a return to ſnuffing, the pains alſo recurred; and this alternation of pains of the ſtomach and of ſnuffing having occurred again, the ſnuff was entirely laid aſide, and the pains did not recur for many months after, nor, ſo far as I know, for the reſt of life.

"A ſpecial effect of ſnuffing is its exciting a conſiderable diſcharge of mucus from the noſe; and there have been ſeveral inſtances of head-achs, tooth-aebs, and ophthalmias relieved by this means: and this is to be particularly remarked, that when this diſcharge of mucus is conſiderable, the ceaſing or ſuppreſſion of it by abſtaining from ſnuff, is ready to occaſion the very diſorders of head-ach, tooth-ach, and ophthalmia, which it had formerly relieved.

"Another effect of ſnuffing to be taken notice of is, that as a part of the ſnuff is often carried back into the fauces, ſo a part of this is often carried down into the ſtomach, and then more certainly produces the dyſpeptic ſymptoms mentioned. Theſe are the conſiderations that relate to ſnuffing; and ſome of them will readily apply to the other modes of uſing this drug.

"Smoking, when firſt practiſed, ſhows very ſtrongly the narcotic, vomiting, and even purging powers of tobacco, and it is very often uſeful as an anodyne; but by repetition theſe effects diſappear, or only ſhow themſelves when the quantity ſmoked is beyond what habit had before admitted of; and even in perſons much accuſtomed to it, it may be carried ſo far as to prove a mortal poiſon. From much ſmoking all the ſame effects may ariſe which we ſaid might ariſe from exceſs in ſnuffing.

"With reſpect to the evacuation of mucus which is produced by ſnuffing, there are analogous effects produced by ſmoking, which commonly ſtimulates the mucous follicles of the mouth and fauces, particularly the excretories of the ſalivary glands. By the evacuation from both ſources, with the concurrence of the narcotic power, the tooth-ach is often relieved by it; but we have not found ſmoking relieve head-achs and ophthalmias ſo much as ſnuffing often does. Sometimes ſmoking dries the mouth and fauces, and occaſions a demand for drink; but as commonly the ſtimulus it applies to the mucous follicles and ſalivary glands draws forth their liquids, it occaſions, on the other hand, a frequent ſpitting.

"So far as this is of the proper ſaliva, it occaſions a waſte of that liquid ſo neceſſary in the buſineſs of digeſtion; and both by this waſte, and by the narcotic power at the ſame time applied, the tone of the ſtomach is often weakened, and every kind of dyſpeptic ſymptoms are produced. Though in ſmoking, a great part of the ſmoke is again blown out of the mouth, ſtill a part of it muſt neceſſarily paſs into the lungs, and its narcotic power applied there often relieves ſpaſmodic aſthma; and by its ſtimulant power it there alſo ſometimes promotes expectoration, and proves uſeful in catarrhal or pituitous difficulty in breathing.

"Smoking has been frequently mentioned as a means of guarding men againſt contagion. In the caſe of the plague, the teſtimony of Diemerbroek is very ſtrong; but Riverius and others give us many facts which contradict this; and Chenot gives a remarkable inſtance of its inutility. We cannot, indeed, ſuppoſe that tobacco contains an antidote of any contagion, or that, in general, it has any antiſeptic power; and therefore we cannot allow that it has any ſpecial uſe in this caſe: but it is very probable, that this and other narcotics, by diminiſhing ſenſibility, may render men leſs ſenſible of contagion; and, by rendering the mind leſs active and anxious, it may alſo render men leſs liable to fear, which has ſo often the power of exciting the activity of contagion. The antiloimic powers of tobacco are, therefore, on the ſame footing with thoſe of wine, brandy, and opium.

"The third mode of uſing tobacco is that of chewing it, when it ſhows its narcotic qualities as ſtrongly as in any other way of applying it; though the nauſeous taſte of it commonly prevents its being carried far in the firſt practice. When the practice, however, is continued, as it is very difficult to avoid ſome part of it, diſſolved in the ſaliva, from going down into the ſtomach, ſo this, with the nauſea excited by the taſte, makes vomiting more readily occaſioned by this than the other modes of applying it. They are the ſtrong, and even diſagreeable, impreſſions repeated, that give the moſt durable and tenacious habits; and therefore the chewing of tobacco is apt to become one of theſe; and it is therefore in this way that it is ready to be carried to the greateſt exceſs, and to ſhow all the effects of the frequent and large uſe of narcoties. As it commonly produces a conſiderable evacuation from the mouth and fauces, ſo it is the moſt powerful in relieving the rheumatic affection of tooth-ach. This practice is alſo the occaſion of the greateſt waſte of ſaliva; and the effects of this in weakening digeſtion, and perhaps from thence, eſpecially, its noted effect of producing emaciation may appear.

"Theſe are the effects of the different modes of employing tobacco, when it comes to be of habitual uſe and an article of living. Theſe effects depend eſpecially upon its narcotic power, and certain circumſtances accidentally attending its application, and the noſe and mouth; but as we have obſerved before, that beſide its narcotic it poſſeſſes alſo a ſtimulant power, with reſpect to the alimentry canal—by this it is frequently employed as a medicine for exciting either vomiting or purging, which it does as it happens to be more immediately applied to the ſtomach or to the inteſtines.

"An infusion of from half a drachm to a drachm of the dried leaves, or of these as they are commonly prepared for chewing, for an hour or two, in four ounces of boiling water, affords an emetic which has been employed by some practitioners, but more commonly by the vulgar only. As it has no peculiar qualities as an emetic, and its operation is commonly attended with severe sickness, it has not been, nor is it likely ever to come into common practice with physicians.

"It is more commonly employed as a purgative in clysters; and, as generally very effectual, it is employed in all cases of more obstinate costiveness; and its powers have been celebrated by many authors. I have known it to be in frequent use with some practitioners; and it is, indeed, a very effectual medicine; but attended with this inconvenience, that, when the dose happens to be in any excess, it occasions severe sickness at the stomach; and I have known it frequently occasion vomiting.

"It is well known that in cases of obstinate costiveness, in ileus, and incarcerated hernia, the smoke of burning tobacco has been thrown into the anus with great advantage. The smoke operates here by the same qualities that are in the infusions of it above mentioned; but as the smoke reaches much farther into the intestines than injections can commonly do, it is thereby applied to a larger surface, and may therefore be a more powerful medicine than the infusions. In several instances, however, I have been disappointed of its effects, and have been obliged to have recourse to other means.

"The infusion of tobacco, when it is carried into the blood-vessels, has sometimes shown its stimulant powers exerted in the kidneys; and very lately we have had it recommended to us as a powerful diuretic of great service in dropsy. Upon the faith of these recommendations we have now employed this remedy in various cases of dropsy, but with very little success. From the small doses that are proper to begin with we have hardly observed any diuretic effects; and though from larger doses they have in some measure appeared, we have seldom found them considerable; and when, to obtain these in a greater degree, we have gone on increasing the doses, we have been constantly restrained by the severe sickness at the stomach, and even vomiting, which they occasioned; so that we have not yet learned the administration of this remedy so as to render it a certain or convenient remedy in any cases of dropsy.

"The same circumstances have occurred to several other practitioners of this city and neighbourhood; and of late the trials of it have been very generally omitted, owing, perhaps, to our practitioners being directed at the ſame time to the uſe of the digitalis, with which they have had ſome more ſucceſs.

"From ſome experiments we are certain that tobacco contains a quantity of volatile parts that may be diſſipated by long boiling in water; and that by ſuch a practice its emetic, purgative, and narcotic qualities may be greatly diminiſhed; and we are of opinion that the preparation in extract, as preſcribed in the Wirtemberg Diſpenſatory, is upon a good foundation, and may be employed in pectoral caſes with more advantage and ſafety than the ſimple infuſion or decoction made by a ſhort boiling only.

"When we were reſtrained in employing the infuſion of tobacco as a diuretic as mentioned, we expected to ſucceed better with the decoction; and I have found that, by long boiling, this might be given in much larger doſes than the infuſion; but we ſtill found it retaining ſo much of the emetic quality that we could not employ it as a diuretic without being interrupted in its uſe by the ſame emetic quality that had interrupted the uſe of the infuſion.

"Beſides the internal uſes of tobacco mentioned, I muſt now remark that it has likewiſe been commended for its virtues as externally employed. I have known the infuſion employed with advantage as a lotion for ſome obſtinate ulcers; but the many inſtances of its being abſorbed, and proving thereby a violent poiſon, diſſuade from ſuch a practice, eſpecially as there are other medicines of as much efficacy that may be employed with much more ſafety. Bergius recommends it to be employed as a fomentation in the paraphymoſis; but we have had no opportunity of employing it."

## *Tormentil.*

This plant is found wild in woods and on commons. The root is the only part which is uſed medicinally: it has a ſtrong ſtyptic taſte, but accompanied with a ſlight aromatic flavour. As a proof of its powerful aſtringency, it has been ſubſtituted for oak bark in the proceſs of tanning. This root has been long held in great eſtimation by phyſicians as a uſeful aſtringent; and as it contains but a very inconſiderable portion of reſin, it is more particularly adapted to thoſe caſes where the heating and ſtimulating medicines of this claſs are leſs proper, ſuch as phthiſical diarrhœas, bloody diarrhœas, &c. Dr. Cullen thinks it has been juſtly commended for every virtue that is competent to aſtringents, and ſays,—"I myſelf have had ſeveral inſtances of its virtues in this reſpect; and particularly I have found it, both by itſelf and as joined with gentian, cure intermittent fevers; but it muſt be given in ſubſtance, and in large quantities."

This root may be given in powder, from half a drachm to one drachm or more for a dofe; but it is more generally given in decoction. For this purpofe an ounce and a half of the powdered root is directed to be boiled in three pints of water to a quart, adding, towards the end of the boiling, a drachm of cinnamon. Of the ftrained liquor, fweetened with an ounce of any agreeable fyrup, two ounces or more may be taken four or five times a day.

## *Turpentine.*

This is a refinous juice extracted from certain fpecies of the fir-tree. There are four kinds of turpentine diftinguifhed in the fhops; viz. Chio or Cyprus turpentine, Venetian turpentine, Strafburg turpentine, and common turpentine.

The firft of thefe turpentines is generally about the confiftence of thick honey, very tenacious, clear, and almoft tranfparent, of a white colour, with a caft of yellow, and frequently of blue. It has a warm, pungent, bitterifh tafte, and a fragrant fmell, more agreeable than any of the other turpentines.

The Venetian turpentine is ufually thinner than any of the other forts, of a clear whitifh or pale yellowifh colour, a hot pungent, bitterifh, difagreeable tafte, and a ftrong fmell, without any thing of the fine aromatic flavour of the Chian kind.

The Strafburg turpentine, as generally met with, is of middle confiftence betwixt the two foregoing, more tranfparent and lefs tenacious than either; its colour a yellowifh brown. Its fmell is very fragrant, and more agreeable than that of any of the other turpentines except the Chian. In tafte it is the bittereft, yet the leaft acrid.

Common turpentine is the coarfeft and heavieft, in tafte and fmell the moft difagreeable, of all the forts. It is about the confiftence of honey, of an opake, brownifh white colour.

All thefe juices yield, in diftillation with water, a very penetrating effential oil,—a brittle infipid refin remaining behind. With regard to their medical virtues, they promote urine, cleanfe the urinary paffages, and deterge internal ulcers in general; and at the fame time, like other bitter hot fubftances, ftrengthen the tone of the veffels. They have an advantage above moft other acrid diuretics, that they gently loofen the belly. Half an ounce or an ounce of Venice turpentine, triturated with the yolk of an egg, and diffufed in water, may be employed in the form of an injection, as the moft certain laxative in colics, and other cafes of obftinate coftivenefs. They are principally recommended in gleets and the *fluor albus*. By fome, alfo, they are confidered as ufeful in calculous complaints: where thefe proceed from fand or gravel, formed into a mafs by vifcid mucous matter, the turpentines, by diffolving the mucus, promote the expulfion of the fand; but where a ftone is formed they can do no fervice, and only ineffectually irritate and inflame the parts. In all cafes accompanied with inflammation thefe juices prove hurtful, as this fymptom is increafed and not unfrequently occafioned by them. It is obfervable that the turpentines impart, foon after taking them, a violet fmell to the urine; and have this effect, though applied only externally to the remote parts, particularly the Venice fort. The latter is accounted the moft powerful as a diuretic and detergent, and the Chian and that of Strafburg as corroborants. The common turpentine, as being the moft offenfive, is rarely given internally—its principal ufe being in plafters and ointments among farriers, and for the diftillation of the oil, or fpirit, as it is called.

The dofe of the turpentine is from a fcruple to a drachm and a half. They are moft commodioufly taken in the form of a bolus, or diffolved in watery liquors by means of the yolk of an egg or mucilage. Of the diftilled oil a few drops are a fufficient dofe. This is an extremely powerful, ftimulating, detergent diuretic, and requires the utmoft caution in its exhibition. When recourfe is had to it, it fhould therefore be given at firft in very fmall dofes, and gradually increafed.

## *Valerian, Wild.*

This grows on open, dry, and mountainous places; and, taken up in autumn or winter, has much ftronger fenfible qualities than that collected in fpring and fummer. The root is a medicine of great ufe in nervous diforders, and is particularly ferviceable in epilepfies proceeding from a debility of the nervous fyftem. It is faid, however, that in fome cafes of epilepfy, at the Edinburgh Difpenfary, it was given to the extent of two ounces a day without effect. It has been employed with fuccefs in feveral other complaints termed nervous, particularly thofe produced by increafed mobility and irritability of the nervous fyftem. Bergius ftates its virtues to be antifpafmodic, diaphoretic, emmenagogue, diuretic, and anthelmintic. Dr. Cullen fays,—"Its antifpafmodic powers are very well eftablifhed, and I truft to many of the reports that have been given of its efficacy; and if it has fometimes failed, I have juft now accounted for it*: adding only this, that it feems to me, in almoft all cafes, it fhould be given in larger dofes than is commonly done. On this footing I have frequently found it ufeful in epileptic, hyfteric, and other fpafmodic affections." In dim-

* From the disease depending upon different causes, and from the root being frequently employed in an improper condition.

nefs of fight Dr. Fordyce recommends it very highly. It fhould be given in dofes from a fcruple to two drachms or more: in infufion from one to two drachms. Its unpleafant flavour is moft effectually concealed by the addition of a little mace.

*Vine, Common.*

The vine is a native of moft of the temperate parts in the different quarters of the world, and is fuccefsfully cultivated in our hemifphere between the thirtieth and fifty-firft degrees of latitude. By the difference of foil and climate numerous varieties of grapes are produced, affording wines extremely various in colour, tafte, and other qualities. The leaves and tendrils of the vine have an aftringent tafte, and were formerly ufed in diarrhoeas, hæmorrhages, and other diforders requiring cooling and ftyptic medicines, but have for a long time been difufed. The trunk of the tree, wounded in the fpring, yields a limpid juice, which has been recommended in calculous diforders, and is faid to be an excellent application to weak eyes and fpecks in the cornea. The unripe fruit has a rough four tafte: its expreffed juice, called verjuice, was much efteemed by the ancients, but is now fuperfeded by the juice of lemons For external ufe, however, particularly in bruifes and ftrains, verjuice continues to be employed, and is generally regarded as a very ufeful application.

The dried fruit conftitutes an article of the Materia Medica, under the name of Uva Paffa, of which the difpenfatories formerly mentioned two kinds, viz. uvæ paffæ majores et minores, or raifins and currants; the latter being a variety of the former. The manner in which they are prepared is by immerfing them in a folution of alkaline falt, and foap ley made boiling hot; to which is added fome olive oil, and a fmall quantity of common falt; and afterwards drying them in the fhade. Thefe fruits are ufed as agreeable, lubricating, acefcent fweets, in pectoral decoctions; and for obtunding the acrimony of other medicines, and rendering them grateful to the palate and ftomach.

From this tree is obtained wine, or the fermented juice of the grape, of which there is a great variety. By medical writers it has principally been confined to four forts, as fufficient for the purpofes of pharmacy: thefe are, white Spanifh wine, or Mountain; Canary, or fack; Rhenifh wine; and red Port.

It appears from chemical inveftigation, that all wines confift chiefly of water, alcohol, a peculiar acid, the aërial acid, tartar, and an aftringent, gummy, refinous matter, in which the colour of red wines refides, and which is expreffed from the hufks of the grapes. They differ from each other in the proportion of these ingredients, and particularly in that of the alcohol which they contain.

The qualities of wines depend not only upon the difference of the grapes, as containing more or lefs faccharine juice, and of the acid matter which accompanies it, but alfo upon circumftances attending the procefs of fermentation. Thus, if the fermentation be incomplete, the wine may contain a portion of *muft*, or unaffimilated juice; or if it be too active, or too long protracted, it may be converted into vinegar.

New wines, when taken into the ftomach, are liable to contract a ftrong degree of acefcency, and thereby occafion much flatulence and acid eructations. Heartburn and violent pains of the ftomach, from fpafms, are alfo frequently produced; and the acid matter, by paffing into the inteftines, and mixing with the bile, is apt to occafion colics, or excite diarrhœas. Sweet wines are likewife more difpofed to become acefcent in the ftomach than others: but as the quantity of alcohol which they contain is more confiderable than appears fenfibly to the tafte, their acefcency is thereby in a great meafure counteracted. Red port, and moft of the red wines, have an aftringent quality, by which they ftrengthen the ftomach, and prove ufeful in reftraining immoderate evacuations: on the contrary, thofe which are of an acid nature, as Rhenifh, pafs freely by the kidneys, and gently loofen the belly. But this, and perhaps all the thin or weak wines, though of an agreeable flavour, yet, as containing little alcohol, are readily difpofed to become acetous in the ftomach, and thereby to aggravate all arthritic and calculous complaints, as well as to produce the effects of new wine.

The general effects of wine are, to ftimulate the ftomach, exhilirate the fpirits, warm the habit, quicken the circulation, promote perfpiration, and, in large quantities, to prove intoxicating and powerfully fedative.

In many diforders wine is admitted to be of important fervice, and efpecially in fevers of a putrid tendency, in which it is found to raife the pulfe, fupport the ftrength, promote a diaphorefis, and to refift putrefaction. In many cafes it proves of more immediate advantage than the Peruvian bark. Delirium, which is the confequence of exceffive irritability, and a defective ftate of nervous energy, is often entirely removed by the free ufe of wine. It is alfo a well-founded obfervation, that thofe who indulge in the ufe of wine are lefs fubject to fevers, both of the malignant and intermittent kind. In the putrid fore throat, in the fmall-pox, when attended with great debility and fymptoms of putrefcency, in gangrenes, and in the plague, wine deferves to be confidered as a principal remedy. In all cafes of languors, likewife, and of great proſtration of ſtrength, wine is experienced to be a more grateful and efficacious cordial than can be furniſhed from the whole claſs of aromatics.

Another article connected with the preſent ſubject is vinegar, the beſt kind of which is made from wine. It is eſteemed of great uſe in all inflammatory and putrid diſorders, whether internal or external. In ardent, bilious fevers, peſtilential, and other malignant diſtempers, it is recommended by Boerhaave as one of the moſt certain ſudorifics. Weakneſs, fainting, vomiting, hyſterical and hypochondriacal complaints, have been frequently relieved by vinegar applied to the mouth or noſe, or received into the ſtomach. It is very efficacious in counteracting the effects of vegetable poiſons, eſpecially thoſe of the narcotic kind. Inhaled in the form of vapour, it is found uſeful in the putrid ſore throat: vinegar likewiſe has been given ſucceſsfully in maniacal caſes, and the ſymptoms uſually conſequent to the bite of a mad dog.

### *Wake-robin.*

This plant, otherwiſe called arum, grows wild under hedges, and by the ſides of banks, in moſt parts of England. All the parts of the arum, in a recent ſtate, are extremely pungent and acrimonious, but the root only is employed medicinally. If but lightly chewed, it excites an intolerable ſenſation of heat and pungency for ſome hours, accompanied with conſiderable thirſt; and when cut in ſlices and applied to the ſkin, it has been known to produce bliſters. This acrimony, however, is gradually loſt by drying, and may be ſo far diſſipated by the application of heat, as to leave the root a mild farinaceous aliment.* Arum is doubtleſs a very powerful ſtimulant, and, by promoting the ſecretions, may be advantageouſly employed in cachectic and chlorotic caſes, in rheumatic affections, and various other complaints of phlegmatic and torpid conſtitutions; but particularly in a relaxed ſtate of the ſtomach, occaſioned by the prevalence of viſcid mucus. When the root is given in powder, great care ſhould be taken that it be young and newly dried. In ſuch a ſtate, it may be uſed in the doſe of a ſcruple or more twice a day; but in rheumatiſms, and other diſorders requiring the full effect of this medicine, the root ſhould be given in a recent ſtate; and, to cover the intolerable pungency it diſcovers on the tongue, Dr Lewis adviſes to adminiſter it in the form of emul-

* In this state it has been made into a wholesome bread. It has also been prepared as starch The root, dried and powdered, is used by the French to wash the skin with, and is sold at a high price, under the name of *Cypress-powder*, which is a good and innocent cosmetic.

ſion, with gum-arabic, and ſpermaceti, increaſing the doſe from ten grains to upwards of a ſcruple three or four times a day. In this way, it generally occaſions a ſenſation of ſlight warmth about the ſtomach, and afterwards in the remoter parts, manifeſtly promotes perſpiration, and frequently produces a plentiful ſweat.

## *Water-Creſſes.*

This plant grows wild in rivulets, and the clearer ſtanding waters; its leaves remain green all the year, but are in greateſt perfection in the ſpring. They have a pungent ſmell, when rubbed betwixt the fingers, and an acrid taſte, ſimilar to that of ſcurvy-graſs, but weaker. In reſpect of medicinal qualities, they are ranked among the milder apperient antiſcorbutics. Hoffman entertained a high opinion of this plant, aud has recommended it as of ſingular efficacy for accelerating the circulation, ſtrengthening the viſcera, opening obſtructions of the glands, promoting the fluid ſecretions, and purifying the blood and humours. For theſe purpoſes the expreſſed juice, which contains the peculiar taſte and pungency of the herb, may be taken in doſes of an ounce or two, and continued for a conſiderable time. It is obſerved that the juice of Seville oranges or other acids, when joined to that of water-creſſes, ſcurvy graſs, and plants of the ſame nature, renders their operation more ſucceſsful, by determining them more powerfully to an aſceſcent fermentation.

The water creſſes are frequently eaten as ſallad, and taken in this way daily for a conſiderable time, under the idea of their being a good corrector of the blood and humours. The garden-creſſes poſſeſs the ſame virtues, but in a much weaker degree.

## *Wolfs'-Bane.*

This plant, the aconitum of the ancients, is a native of the mountainous and woody parts of Germany, France, and Switzerland; but ſince the time of Gerard, it has been cultivated for ornament in moſt of the flower-gardens in this country. Wolfs'-Bane, when firſt gathered, has a ſtrong ſmell, but no peculiar taſte. Every part of the freſh plant is ſtrongly poiſonous, but the root is unqueſtionably the moſt powerful, and when firſt chewed imparts a ſlight ſenſation of acrimony, but afterwards an inſenſibility, or ſtupor at the apex or point of the tongue; and a pungent heat of the lips, gums, palate, and fauces, is perceived, followed with a general tremor and ſenſation of chilneſs. Though the plant loſes much of its power by drying, yet Stoerck obſerves that, when powdered and put upon the tongue, it excites a durable ſenſe of heat, and ſharp, wandering pains, but without redneſs or inflammation. The juice applied to the wound ſeemed to affect the whole nervous ſyſtem; even by keeping it long in the hand, or in the boſom, we are told that unpleaſant ſymptoms have been produced. That the ancients conſidered the aconitum as the moſt deſtructive of vegetable productions, appears from their fanciful derivation of its origin, which they aſcribed to the invention of Hecate, or the foam of Cerberus. The deleterious effects of this plant, like thoſe of moſt vegetable poiſons, are produced by its immediate action upon the nervous energy. It occaſions giddineſs convulſions, violent purging both upwards and downwards, faintings, cold ſweats, and even death itſelf.

Dr. Stoerck appears to be the firſt who gave the wolfs'-Bane internally; and ſince his experiments were publiſhed, in 1762, it has been generally and often ſucceſsfully employed in Germany, and the northern parts of Europe, particularly as a remedy for obſtinate rheumatiſms; and many caſes are related where this diſeaſe were of ſeveral years duration, and had withſtood the efficacy of other powerful medicines, as mercury, opium, antimony, cicuta, &c. yet in a ſhort time were entirely cured by the aconitum. Inſtances are alſo given of its good effects in gout, ſcrofulous ſwellings, venereal nodes, decays, or loſs of ſight, intermittent fevers, &c.

Wolfs'-Bane has been generally adminiſtered in extract, or inſpiſſated juice. Like all virulent medicines, it ſhould be at firſt exhibited in ſmall doſes. Stoerck recommends two grains of the extract to be rubbed into a powder, with two drachms of ſugar, and to begin with ten grains of this powder two or three times a day. We find, however, that the extract is often given from one grain to ten for a doſe, and Stoll, Schenchbecher, and others, increaſed this quantity very conſiderably. Inſtead of the extract a tincture has been made of the dried leaves, macerated in ſix times their weight of ſpirits of wine, and forty drops given for a doſe.

## *Worm-ſeed.*

This is the top of the ſantonicum, a plant of the wormwood or mugwort kind, growing in the Levant. Worm-ſeed is ſmall, light, oval, compoſed as it were of a number of thin membranous coats, of a yellowiſh green colour, with a caſt of brown; eaſily friable on being rubbed between the fingers, into a fine, chaffy kind of ſubſtance. It has a moderately ſtrong and not agreeable ſmell, ſomewhat of the wormwood kind; and a very bitter, ſubacrid taſte.

The ſeeds are eſteemed to be ſtomachic, emmenagogue, and anthelmintic; but it is for the laſt-mentioned power in particular that they are uſually adminiſtered; and from their efficacy in this way they obtained the name of wormſeed. Their quality of deſtroying worms has been aſcribed ſolely to their bitterneſs; but it appears from Baglivi, that worms immerſed in a ſtrong infuſion of theſe ſeeds were killed in five, and according to Redi, in ſeven or eight hours, while in the infuſion of wormwood, and in that of agaric, the worms continued to live more than thirty hours; and hence it has been inferred that their vermifuge effects could not wholly depend upon the bitterneſs of this ſeed. To adults the doſe in ſubſtance is from one to two drachms twice a-day. Lewis thinks that the ſpirituous extract is the moſt eligible preparation of the ſantonicum for the purpoſes of an anthelmintic.

## *Wormwood, Common.*

The leaves of this ſort of wormwood are divided into roundiſh ſegments, of a dull green colour above, and whitiſh underneath. It grows wild in ſeveral parts of England; but about London large quantities are cultivated for medicinal uſe. It flowers in June and July; and, after having ripened its ſeeds, dies down to the ground, except a tuft of the lower leaves, which generally abides the winter.

The leaves of wormwood have a ſtrong, diſagreeable ſmell; their taſte is nauſeous, and ſo intenſely bitter as to be proverbial. The flowers are more aromatic and leſs bitter than the leaves; and the roots diſcover an aromatic warmth without any bitterneſs.

Wormwood was formerly much uſed as a bitter, againſt weakneſs of the ſtomach, and dyſpeptic complaints, in medicated wines and ales. At preſent it is rarely employed in theſe intentions, on account of the ill reliſh and offenſive ſmell with which it is accompanied: but from theſe it may be in part freed by keeping, and totally by long coction, the bitter remaining entire. An extract made by boiling the leaves in a large quantity of water, and evaporating the liquor with a ſtrong fire, proves a bitter ſufficiently grateful, and void of the nauſeous flavour of the herb.

This ſpecies of wormwood may be conſidered as the principal of the herbaceous bitters; and though it is now chiefly employed as a tonic and ſtomachic, yet we are told of its good effects in a great variety of diſeaſes, ſuch as intermittent fevers, hypochondriac diſorders, obſtructions of the liver and ſpleen, gout, the ſtone, the ſcurvy, dropſy, worms, &c. Lindeſtolphe has aſſerted, that a continued uſe of this herb is extremely hurtful to the nervous ſyſtem, from its narcotic and debilitating effects, which he experienced upon himſelf; obſerving alſo, that he could never taſte the extract or eſſence of wormwood without being immediately affected with head-ach and inflammation of the eyes; and it is added both by him and his commentator, Stenzelius, that this herb produced ſimilar effects on many others. Theſe narcotic effects of wormwood have, however, been attributed to a peculiar idioſyncraſy, as numerous inſtances have occurred in which this plant produced a contrary effect, though taken daily for the ſpace of ſix months. Dr. Cullen, ſpeaking on this ſubject, ſays, "I have not had an opportunity of making proper experiments; but to me, with Bergius and Gleditſch, the odour of wormwood ſeems temulentans, that is, giving ſome confuſion of head: and formerly, when it was a faſhion with ſome people in this country to drink purl, that is, ale, in which wormwood is infuſed, it was commonly alleged to be more intoxicating than other ales. This effect is improperly ſuppoſed to be owing to its volatile parts: but I am more ready to admit the general doctrine of a narcotic power; and I believe, from ſeveral conſiderations, particularly from the hiſtory of the Portland powder, that there is in every bitter, when largely employed, a power of deſtroying the ſenſibility and irritability of the nervous power.

Externally wormwood is uſed in diſcutient and antiſeptic fomentations. This plant may be taken in powder, but it is more commonly preferred in infuſion. The Edinburgh Pharmacopœia directs a tincture of the flowers, which is, in the opinion of Dr. Cullen, a light and agreeable bitter, and at the ſame time a ſtrong impregnation of the wormwood.

### *Yarrow.*

This plant is frequent about the ſides of fields, and on dry commons, maintaining its flowers during the greater part of ſummer. The leaves have a rough, bitteriſh taſte, and a faint, aromatic ſmell. The virtues of the millefolium are thoſe of a mild aſtringent, for which it was held in eſteem among the ancient Greek writers. Inſtances of its good effects in hæmorrhagic complaints are likewiſe mentioned by ſeveral eminent German phyſicians, particularly by Stahl and Hoffman, who alſo recommended it as an efficacious remedy in various other diſeaſes. The former found it not only an aſtringent, but alſo a powerful tonic, antiſpaſmodic, and ſedative. In proof of the laſt mentioned quality, we find that in ſome parts of Sweden the millefolium is uſed in making beer, for the purpoſe of rendering it more intoxicating: and Sparrman has obſerved, that it is employed with the ſame intention in ſome parts of Africa. The leaves and flowers of milfoil are both directed for medicinal uſe in the Edinburgh Pharmacopœia. In the preſent practice, however, this plant is not regarded in any degree conformable to its reputed qualities and effects.

# GENERAL RULES

FOR THE

## COLLECTION AND PREPARATION OF SIMPLES.

### ROOTS.

ANNUAL ROOTS ought to be taken up before they ſhoot out ſtalks or flowers: *biennial roots*, chiefly in the autumn of the ſame year in which the ſeeds are ſown; the *perennial*, when the leaves fall off, and therefore generally in the autumn. After waſhing them clean from dirt, and cutting off the rotten and decayed fibres, they are to be hung up in a covered airy place, till ſufficiently dried. The thicker roots require to be ſlit longitudinally, or cut tranſverſely into thin ſlices. Such roots as loſe their virtues by exſiccation (or are deſired to be preſerved in a freſh ſtate, for the greater conveniency of uſing them in certain forms) are to be kept buried in dry ſand.

There are two ſeaſons in which the biennial and perennial roots are reckoned the moſt vigorous, viz. the autumn and ſpring; or rather the time when the ſtalks or leaves have fallen off, and that in which the vegetation is juſt going to revive, or ſoon after it has begun. Theſe ſeaſons are found to differ conſiderably in different plants.

The generality of roots appear to be moſt efficacious in the ſpring: but as at this ſeaſon they are alſo the moſt juicy, and conſequently ſhrivel much in drying, and are rather more difficultly preſerved, it is commonly thought moſt adviſeable to take them up in autumn. No rule, however, can be given, that ſhall obtain univerſally: for *arum-root* taken up even in the middle of ſummer is equally active as at any other ſeaſon: while angelica-root, in the ſummer, is in no degree comparable, in point of activity, to what it is in the autumn, ſpring, or winter.

## HERBS AND LEAVES.

Herbs are to be gathered when the leaves have come to their full growth, before the flowers unfold; but of ſome plants the flowery tops are preferred. They are to be dried in the ſame manner as roots.

For the gathering of leaves, perhaps no univerſal rule can be laid down, any more than for roots; for though moſt herbs appear to be in their greateſt vigour about the time of their flowering, or a little before, there are ſome in which the medicinal parts are more abundant at an earlier period. Thus mallow and marſh mallow leaves are moſt mucilaginous when young, and by the time of flowering approach more to a woody nature. A difference of the ſame kind is more remarkable in the leaves of certain trees and ſhrubs.

Moſt writers on pharmacy have directed that herbs ſhould be dried in the ſhade. It is not however, to be underſtood by this rule, that they are to be excluded from the ſun's heat, but from the ſtrong action of the ſolar rays, by which laſt their colours are very liable to be altered or deſtroyed, much more than thoſe of the roots.

The method of ſlowly drying herbs in a cool place is far from being of any advantage. Both their colours and virtues are preſerved in greateſt perfection, when they are dried haſtily by a heat of common fire as great as that which the ſun can impart. The very ſucculent or juicy herbs, in particular, require to be dried by heat, being otherwiſe liable to turn black.

Odoriferous herbs, dried by the fire till they become friable, diſcover, indeed, in this arid ſtate, very little ſmell, not that the odorous matter is diſſipated; but on account of its not been communicated from the perfectly dry ſubject to dry air; for as ſoon as an aqueous vehicle is ſupplied, whether by infuſing the plant in water, or by expoſing it for a little time to moiſt air, the odorous parts begin to be extracted, and diſcover themſelves in their full force.

## FLOWERS.

Flowers ought to be gathered when moderately expanded, on a clear dry day, before noon. Red roſes, however, are taken before they open, and the white heels clipped off and thrown away.

The quick drying, above recommended for the leaves of plants, is more particularly proper for flowers; in moſt of which, both the colour and ſmell are more periſhable than in leaves, and more ſubject to be impaired by ſlow exſiccation.

It is not unworthy of being obferved, that the virtues of flowers are confined to different parts of the flower in different plants. Not to mention faffron, which is a fingular production, the active part of chamomile flowers is the yellowifh difk, or button in the middle; that of lilies, rofes, clove, July-flowers, violets, and many others, the *petala* or flower-leaves; while rofemary has little virtue in any of thefe parts, the fragrance of this plant refiding chiefly in the cups.

## SEEDS AND FRUITS.

Seeds fhould be collected when ripe, and beginning to grow dry, before they fall off fpontaneoufly. Fruits alfo are to be gathered when ripe, unlefs they are ordered to be otherwife.

Of the fruits collected for medicinal ufe, very few are employed in an unripe ftate. The principal is the floe, the virtue of which, as a mild aftringent, is greatly diminifhed by maturation.

The rule for collecting feeds is more general than any of the others; all the officinal feeds being in their greateft perfection at the time of their maturity. As feeds contain little watery moifture, they require no other warmth for drying them than that of the temperate air in autumn. Such as abound with a grofs expreffible oil, as thofe commonly called the cold feeds, fhould never be expofed to any confiderable heat; for this would haften the rancidity, which, however carefully kept, they are very liable to contract. Seeds are beft preferved in their natural hufks, or coverings, which fhould be feparated only at the time of ufing; this part ferving to defend the feed from being injured by the air.

## WOODS AND BARKS.

The moft proper feafon for the felling of woods, or fhaving off their barks, is generally the winter; but there are fo few of thofe of our own country preferved for medicinal ufe, that it is here unneceffary to fay any thing of them. It may, however, be doubted whether barks be not generally more replete with a medicinal matter in the fummer and fpring than in winter. The barks of many trees are in fummer, fo much loaded with refin and gum, as to burft fpontaneoufly, and difcharge the redundant quantity. It is faid that the bark of the oak anfwers heft for the tanners, at the time of the rifing of the fap in the fpring; and as its ufe in tanning depends on the fame aftringent quality for which it is ufed in medicine, it fhould feem to be beft fitted for medicinal purpofes alfo in the fpring. It may farther be obferved, that it is in the latter feafon that barks in general are moft conveniently peeled off.

# MEDICINAL PREPARATIONS.

## BALSAMS.

BY this denomination is not underſtood the natural balſams, ſuch as thoſe of Gilead, Peru, &c. but certain compoſitions which have received the name, from an opinion of their being endowed with balſamic qualities. Theſe reputed balſams were formerly very numerous, but are now reduced to a ſmall number, which conſiſts of the following:

### *Anodyne Balſam*, commonly called *Bate's Balſam.*

Take of Spaniſh ſoap, one ounce; crude opium, two drachms; eſſential oil of roſemary, one drachm; rectified ſpirit of wine, half a pint. Digeſt them together in a gentle heat for three days; then ſtrain off the liquor, and add to it half an ounce of camphor.

This balſam, as intimated by its title, is deſigned to allay pain. It is uſeful in ſtrains, bruiſes, and rheumatic complaints, when not attended with inflammation. It ought to be rubbed with a warm hand on the part affected; or a linen rag moiſtened with it may be applied to the part, and renewed every two or three hours, till the pain abates. If the opium be left out, it will be the *ſaponaceous balſam* otherwiſe named *oppodeldoch.*

### *Locatelli's Balſam.*

Take of olive oil, one pint; Straſburg turpentine and yellow wax, of each half a pound; red ſaunders, ſix drachms. Melt the wax with ſome part of the oil over a gentle fire; then add the remaining part of the oil and the turpentine; afterwards the ſaunders, previouſly reduced to a powder, and continue ſtirring them together till the balſam is cold.

This balſam is recommended in the dyſentery, eroſions of the inteſtines, internal bruiſes, and in complaints of the breaſt proceeding from ſharp humours. Outwardly it is employed in the cure of wounds and ulcers. When taken internally, the doſe is from two ſcruples to two drachms.

### *Vulnerary Balsam.*

Take of the resinous juice called benzoin, powdered, three ounces; balsam of Peru, two ounces; hepatic aloes, powdered, half an ounce; rectified spirit of wine, two pints. Digest them in a gentle heat for three days, and then strain the balsam.

This medicine is applied externally to heal wounds and bruises; and is used internally against coughs, asthmas, and other complaints of the breast; besides which, it is said to have been given with advantage in the colic, and for healing internal ulcers, &c.

The dose is from twenty to sixty drops.

This has long been celebrated under the different names of the Persian balsam, Wade's balsam, Friar's balsam, Jesuit's drops, Turlington's drops, &c. But though the encomiums bestowed upon it may justly be deemed extravagant, it is a medicine not destitute of utility.

## BOLUSES.

A bolus is very little different from an electuary, only that it is made for a single dose, and is rather of a firmer consistence, but such as to be easily swallowed. As it is intended for immediate use, it admits into its composition volatile salts, and other ingredients, the virtues of which are liable to perish in a little time; and it is a form well calculated for powerful medicines, which require their dose to be adjusted with suitable precision. Boluses are generally composed of powders, with a proper quantity of syrup, conserve, or mucilage. The lighter powders are commonly made up with syrup. A scruple, or twenty six grains of the powder, with as much syrup as will bring it to a due consistence, makes a bolus sufficiently large. The more ponderous powders, such as the mercurial, are commonly made up with conserve, but both the light and ponderous powders may be conveniently made up with mucilage, which increases the bulk less than the other additions, and occasions the bolus to pass down more freely.

### *Astringent Bolus.*

Take of alum, in powder, fifteen grains; gum-kino, five grains; simple syrup, a sufficient quantity to make a bolus.

This bolus, given every four or five hours, proves an efficacious remedy in an excessive flow of the *menses*, and other discharges of blood, proceeding from relaxation, and which required to be speedily restrained.

### *Diaphoretic Bolus.*

Take of gum-guaiacum, in powder, ten grains; crude ſal ammoniac, and flowers of ſulphur, of each one ſcruple; ſimple ſyrup, a ſufficient quantity to make the ingredients into a proper conſiſtence.

This bolus may be taken with advantage twice a day, in rheumatic complaints, and diſorders affecting the ſkin.

### *Pectoral Bolus.*

Take of ſpermaceti, fifteen grains; gum-ammoniac, ten grains; ſalt of hartſhorn, five grains; ſimple ſyrup, as much as is ſufficient to make them into a bolus.

In colds and coughs of long ſtanding, aſthmas, and beginning conſumptions, this bolus may be given with ſucceſs; but it is generally proper that the uſe of it ſhould be preceded by bleeding.

### *A Purging Bolus.*

Take of rhubarb, in powder, twenty-five grains; calomel, five grains; ſimple ſyrup, a ſufficient quantity to make a bolus.

This is particularly ſerviceable for expelling worms. If a ſtronger purge be neceſſary, as in a dropſy, half a drachm of jalap may be ſubſtituted for the rhubarb.

## CATAPLASMS AND SINAPISMS.

Cataplaſms are chiefly intended to act as diſcutients, or to promote ſuppuration. Their place may in general be ſupplied by a poultice, but as they may prove ſerviceable in ſome caſes, it is proper to give an example of each kind.

### *Diſcutient Cataplaſm.*

Take of barley meal, ſix ounces; freſh hemlock, well bruiſed, two ounces; crude ſal ammoniac, half an ounce; vinegar, a ſufficient quantity. Boil the meal and the hemlock leaves for a little time in the vinegar; and then mix with them the ſal ammoniac.

### *Ripening Cataplaſm.*

Take of white lily, or marſh-mallow root, four ounces; fat figs, an ounce; raw onions, bruiſed, ſix drachms; galbanum, half an ounce; yellow basilicon ointment, one ounce; linseed meal, as much as is sufficient. Boil the roots and figs together in a sufficient quantity of water: then bruise, and add to them the other ingredients; previously dissolving the galbanum with the yolk of an egg. In this manner the whole mass is to be made into a soft cataplasm.

Such is the form of a ripening cataplasm elaborately made; but the purpose may be equally well answered by a poultice of bread and milk, to which is added a portion of onions either boiled or raw, and some oil or fresh butter to soften it.

### *Sinapisms.*

Sinapisms act as stimulants, and with this intention may be applied to different parts of the body. In a palsy, or decay of any part, they are employed to solicit the return of the blood and animal spirits into the vessels. With a similar view they are applied to the feet, when the gout has seized the head or stomach. They are also frequently applied to the patient's soles in the low state of fevers, for the purpose of raising the pulse, and relieving the head. Besides the several uses now mentioned, they are serviceable in deep-seated pains, such as the sciatica. They often inflame the part, and raise blisters, though not so perfectly as the cantharides or Spanish flies; but this not being the effect which they are intended to produce, the use of them should only be continued till the parts have become red, and preserve that colour when pressed with the finger.

A sinapism is nothing more than a poultice made with vinegar instead of milk, and rendered stimulating by the addition of warm materials, such as mustard, horse-radish, or garlic.

To make a common sinapism, take crumb of bread, and mustard-seed, in powder, of each equal quantities; strong vinegar as much as is sufficient. Mix them so as to make a poultice. It may be rendered more stimulating, if necessary, by the addition of an eighth part of garlic, bruised.

## CLYSTERS.

Whatever prejudice may be entertained against clysters, they are of extensive utility in the cure of various diseases. They not only serve to evacuate the contents of the belly, but also to convey into the system very active medicines, which in some cases will not sit upon the stomach, and to introduce a supply of aliment, when patients are incapable of ſwallowing. By acting likewiſe in the way of fomentation, they prove highly ſerviceable in inflammations of the bladder, and the lower inteſtines, &c.

### *Emollient Clyſter.*

Take of linſeed tea and new milk, each ſix ounces. Mix them. If to this there be added a tea-ſpoonful of laudanum, it will ſupply the place of the *anodyne clyſter.*

### *Laxative Clyſter.*

Take of milk and water, each ſix ounces; ſweet oil or freſh butter, and brown ſugar, of each two ounces; common ſalt, one ſpoonful. Mix them.

If it be deſired more purgative, another ſpoonful of common ſalt may be added.

### *Carminative Clyſter.*

Take of chamomile-flowers, an ounce; aniſe-ſeeds, or the ſeeds of ſweet fennel, half an ounce. Boil them in a pint and a half of water to one pint.

In hyſteric and hypochondriac complaints, as well as the tympany, this may be adminiſtered with great advantage.

### *Starch Clyſter.*

Take of jelly of ſtarch, four ounces; linſeed oil, half an ounce. Warm the jelly over a gentle fire, and afterwards mix it with the oil. In the dyſentery, or bloody flux, this clyſter, adminiſtered after every looſe ſtool, will blunt the ſharpneſs of the corroding humours, and conduce to heal the ulcerated inteſtines. With the addition of forty or fifty drops of laudanum, it will act as an aſtringent clyſter.

### *Turpentine Clyſter.*

Take of a decoction of chamomile-flowers, ten ounces; Venice turpentine, diſſolved in the yolk of an egg, half an ounce; ſweet oil, one ounce. Mix them.

This clyſter is uſeful in obſtructions of the urinary paſſages, and in pains of the bowels, occaſioned by gravel.

# COLLYRIA, OR EYE-WATERS.

Extremely numerous are the waters recommended by different perſons for the cure of ſore eyes, but, in general, the baſis of them is alum, vitriol, or lead; the effects of which are to brace the parts, and thereby remove the complaints proceeding from relaxation.

*Collyrium of Alum.*

Take of alum, half a drachm; agitate it well together with the white of an egg.

This collyrium, which is made according to the preſcription of Riverius, is uſed in inflammation of the eyes, to allay heat, and reſtrain the flux of humours. In applying it to the eyes, it is to be ſpread upon linen; but ſhould not be kept on above three or four hours at a time.

*Collyrium of Vitriol.*

Take of white vitriol, half a drachm; roſe-water, ſix ounces. Diſſolve the vitriol in the water, and filter the liquor.

This may juſtly be regarded as one of the moſt efficacious remedies in the claſs of the collyria. It is an excellent application in weak, watery, and inflamed eyes; though, where the inflammation is of an obſtinate nature, it will be neceſſary to aſſiſt the medicine by the conjunct reſources of bleeding and bliſtering.

When a ſtrong aſtringent is judged proper, the quantity of vitriol may be increaſed to double or triple the proportion above mentioned.

*Collyrium of Lead.*

Take of acetated ceruſſe or ſugar of lead, and crude ſal ammoniac, each four grains; and diſſolve them in eight ounces of common water.

When the eyes are much pained, forty or fifty drops of laudanum may be occaſionally added to this collyrium.

Similar to this in its effects, is the collyrium of lead recommended by Goulard; which is made by putting twenty-five drops of his *extract of lead* to eight ounces of water, and adding a tea-ſpoonful of brandy.

Even common water and brandy, without any other addition, is a uſeful application to weak eyes. It may be employed in the proportion of an ounce of the latter to five or ſix ounces of the former; and the eyes be bathed with it night and morning.

## CONSERVES.

Conſerves are made of freſh vegetables and ſugar, beaten together into an uniform maſs. In preparing theſe compoſitions, the leaves of vegetables muſt be freed from their ſtalks, the flowers from their cups, and the yellow part of orange-peel taken off with a raſp. They are then to be pounded in a marble mortar, with a wooden peſtle, into a ſmoth maſs; after which, thrice their weight of fine ſugar is commonly added by degrees, and the beating continued till they are uniformly mixed. But the conſerve will be better, as well as keep longer, if only twice its weight of ſugar be added.

*Conſerve of red Roſes.*

Take a pound of red roſe buds, cleared of their heels; beat them well in a mortar; adding by degrees two pounds of double-refined ſugar.

The conſerve of roſes is one of the moſt agreeable and uſeful preparations belonging to this claſs. Half an ounce, or an ounce of it, diſſolved in warm milk, is an excellent medicine in conſumptive coughs and ſpitting of blood.

In the ſame manner are prepared the conſerves of orange-peel, roſemary-flowers, leaves of wood-ſorrel, &c.

## DECOCTIONS.

Though moſt vegetables yield their virtues to water, as well by infuſion as decoction, yet the latter is often neceſſary, as it ſaves time, and performs in a few minutes what the other would require hours, and ſometimes days to effect. Odorous ſubſtances, however, and thoſe in general the virtues of which depend on their volatile parts, are unfit for this treatment. In ſome caſes, nevertheleſs, this inconvenience may be obviated, by infuſing ſuch materials in the decoction.

*Decoction of Althæa.*

Take of the roots of marſh-mallows, moderately dried, three ounces; raiſins of the ſun, one ounce; water, three pints.—Boil the ingredients in the water till one third of it be conſumed; afterwards ſtrain the decoction, and let it ſtand for ſome time to ſettle. If the roots be thoroughly dried, they muſt be boiled till one half of the water is conſumed.

In coughs, and ſharp defluxions upon the lungs, and in pains ariſing from gravel in the urinary paſſages, this decoction may be uſed for ordinary drink.

### *The common Decoction.*

Take of chamomile-flowers, one ounce; elder-flowers, and ſweet fennel ſeeds, of each half an ounce; water, two quarts. Boil them for a little, and then ſtrain the decoction.

This decoction is chiefly intended as the baſis of clyſters, to which other ingredients may be occaſionally added. It may likewiſe be employed as a common fomentation; adding to it ſpirit of wine, and other things, in ſuch quantity as may be judged ſuitable to the caſe of the patient.

### *Decoction of Barley, or Barley-water.*

Take of pearl barley, waſhed from the impurities with cold water, two ounces. Firſt boil it a little with about half a pint of freſh water; then throwing away this, add to the barley four pints of boiling water, and boil it till half the water be waſted; after which ſtrain it.

This is the liquor ſo often mentioned in the courſe of the preſent work, to be drunk freely as a diluter, in fevers and other diſorders.

### *Decoction of the Peruvian Bark.*

Boil an ounce of the bark, groſsly powdered, in a pint and a half of water to one pint; then ſtrain the decoction. This decoction will be rendered both more agreeable and efficacious, by adding to it a tea-ſpoonful of the weak ſpirit of vitriol.

### *Compound Decoction of the Peruvian Bark.*

Take of Peruvian bark, and Virginian ſnake-root, groſsly powdered, each three drachms. Boil them in a pint of water to one half; and to the ſtrained liquor add an ounce and a half of aromatic water.

This decoction is recommended towards the decline of malignant fevers, when the pulſe is low, the voice weak, and the head affected with a ſtupor or inſenſibility, but with little delirium.

The doſe is four table-ſpoonfuls every four or ſix hours.

### *Decoction of Logwood.*

Take of the chips of logwood, three ounce; water, four pints: boil them till one half of the liquor be wasted. It will be improved in taste by adding to it four ounces of simple cinnamon water.

In fluxes of the belly, a tea-cupful of this decoction may be taken, as a moderate and safe astringent, three or four times a day.

### *Decoction of Sarsaparilla.*

Take of fresh sarsaparilla root, sliced and bruised, two ounces; shavings of guaiacum wood, one ounce. Boil them over a slow fire in three quarts of water to one; adding, towards the end, two drachms of liquorice: then strain the decoction.

This decoction may be used with great advantage in disorders of the skin, as well as to assist the operation of mercurial alteratives. It may be taken from a pint and a half to two quarts in the day.

### *Decoction of Seneka.*

Take of seneka rattle-snake root, one ounce; water, a pint and a half. Boil it to one pint, and strain.

This decoction is recommended in the pleurisy, rheumatism, dropsy, and some obstinate cutaneous disorders.

The dose is two ounces, three or four times a day, or oftener, if the stomach will bear it.

### *White Decoction.*

Take of the purest chalk, in powder, two ounces; gum-arabic, half an ounce; water, three pints. Boil to one quart, and strain the decoction.

This is a proper drink in acute diseases, attended with a looseness, and where acidities prevail in the stomach or bowels. It is particularly well adapted for children, when subject to such disorders in the stomach, and to persons troubled with the heart-burn. It may be sweetened with sugar, as it is used; and will be rendered more pleasant, as well as more efficacious, by the addition of two or three ounces of simple cinnamon water.

The place of this decoction, and also of the chalk-julep, may be supplied by an ounce of powdered chalk, mixed with two pints of water.

### *Decoction of Burdock-root.*

Take of burdock-root, half an ounce: boil it in a pint and a half of water to one pint, and strain the liquor.

This decoction is used as a diuretic and ſweetener of the blood, in ſcorbutic and rheumatic complaints. It is drunk in the quantity of a pint a day.

### *Decoction of Mezereon.*

Take of the bark of the root of mezereon, two drachms; boil it in three pints of water to two pints; adding towards the end of the boiling, half an ounce of bruiſed liquorice.

From half a gill to a gill is taken four times a day, for curing the remains of the venereal diſeaſe, and obſtinate ulcerations in different parts of the body.

## DRAUGHTS.

This is a proper form for exhibiting ſuch medicines as are intended to operate immediately, and which do not require to be frequently repeated, ſuch as vomits, purges, and a few others, which are to be taken at one doſe. Where a medicine muſt be uſed for ſome length of time, it is better to make up a larger quantity at once, which ſaves both trouble and expence.

### *Anodyne Draught.*

Take of laudanum, twenty-five drops; ſimple cinnamon water, an ounce; common ſyrup, two drachms; or, in place of it, a bit of ſugar. Mix them.

In great reſtleſſneſs, or exceſſive pain, where bleeding is not neceſſary, this compoſing draught may be taken and repeated occaſionally.

### *Sweating Draught.*

Take of ſpirit of Mindererus, two ounces; ſalt of hartſhorn, five grains; ſimple cinnamon water, and ſyrup of poppies, of each half an ounce. Make them into a draught.

This draught is of ſervice in recent colds, and rheumatic complaints. But to promote its effects, the patient ought to drink freely of warm water-gruel, or ſome other diluting liquor.

## ELECTUARIES.

These are generally composed of the lighter powders, mixed with syrup, conserve, mucilage, or honey, into such a consistence that the powders may neither separate by keeping, nor the mass prove too stiff for swallowing. They receive chiefly the milder alterative medicines, and such as are not ungrateful to the palate.

Astringent electuaries, and such as have pulp of fruits in their composition, should only be prepared in small quantities at a time; for astringent medicines lose much of their virtues by being kept in this form, and the pulp of fruits is apt to ferment. Where the common syrups are employed, it is proper to add likewise a little conserve, to prevent the compound from drying too soon; which is particularly the case with respect to electuaries made of the Peruvian-bark.

*Lenitive Electuary, or Electuary of Senna.*

Take of Senna, in fine powder, eight ounces; coriander-seed, also in powder, four ounces; pulp of tamarinds and of French prunes, each a pound. Mix the pulps and powders together, with a sufficient quantity of simple syrup; reduce the whole into an electuary.

A tea-spoonful of this electuary, taken two or three times a day, generally proves an agreeable laxative. It likewise serves as a convenient vehicle for stronger purgatives.

*Electuary of the Bark.*

Take of Peruvian-bark, in powder, two ounces; crude sal ammoniac, two drachms; syrup of ginger enough to make an electuary.

This is a convenient form for giving the bark in intermittent fevers or agues. A large tea-spoonful of it may be taken every two or three hours, according as the intermissions are longer or shorter.

*Electuary for the Dysentery.*

Take of the japonic confection, two ounces; Locatelli's balsam, one ounce; rhubarb, in powder, half an ounce; syrup of marshmallows, enough to make an electuary.

It being often dangerous in dysenteries to give opiates and astringents, without interposing purgatives, these three classes of medicines are conveniently joined in this composition, which is thereby rendered equally useful and safe.

The dose is about the bulk of a nutmeg twice or thrice a day, according as the symptoms and constitution of the patient may require.

*Electuary for the Gonorrhoea.*

Take of lenitive electuary, three ounces; jalap and rhubarb, in powder, of each two drachms; nitre, half an ounce; simple syrup, enough to make an electuary.

This is a useful laxative during the inflammation and tension of the urinary passages, which accompany a virulent gonorrhoea.

The dose is about the bulk of a nutmeg, two or three times a day; more or less as may be necessary to keep the body gently open.

When the inflammation is gone off, the following electuary may be used:

Take of lenitive electuary, two ounces; balsam of copaiba, otherwise named capivi, one ounce; gum-guaiacum and rhubarb, in powder, of each two drachms; simple syrup, enough to make an electuary.

This may be taken in the same manner as the preceding.

*Electuary for the Piles.*

Take of lenitive electuary one ounce; flowers of sulphur, half an ounce; simple syrup enough to make an electuary.

A tea-spoonful of this may be taken three or four times a day.

## EMULSIONS.

These are mixtures of oily, resinous, and similar substances, with water, in a liquid form, of a white colour resembling milk, and hence called emulsions, or milks. They are generally prepared by grinding the oily seeds of plants, or kernels of fruits, with common water, or any agreeable simple distilled water. In this process, the oil of the subject is, by the mediation of the other matter, united with the water; on which account, they partake of the emollient virtue of pure oil. They have, besides, this advantage, that they are agreeable to the palate, and not apt to turn rancid or acrimonious by the heat of the body, as may be the case with pure oils in some inflammatory diseases. Emulsions, exclusive of their own quality as medicines, are good vehicles for certain substances, which cannot otherwise be taken so conveniently in a liquid form. Thus camphor, triturated with almonds, readily unites with water into an emulſion. In the ſame way alſo, oils, balſams, and reſins, are rendered miſcible with water by the intervention of mucilages.

*Common Emulſion.*

Take of ſweet almonds, an ounce; water, two pints.

Let the almonds be blanched, and beat up in a marble mortar; gradually pouring upon them the water, ſo as to make an emulſion. Afterwards let it be ſtrained.

*Arabic Emulſion.*

This is made exactly in the ſame manner as the preceding; adding to the almonds, while beating, two ounces of the mucilage of gum-arabic.

Where ſoft and cooling liquors are required, theſe emulſions may be uſed as ordinary drink.

*Camphorated Emulſion.*

Take of camphor, half a drachm; ſweet almonds, half a dozen; loaf ſugar, half an ounce; mint-water, eight ounces. Grind the camphor and almonds well together in a ſtone mortar, and add by degrees the mint-water: then ſtrain the liquor, and diſſolve in it the ſugar.

In fevers, and other diſorders which require the uſe of camphor, a table-ſpoonful of this emulſion may be taken every two or three hours.

*Emulſion of Gum-Ammoniac.*

Take of gum-ammoniac, two drachms; water, eight ounces. Grind the gum with the water poured gradually upon it, till it is diſſolved.

This emulſion is uſed for attenuating tough phlegm, and promoting expectoration. In obſtinate coughs, two ounces of the ſyrup of poppies may be added to it with advantage. The doſe is two table-ſpoonfuls three or four times a day.

## FOMENTATIONS.

Fomentations are calculated either to eaſe pain, by taking off tenſion and ſpaſm; or to reſtore the tone and vigour of parts which have become relaxed. Both these intentions may generally be answered by very simple means; the former, by the application of warm water alone, and the latter by that of cold water. With a view, however, to increase the effect of the water, it is a usual practice to impregnate it with other substances, the qualities of which are conducive to the purpose intended. These may be distinguished into anodynes, aromatics, astringents, &c.

*Anodyne Fomentation.*

Take of white poppy-heads, two ounces; elder-flowers, half an ounce; water, three pints. Boil in an open vessel till one pint is evaporated, and strain out the liquor.

This fomentation, as its title expresses, is used for relieving acute pain.

*Common Fomentation.*

Take tops of wormwood, and chamomile-flowers, dried, of each two ounces; water, two quarts. Boil them for a very little, and pour off the liquor.

A portion of brandy may occasionally be added to this fomentation, in such a quantity as the circumstances of the case shall require.

*Strengthening Fomentation.*

Take of oak bark, one ounce; alum, half an ounce; smith's forge-water, three pints. Boil the water with the bark till one third is consumed; then strain the decoction, and dissolve in it the alum.

This is generally employed as a fomentation to weak parts; but may also be used internally, in the quantity of four table-spoonfuls three or four times a day.

## GARGARISMS, OR GARGLES.

This class of medicines, though confined to local and subordinate operation, are far from being unworthy of a place in the province of physic. They are peculiarly useful in fevers and sore throats, by alleviating the dryness of the mouth, and removing the foulness of the tongue and fauces, &c. They have likewise the advantage of being easily prepared. A very useful gargle for cleanſing the mouth may be made with a little barley-water and honey, to which is added as much vinegar as will give them an agreeable ſharpneſs.

Gargles act moſt powerfully when injected with a ſyringe.

### *Common Gargle.*

Take of roſe water, ſix ounces; ſyrup of clove, July-flowers, half an ounce; ſpirit of vitriol, a ſufficient quantity to give it an agreeable ſharpneſs. Mix them.

This gargle, beſides cleanſing the tongue and fauces, acts as a gentle repellent, and will ſometimes remove a ſlight quinſey.

### *Detergent Gargle.*

Take of the emollient gargle, a pint; tincture of myrrh, an ounce; honey, two ounces. Mix them. This gargle is well adapted for cleanſing exulcerations, and promoting the excretion of tough ſaliva from the glands of the mouth.

### *Emollient Gargle.*

Take an ounce of marſh-mallow roots, and two or three figs: boil them in a quart of water till near one half of it be conſumed; then ſtrain out the liquor.

This gargle is of ſervice in fevers, both by ſoftening all the parts of the mouth, and promoting the diſcharge of ſaliva.

It is remarked by the learned ſir John Pringle, that, in the inflammatory quinſey, or ſtrangulation of the fauces, little benefit ariſes from the common gargles; that ſuch as are of an acid nature do more harm than good, by contracting the emunctories of the ſaliva and mucus, and by thickening thoſe humours; that a decoction of figs in milk and water has a contrary effect, eſpecially if ſome ſal-ammoniac be added; by which the ſaliva is made thinner, and the glands brought to ſecrete more freely—a circumſtance always greatly conducive to the cure.

## INFUSIONS.

Vegetables in general yield their virtues to an infuſion in boiling water, and ſome even to cold water, though in the latter they require a longer time. Water is naturally adapted to extract the gummy and ſaline parts of vegetables, but its action is not limited to theſe: for the reſinous and oily principles are, in moſt vegetables, ſo intimately blended with the gummy and ſaline, as to be in a great part taken up along with them.

Of pure ſalts, water diſſolves only certain determinate quantities. By applying heat, however, it is generally enabled to take up more than it can do in the cold, and this in proportion to the degree of the heat. But as the liquor cools, this additional quantity ſeparates, and the water retains no more than it would have diſſolved without heat.

With gummy ſubſtances, on the other hand, it unites without limitation, diſſolving more and more of them till it loſes its fluidity.

It has been imagined that vegetables in a freſh ſtate, while their oily, reſinous, and other active parts, are already blended with a watery fluid, would yield their virtues to water more freely and more plentifully than when their native moiſture has been diſſipated by drying. Experience however evinces, that dry vegetables, in general, give out more than ſuch as are freſh; water ſeeming to have little action upon them in their recent ſtate. In making infuſions, therefore, it is always better to uſe the vegetables in a dry ſtate; and it deſerves to be remarked, that even from thoſe vegetables, which are weak in virtue, rich infuſions may be obtained, by returning the liquor upon freſh quantities of the ſubject, the water thence becoming ſtill more impregnated with the active parts.

*Bitter Infuſion.*

Take of gentian root, half an ounce; Seville orange peel, dried, and carefully freed from the inner white part, two drachms. Cut them in ſmall pieces, and infuſe them in a quart of boiling water for ſome hours; after which ſtrain off the liquor.

For want of appetite, or complaints of the ſtomach ariſing from indigeſtion, a tea-cupful of this infuſion may be taken two or three times a day.

*Infuſion of Peruvian-bark.*

To an ounce of the bark, in powder, add four table-ſpoonfuls of brandy, and a pint of boiling water. Let them infuſe for twenty-four hours, or even double that time; after which ſtrain the liquor.

This is a light and ſtrengthening preparation of the bark for weak ſtomachs; and may be taken in the quantity of a tea-cupful, two or three times a dry.

The infuſion may likewiſe be made with cold water.

### *Infuſion of Linſeed.*

Take of linſeed, two table-ſpoonfuls; liquorice-root, ſliced, half an ounce; boiling water, three pints. Let them infuſe in a gentle heat for ſome hours, and then ſtrain off the liquor.

If an ounce of the leaves of colt's-foot be added to theſe ingredients, it will then be the *pectoral infuſion.* Both theſe, taken as ordinary drink, are ſerviceable not only in coughs and other complaints of the breaſt, but in difficulty of making water, when occaſioned by a ſpaſm which has its foundation in an acrimony of the humours.

### *Infuſion of Roſes.*

Take of red roſes, dried, half an ounce; boiling water, a quart; vitriolic acid, commonly called oil of vitriol, half a drachm; loaf ſugar, an ounce.

Infuſe the roſes in the water for four hours, in an unglazed earthen veſſel; afterwards pour in the acid, and, having ſtrained the liquor, add to it the ſugar.

In an exceſſive flow of the *menſes*, vomiting of blood, and other hæmorrhages, a tea-cupful of this infuſion may be taken every three or four hours. It likewiſe makes a good gargle, where a gentle aſtringent is required.

### *Spaniſh Infuſion.*

Take of Spaniſh juice, cut into ſmall pieces, an ounce; ſalt of tartar, three drachms. Infuſe in a quart of boiling water for a night. To the ſtrained liquor add an ounce and a half of the ſyrup of poppies.

In recent colds, coughs, and obſtructions of the breaſt, a tea-cupful of this infuſion may be taken with advantage three or four times a day.

## JULEPS.

By a julep is commonly underſtood an agreeable liquor, deſigned as a vehicle for medicines of greater efficacy, or to be drunk after them, or taken occaſionally as an auxiliary. The baſis of this kind of medicine is uſually common water, or a ſimple diſtilled water, with one-third or one-fourth of its quantity of a diſtilled ſpirituous water, and as much ſyrup or ſugar as will render the mixture agreeable. The compofition is fharpened with vegetable or mineral acids, or impregnated with other medicines fuitable to the particular intention.

### *Camphorated Julep.*

Take of camphor one drachm; rectified fpirit of wine, ten drops; double-refined fugar, half an ounce; boiling, diftilled water, one pint. Rub the camphor firft with the fpirit of wine, then with the fugar; laftly add the water by degrees, and ftrain the liquor.

This julep is adapted to hyfterical and other complaints where camphor is proper, and may be taken in the quantity of a table-fpoonful or two as often as the ftomach will bear it.

### *Cordial Julep.*

Take of fimple cinnamon-water four ounces; Jamaica-pepper water, two ounces; volatile aromatic fpirit and compound fpirit of lavender, of each two drachms; fyrup of orange-peel, an ounce. Mix them.

In diforders accompanied with great weaknefs and depreffion of fpirits this is given in the quantity of two fpoonfuls three or four times a day.

### *Mufk Julep.*

Take of mufk half a drachm; double-refined fugar, half an ounce; fimple cinnamon-water, four ounces; volatile aromatic fpirit, two drachms. Grind the mufk well with the fugar, and then add gradually the other ingredients.

In the low ftate of nervous fevers, hiccup, convulfions, and other fpafmodic affections, two table-fpoonfuls of this julep may be taken every two or three hours.

### *Saline Julep.*

Diffolve two drachms of the falt of tartar in three ounces of frefh lemon-juice ftrained: when the effervefcence is over, add of mint-water and common water each two ounces; double-refined fugar, fix drachms.

This julep, by abating ficknefs at the ftomach, tends to relieve vomiting; and, by promoting perfpiration, may likewife be ferviceable in fevers, efpecially thofe of the inflammatory kind.

For anfwering the former intention, however, the medicine is more effectual when taken during the act of effervefcence, and ought, therefore, to be adminiſtered in the form of a draught, conſiſting of a ſcruple of the ſalt, a table-ſpoonful of the juice of lemon, an ounce of mint-water, half that quantity of common water, and a bit of loaf ſugar.

## MIXTURES.

The difference between a mixture and a julep is, that the former receives into its compoſition not only ſalts, extracts, and other ſubſtances diſſoluble in water, but alſo earths, powders, and ſuch ſubſtances as cannot be diſſolved. A mixture is ſeldom agreeable either to the eye or taſte, but may, notwithſtanding, be a very uſeful medicine; and there are ſubſtances which have greater effect when adminiſtered in this than in any other form.

### *Aſtringent Mixture.*

Take of the electuary of catechu, commonly called japonic confection, half an ounce; ſimple cinnamon-water and common-water, of each three ounces; ſpirituous cinnamon-water, an ounce and a half. Mix them.

This mixture is uſeful in dyſenteries which are not of long ſtanding. After the neceſſary evacuations, a ſpoonful or two of it may be taken every four hours, interpoſing a doſe of rhubarb every ſecond or third day.

### *Squill Mixture.*

Take of ſimple cinnamon-water five ounces; vinegar of ſquills, one ounce; ſyrup of marſh-mallows, an ounce and a half. Mix them.

This mixture is beneficial in aſthmatic complaints from tough phlegm, and for promoting a diſcharge of urine in dropſical perſons.

A table-ſpoonful of it may be taken every two hours, or oftener.

## OINTMENTS, LINIMENTS, AND CERATES.

Extraordinary virtues have been aſcribed to preparations of this kind in the cure of wounds, ſores, &c. but the principal uſe of them is to defend from the external air, and to retain ſuch ſubſtances as may be neceſſary for drying and cleanſing wounds and ulcers, deſtroying proud fleſh, &c.

### *Yellow Basilicon Ointment.*

Take of yellow wax, white resin, and frankincense, each a quarter of a pound; melt them together over a gentle fire; then add, of hog's lard prepared, one pound. Strain the ointment while warm.

This ointment is generally employed for cleansing and healing wounds and ulcers.

### *Ointment of Calamine.*

Take of olive oil a pint and a half; white wax, and calamine-stone levigated, of each half a pound. Let the calamine-stone, reduced into a fine powder, be rubbed with some part of the oil, and afterwards added to the rest of the oil and wax previously melted together, continually stirring them till quite cold.

This ointment, commonly known by the name of *Turner's Cerate*, is a very beneficial application in burns, scalds, and excoriations, from whatever cause.

### *Emollient Liniment.*

Take of palm oil, two pounds; olive oil, a pint and a half; yellow wax, half a pound; Venice turpentine, a quarter of a pound. Melt the wax and the oils over a gentle fire; then mix with them the turpentine, and strain the ointment.

This is used for anointing inflamed parts, hard tumors, &c.

### *Eye-Ointment.*

Take of hog's lard prepared, four ounces; white wax, two drachms; tutty prepared one ounce. Melt the wax with the lard over a gentle fire, and then sprinkle in the tutty, continually stirring them till the ointment be cold.

### *Issue Ointment.*

Mix half an ounce of Spanish flies, finely powdered, with six ounces of yellow basilicon ointment.

This ointment is chiefly intended for dressing blisters, in order to keep them open during pleasure.

### *Mercurial Ointment.*

Take of quicksilver two ounces; hog's lard three ounces; mutton suet, one ounce. Rub the quicksilver with an ounce of the hog's lard in a warm mortar till the globules be perfectly extinguiſhed; then rub it up with the reſt of the lard and ſuet, previouſly melted together.

The principal uſe of this ointment is to convey mercury into the body by being rubbed upon the ſkin.

*Ointment of Sulphur.*

Take of hog's lard, prepared, four ounces; flour of ſulphur, an ounce and a half; crude ſal-ammoniac, two drachms; eſſence of lemon, ten or twelve drops. Make them into an ointment.

This is the ſafeſt, beſt, and leaſt, offenſive, application for the itch, which it cures with certainty by being rubbed upon the parts affected.

*White Ointment.*

Take of olive oil, one pint; white wax and ſpermaceti, of each three ounces. Melt them with a gentle heat, and keep them conſtantly and briſkly ſtirring together till quite cold.

If two drachms of camphor, previouſly rubbed with a ſmall quantity of oil be added to the above, it will make the *white camphorated liniment.*

Theſe are uſeful cooling ointments, ſerviceable in excoriations and ſimilar frettings of the ſkin.

*Liniment for Burns.*

Take equal parts of Florence oil, or of freſh-drawn lint-ſeed oil, and lime-water: ſhake them well together in a wide mouthed bottle, ſo as to form a liniment.

This is a very proper application for recent ſcalds or burns. It may either be ſpread upon a cloth, or the parts affected may be anointed with it two or three times a day.

*Liniment for the Piles.*

Take of emollient ointment two ounces; Laudanum, half an ounce. Mix theſe ingredients with the yolk of an egg, and work them well together.

*Volatile Liniment.*

Take of water of ammonia, or ſpirit of hartſhorn, half an ounce; olive oil, one ounce and a half. Cork the phial, and ſhake them together.

This excellent compoſition was introduced by ſir John Pringle, who observes that, in the inflammatory quinsey, a flannel, moistened with this liniment and applied to the throat, to be renewed every four or five hours, is one of the most efficacious remedies; and that it seldom fails, after bleeding, either to lessen or carry off the complaint. Where the skin cannot bear the acrimony of this mixture, a larger proportion of oil may be added.

The great utility of this application is now universally acknowledged.

*Camphorated Oil.*

Rub an ounce of camphor, with two ounces of olive oil in a mortar till the camphor be entirely dissolved.

This liniment is used in obstinate rheumatisms, and in some other cases accompanied with great pain and tension of the parts.

## PILLS.

This form is peculiarly adapted to such medicines as operate in a small dose, and, by their disagreeable taste or smell, require to be concealed from the palate; but it is not calculated for medicines which are intended to operate quickly, as pills may lie a considerable time on the stomach before they are sufficiently dissolved to produce any effect. Light dry powders require syrup or mucilages to make them into pills; and the more ponderous, such as the mercurial and other preparations, thick honey, conserve, or extracts.

*Fœtid Pill.*

Take of asafœtida half an ounce; simple syrup, as much as is necessary to form into pills.

In hysteric complaints four or five pills of an ordinary size may be taken two or three times a day.

This medicine is likewise serviceable in the dry asthma.

When it is necessary that the body be kept open, a proper quantity of rhubarb, aloes, or jalap, may occasionally be added to the above mass.

*Mercurial Pill.*

Take of purified quicksilver two drachms; conserve of roses three drachms; liquorice finely powered, one drachm. Rub the quicksilver with the conserve till the globules of mercury be perfectly extinguished; then add the liquorice powder, and mix them together.

The dose of these pills is different, according to the intention with which they are given. As an alterative, two or three may be taken daily. To raise a salivation four or five will be necessary.

## *Plummer's Pill.*

Take of calomel or sweet mercury, and precipitated sulphur of antimony, each three drachms; extract of liquorice, two drachms. Rub the sulphur and mercury well together; afterwards add the extract, and, with a sufficient quantity of the mucilage of gum-arabic, make them into pills.

This pill, which receives its name from a late professor of chemistry in the university of Edinburgh, has been found a powerful yet safe alterative in obstinate cutaneous disorders, and has completed a cure after salivation had failed. In venereal cases it has likewise been employed with great advantage. Two or three pills of an ordinary size may be taken night and morning, the patient keeping moderately warm, and drinking after each dose a draught of decoction of the woods, or of sarsaparilla.

## *Purging Pills.*

Take of Socotorine aloes and Castile soap, each two drachms; of simple syrup, a sufficient quantity to make them into pills.

Four or five of these pills will generally prove a sufficient purge. For keeping the body gently open, one may be taken night and morning. They are accounted both deobstruent and stomachic, and answer all the purposes of Dr. Anderson's pills, of which the principal ingredient is aloes.

Where aloetic purges are improper, as in sanguine and plethoric constitutions, the following pills may be used:

Take extract of jalap and vitriolated kali, of each two drachms; syrup of ginger, as much as will make them of a proper consistence for pills. These pills may be taken in the same quantity as the aloetic above mentioned.

## *Pills for the Jaundice.*

Take of Castile soap, Socotorine aloes, and rhubarb, each one drachm; simple syrup, as much as will make them into pills.

Five or six of them may be taken twice a-day, more or less, as is necessary to keep the body open. During the use of them, however, it will be proper to interpose now and then a vomit of ipecacuanha or tartar emetic.

### *Squill Pills.*

Take of ſquills, dried and finely powdered, a drachm and a half; gum-ammoniac, and cardamom-ſeeds in powder, of each three drachms; ſimple ſyrup, a ſufficient quantity.

In dropſical and aſthmatic complaints two or three of theſe pills may be taken twice a-day, or oftener, if the ſtomach will bear them.

### *Strengthening Pills.*

Take ſoft extract of the Peruvian bark, and vitriolated iron or ſalt of ſteel, each a drachm. Make them into pills of an ordinary ſize.

In diſorders ariſing from great relaxation, ſuch as the *chloroſis*, or green-ſickneſs, two or three pills may be taken twice or thrice a-day.

## PLASTERS.

Plaſters are formed chiefly of oily and unctuous materials, united with powders; but the conſiſtence of them is different, according to the reſpective purpoſes for which they are intended. Such as are deſigned for the breaſt or ſtomach ought to be ſoft and yielding, while thoſe adapted to the limbs are made more firm and adheſive.

An opinion has been entertained that plaſters might be impregnated with the virtues of different vegetables, by boiling the freſh vegetables with the oil employed in the compoſition of the plaſter; but it is found that this expedient, however apparently promiſing, does not communicate to the oils any valuable qualities.

The *calces* of lead, boiled with oils, unite with them into a plaſter of a proper conſiſtence, which forms the baſis of ſeveral other plaſters. During the proceſs of boiling theſe compoſitions, a quantity of hot water muſt be added from time to time, to prevent the plaſter from burning and becoming black: but this muſt be done gradually and with great care, leſt it cauſe the matter to explode, to the danger of the operator; an accident which is liable to happen, if the plaſter be extremely hot.

### *Common Plaſter.*

Take of common olive oil, ſix pints; litharge, reduced to a fine powder, two pounds and a half. Boil the litharge and oil together over a gentle fire, continually ſtirring them, and keeping always about half a gallon of water in the veſſel. When they have boiled about three hours, a little of the plaſter may be taken out and put into cold water, to try whether it be of a proper conſiſtence. As ſoon as that is the caſe, the whole may be ſuffered to cool, and the water well preſſed out of it with the hands.

This plaſter is generally applied in ſlight wounds and excoriations of the ſkin. Its effect is to keep the part ſoft and warm, and defend it from the air; but its principal uſe is to ſerve as a baſis for other plaſters.

### *Adheſive Plaſter.*

Take of common plaſter, half a pound; of Burgundy pitch, a quarter of a pound; melt them together.

This plaſter is principally uſed for retaining other dreſſings.

### *Anodyne Plaſter.*

Melt an ounce of adheſive plaſter, and, when it is cooling, mix with it a drachm of opium powdered, and the ſame quantity of camphor, previouſly rubbed up with a little oil.

This plaſter is employed in acute pains, eſpecially of the nervous kind, and generally gives eaſe.

### *Bliſtering Plaſter.*

Take of Venice turpentine, ſix ounces; yellow wax, two ounces; Spaniſh flies, in fine powder, three ounces; powdered muſtard, one ounce. Melt the wax, and, while it is warm, add to it the turpentine, taking care not to evaporate it by too much heat. After the turpentine and wax are ſufficiently incorporated, ſprinkle in the powders, continually ſtirring the maſs till it be cold.

This plaſter being made in a variety of ways, it is found to vary greatly in conſiſtence. When compounded with oils and other greaſy ſubſtances, its efficacy is diminiſhed, and it is apt to run; while, on the other hand, pitch and reſin render it too hard, and very inconvenient for uſe.

When the bliſtering plaſter is not at hand, its place may be ſupplied by mixing with any ſoft ointment a ſufficient quantity of powdered flies, or by forming them into a paſte with flower and vinegar.

### *Gum Plaſter.*

Take of the common plaſter, four pounds; gum-ammoniac and galbanum, ſtrained, of each half a pound. Melt them together, and add of Venice turpentine, ſix ounces.

This plaſter is uſed as a digeſtive, and likewiſe for diſcuſſing indolent tumors.

### *Mercurial Plaſter.*

Take of common plaſter, one pound; of gum-ammoniac, ſtrained, half a pound. Melt them together, and, when cooling, add eight ounces of quickſilver, previouſly extinguiſhed by triture, with three ounces of hog's-lard.

This plaſter is uſed for pains of the limbs ariſing from a venereal cauſe; and likewiſe for tumors, particularly indurations of the glands.

### *Compound Plaſter of Laudanum.*

Take of laudanum, three ounces; frankincenſe, one ounce; cinnamon powdered, and the expreſſed oil of nutmegs, of each half an ounce; oil of ſpearmint, one drachm. Having melted the frankincenſe, add to it firſt the laudanum ſoftened by heat, and then the oil of nutmegs. Afterwards mix theſe with the cinnamon and oil of mint; and beat them together in a warm mortar, into a maſs, which is to be kept in a cloſe veſſel.

This plaſter is uſually applied to the pit of the ſtomach, in a weakneſs of that organ, in vomitings, the diſorder called the heartburn, &c. But the pit of the ſtomach, as Hoffman obſerves, is not always the moſt proper place for applications of this kind. If applied to the five lower ribs of the left ſide, towards the back, the ſtomach will in general receive more benefit from it; the greater part of that organ being ſituated under them.

### *Anti-hyſteric Plaſter.*

Take of common plaſter, and aſafœtida, ſtrained, each two ounces; yellow wax and galbanum, ſtrained, each one ounce. Melt them in a gentle heat, and ſtir them together, ſo as to mix.

In hyſteric caſes, this plaſter is applied over the belly, and ſometimes produces good effects.

# POWDERS.

This form admits only of ſuch materials as are capable of being ſufficiently dried to become pulverable without the loſs of their medicinal virtue. There are, however, many ſubſtances which cannot be conveniently taken in powder. For example, bitter, acrid, fœtid drugs, are too diſagreeable; emollient and mucilaginous herbs and roots are too bulky; pure reſins cohere, and become tenacious in the mouth; fixt alkaline ſalts liquify upon expoſing the compoſition to the air; and volatile alkalis exhale, if not immediately ſwallowed.

The lighter powders may be taken in any agreeable thin liquid, ſuch as tea, or water-gruel. The more ponderous powders, particularly thoſe prepared from metallic ſubſtances, require a more conſiſtent vehicle, as ſyrup, conſerve, honey, or the like. Reſinous ſubſtances, likewiſe, are moſt commodiouſly taken in thick liquors; otherwiſe they are apt to run into lumps, which do not aſterwards eaſily diſſolve.

Gums and ſuch other ſubſtances as are difficult to powder ſhould be pounded along with the drier materials; but thoſe which are too dry, eſpecially aromatics, ought to be ſprinkled during their pulverization, with a few drops of any proper water.

Aromatic powders ought to be prepared only in ſmall quantities at a time, and kept in glaſs veſſels very cloſely ſtopped. Indeed, powders of any kind ſhould not be expoſed to the air, nor kept too long; otherwiſe their virtues will ſuffer a great dimunition.

## *Aſtringent Powder.*

Take of alum, one ounce and a half; gum-kino, three drachms. Rub them together into a fine powder.

In an immoderate flow of the *menſes*, and other hæmorrhages, this powder may be given from five to fifteen grains or more, every four hours.

## *Carminative Powder.*

Take of coriander-ſeed, half an ounce; ginger one drachm; nutmegs, half a drachm; double-refined ſugar, a drachm and a half Reduce them into powder for twelve doſes.

This powder is uſed for expelling flatulencies ariſing from indigeſtion, and particularly troubleſome to hyſteric and hypochondriac conſtitutions. It may likewiſe be given in ſmall quantities to children, in their food, when affected with gripes.

*Compound Powder of Chalk.*

Take of chalk, two ounces; cinnamon, one ounce; tormentil-root and gum-arabic, of each fix drachms; long pepper, one drachm. Reduce thefe ingredients into a fine powder.

*Compound Powder of Chalk with Opium.*

Take of compound powder of chalk, one ounce; hard purified opium, powdered, ten grains. Mix them.

Thefe powders are confidered as warm abforbents, particularly ufeful in diarrhoeas proceeding from acidity. That with opium is employed in cafes of great irritability, where the aromatic abforbents require the affiftance of fuch a medicine.

The powder with opium may be taken in the quantity of two fcruples, repeated every five or fix hours, if neceffary; but the powder without opium, more frequently, and in larger dofes.

*Aromatic Powder.*

Take of cinnamon, cardamom-feeds, and ginger, each half an ounce. Beat them together into a powder.

This may be taken for the fame purpofes as the carminative powder.

*Sudorific Powder.*

Take of ipecacuanha, and purified opium, each one drachm; vitriolated kali, one ounce. Mix thefe ingredients, and reduce them into a fine powder.

This medicine has been much celebrated under the name of Dover's Powder. It is a powerful fudorific, frequently of great advantage in obftinate rheumatifms, and other cafes where a copious fweat is required. Its intention is better promoted by drinking with it fome warm diluting liquor. It may be given in dofes from ten grains to a fcruple, or half a drachm.

*Worm-Powders.*

Take equal parts of worm-feed and tin reduced into fine powder, and mix them together.

Half a drachm of this powder may be taken by an adult twice a-day, in a little honey or treacle; and, after ufing it three or four days, the following purgative powder is to be taken.

Take of rhubarb, a fcruple; calomel, five grains. Mix them.

## SYRUPS.

Syrups were formerly conſidered as of great importance, and almoſt entirely ſuperſeded every other medicine, particularly thoſe of the alterative kind. At preſent, however, they are employed chiefly as vehicles for medicines of greater efficacy; being uſed for ſweetning draughts, juleps, or mixtures; and for reducing the lighter powders into boluſes, pills, and electuaries; all which purpoſes may be anſwered by the ſimple ſyrup alone.

*Simple Syrup.*

This is made by diſſolving in water, either with or without heat, about double its weight of fine ſugar.

If twenty-five drops of laudanum be added to an ounce of the ſimple ſyrup, it will ſupply the place of diacodium, or the ſyrup of poppies, and will be found a more certain medicine.

The lubricating virtues of the ſyrup of marſh-mallows may likewiſe be ſupplied, by adding to the common ſyrup a ſufficient quantity of mucilage of gum-arabic.

The juice of lemons may be preſerved in the form of a ſyrup, by diſſolving in it, with the heat of a warm bath, nearly double its weight of fine ſugar. The juice, however, ought to be previouſly ſtrained, and ſuffered to ſtand till it ſettles.

The ſyrup of ginger, which is ſometimes a uſeful vehicle for giving medicines to perſons troubled with flatulency, may be made by infuſing two ounces of bruiſed ginger in a quart of boiling water for twenty-four hours. After the liquor has been ſtrained, and has ſtood to ſettle for ſome time, it may be poured off, and a little more than double its weight of fine powdered ſugar diſſolved in it.

## TINCTURES, ELIXIRS, &c.

Rectified ſpirit of wine is the appropriate liquid which extracts the reſins and eſſential oils of vegetables, either totally unattainable by water, or yielding to it only in part.

It diſſolves likewiſe thoſe parts of animal ſubſtances in which their peculiar ſmells and taſtes reſide; on which account tinctures prepared with rectified ſpirits poſſeſs many of the moſt eſſential virtues of ſimples, without being clogged with their uſeleſs parts.

Water, however, being the proper menſtruum of the gummy, ſaline, and ſaccharine parts of mediciual ſubſtances, it is neceſſary, in the preparation of ſeveral tinctures, to make uſe of a weak ſpirit, or a compoſition of rectified ſpirit and water.

### *Aromatic Tincture.*

Infuſe two ounces of Jamaica-pepper in two pints of brandy, without heat, for a few days; then ſtrain off the liquor.

This ſimple tincture may anſwer all the purpoſes of the moſt coſtly preparation of aromatics. It is rather too hot to be taken by itſelf; but may very properly be mixed with ſuch medicines as might otherwiſe prove too cold for the ſtomach.

### *Compound Tincture of the Peruvian-bark, commonly called Huxham's Tincture.*

Take of Peruvian-bark, groſsly powdered, two ounces; outer rind of Seville orange, dried, one ounce and a half; Virginian ſnake-root, bruiſed, three drachms; ſaffron, one drachm; cochineal, powdered, two ſcruples; proof ſpirit of wine, twenty ounces by meaſure. Infuſe for a fortnight, and then ſtrain off the liquor.

This is a good ſtomachic and ſtrengthening medicine, very ſuitable in a relaxed ſtate of the digeſtive organ, and when a perſon is recovering from a tedious fever. It may be taken twice a-day, in the quantity of three or four tea-ſpoonfuls, mixt with half a common glaſsful of white wine or water.

### *Tincture of Aſafœtida.*

Take of aſafœtida, one ounce; brandy, half a pint. Infuſe with a gentle heat for five or ſix days, and then ſtrain off the liquor.

This tincture poſſeſſes all the virtues of the aſafœtida, and may be given in hyſterical and nervous complaints, from ten drops to fifty or ſixty, and even more.

### *Volatile Tincture of Gum-Guaiacum.*

Take of gum-guaiacum, four ounces; compound ſpirit of ammonia, a pint and a half. Infuſe in a cloſe veſſel for three or four days, and afterwards ſtrain the tincture.

A tea-ſpoonful of this tincture, taken twice a-day, in a cup of any ſuitable infuſion, ſuch as that of water-trefoil, is an excellent remedy in rheumatic complaints.

For domeſtic uſe, a very good tincture of guaiacum may be made by infuſing the ſame quantity of the gum in a bottle of rum or brandy.

### *Tincture of Black Hellebore.*

Take of the roots of black hellebore, coarſely powdered, two ounces: infuſe them in a pint of proof ſpirit, for a week; then filter the tincture through paper.

If a ſcurple of cochineal be infuſed along with the roots, it will give the tincture an agreeable colour.

In obſtructions of the *menſes* a tea-ſpoonful of this tincture, taken in a cup of chamomile, or penny-royal tea, is a uſeful medicine.

### *Tincture of Opium, or Liquid Laudanum.*

Take of crude opium, two ounces; ſpirituous aromatic water, and mountain wine, of each ten ounces. Diſſolve the opium, ſliced, in the wine, with a gentle heat, frequently ſtirring it: afterwards add the ſpirit, and ſtrain off the tincture.

As twenty drops of this tincture contain about a grain of opium, the common doſe may be from twenty to thirty drops.

### *Tincture of Rhubarb.*

Take of rhubarb, two ounces and a half; leſſer cardamom-ſeeds, half an ounce; brandy two pints. Digeſt for a week, and then ſtrain the tincture.

Thoſe who prefer a vinous tincture of rhubarb, may infuſe the above ingredients in a bottle of Liſbon wine, adding to it about two ounces of proof ſpirits.

If half an ounce of gentian-root, and a drachm of Virginian ſnake-root, be added to the above ingredients, it will make the bitter tincture of rhubarb.

Theſe ſeveral tinctures are deſigned as ſtomachics and ſtrengtheuers as well as purgatives. In weakneſs of the ſtomach or inteſtines, they are frequently of great ſervice. The doſe is from four tea-ſpoonfuls to three or four table-ſpoonfuls, or more, according to the circumſtances of the patient, and the purpoſe for which it is intended.

### *Paregoric Elixir, or Camphorated Tincture of Opium.*

Take of flowers of benzoin, half an ounce; opium, two drachms. Infuse in one pound of the volatile aromatic spirit, for four or five days, frequently shaking the bottle; afterwards strain the elixir.

This is an agreeable and safe composition for administering opium. It eases pain, allays tickling coughs, relieves difficult breathing, and is useful in many disorders of children, particularly the hooping-cough.

The dose to an adult is from fifty to a hundred drops.

### *Sacred Elixir.*

Take of rhubarb cut small, ten drachms; Socotorine aloes, in powder, six drachms; lesser cardamom-seeds, half an ounce; French brandy, two pints. Infuse for two or three days, and then strain the elixir.

This is a useful stomachic purge, and may be taken from one ounce to an ounce and a half.

## CAMPHORATED SPIRIT OF WINE.

Dissolve an ounce of camphor in a pint of rectified spirits.

This medicine is chiefly employed as an embrocation in bruises, palsies, the chronic rheumatism, and for preventing gangrenes.

### *Spirit of Mindererus.*

Take of volatile sal ammoniac, any quantity. Pour upon it gradually distilled vinegar, till the effervescence ceases.

This medicine is useful in promoting a discharge both by perspiration and urine. It is also a good external application in strains and bruises.

When intended to raise a sweat, half an ounce of it in a cup of warm gruel may be given to the patient in bed, every hour, till it has the desired effect.

# VINEGARS.

Vinegar is an acid produced from vinous liquors by a ſecond fermentation. It is a uſeful medicine both in inflammatory and putrid diſorders. It not only cools the blood, but counteracts a tendency to putrefaction, and allays inordinate motions of the vaſcular and nervous ſyſtem. It likewiſe promotes the natural ſecretions, and in ſome caſes excites a copious ſweat, where the warm medicines, called alexipharmic, tend rather to prevent that ſalutary evacuation.

Faintings, vomitings, and other hyſteric affections, are often relieved by vinegar applied to the mouth and noſe, or received into the ſtomach. It is highly ſerviceable in correcting many poiſonous ſubſtances, when taken into the ſtomach, as well as in promoting their diſcharge by the different emunctories, when received into the blood.

Beſides its uſefulneſs as a medicine, vinegar is employed to extract the virtues of ſeveral other medicinal ſubſtances. Moſt of the odoriferous flowers impart to it their fragrance, accompanied with a beautiful purpliſh or red colour. It alſo improves the efficacy of garlic, gum-ammoniac, ſquills, and ſome other valuable medicines.

Theſe effects, however, are only to be expected from vinegar that is genuine, ſound, and well prepared. It is allowed, that the beſt vinegars are thoſe prepared from French wines.

It is neceſſary for ſome purpoſes that the vinegar be diſtilled; but this operation requiring a particular chemical apparatus, we ſhall not detail it.

### *Vinegar of Litharge.*

Take of litharge, half a pound; Strong vinegar, two pints.—Infuſe them together in a moderate heat for three days, frequently ſhaking the veſſel; then filter the liquor.

This medicine is ſeldom employed, from a general notion of its being dangerous; though there is reaſon to believe, that the preparations of lead with vinegar might be uſed in many caſes both with ſafety and advantage: for a preparation of a ſimilar nature has lately been introduced into practice by Goulard, a French Surgeon, who calls it the *Extract of Saturn*, and directs it be made in the following manner:

Take of latharge, one pound; vinegar, made of French wine, two pints. Put them together into a glazed earthen pipkin, and let them boil, or rather ſimmer, for an hour, or an hour and a quarter, taking care to ſtir them all the while with a wooden ſpatula. After the whole has ſtood to ſettle, pour off the liquor which is upon the top into bottles for uſe.

With this extract Goulard makes his *vegeto-mineral water*, which he recommends in various external diforders, fuch as inflammations, burns, bruifes, ftrains, ulcers, &c. He likewife prepares with it a number of other medicinal forms, viz. poultices, plafters, ointments, powders, &c.

*Vinegar of Rofes.*

Take of red rofes, half a pound; ftrong vinegar, half a gallon. Infufe in a clofe veffel for feveral weeks, in a gentle heat; then ftrain off the liquor. This is chiefly ufed as an embrocation for head-achs, &c.

*Vinegar of Squills.*

Take of dried fquills, two ounces; diftilled vinegar, two pints. Infufe for ten days or a fortnight in a gentle degree of heat; afterwards ftrain off the liquor, and add to it about a twelfth part of its quantity of proof fpirits.

This is an efficacious medicine in diforders of the breaft, proceeding from tough phlegm; and likewife in dropfical cafes for promoting a difcharge of urine.

When this medicine is intended for a vomit, it fhould be given in the quantity of an ounce or more; but in other cafes the dofe is from a drachm to half an ounce, mixed with cinnamon-water, or fome other agreeable aromatic liquor, to prevent the naufea which it is apt to occafion.

## WATERS BY INFUSION, &c.

*Lime-water.*

This is directed to be made with different proportions of lime and water. In the Difpenfatory of the London College, the proportion is half a pound of quick-lime to twelve ounces of water; in that of the Edinburgh College, it is half a pound of lime to twelve pounds of water. It does not appear, however, that the different proportions of water occafion any fenfible difference in the ftrength of the product. The quick-lime is far from yielding all its foluble parts to either of the proportions above mentioned; the remainder giving a ftrong impregnation to many frefh quantities of water, though not fo ftrong as to the firft. The method of making lime-water may, therefore, be confidered as arbitrary. By fome it is made in the following manner:

Pour two gallons of water gradually upon a pound of freſh burnt quick-lime; and, when the ebullition ceaſes, ſtir them well together: then ſuffer the whole to ſtand at reſt till the lime has ſettled; after which filter the liquor through paper, and keep it in veſſels cloſely ſtopt.

Calcined oyſter-ſhells may be uſed inſtead of quick-lime.

Lime-water is chiefly uſed in complaints from the gravel; in which caſes it may be taken daily from a pint to two or more. Externally it is employed for waſhing foul ulcers, and removing ſome diſeaſes of the ſkin.

### *Compound-Lime-water.*

Take ſhavings of guaiacum wood, half a pound; liquorice-root, one ounce; ſaſſafras bark, half an ounce; coriander ſeeds, three drachms; ſimple lime-water, ſix pints. Infuſe without heat for two days, and then ſtrain off the liquor.

In the ſame manner may lime-water be impregnated with the virtues of other vegetable ſubſtances. By this means the water is not only rendered more agreeable to the palate, but alſo more efficacious, eſpecially in cutaneous diſorders, and a vitiated ſtate of the fluids.

### *Styptic-water.*

Take of blue vitriol and alum, each an ounce and a half; water, one pint. Boil them until the ſalts are diſſolved; then filter the liquor, and add to it a drachm of the oil of vitriol.

This water is employed for ſtopping a bleeding at the noſe, and other hæmorrhages; for which purpoſe cloths or doſſils dipt in it muſt be applied to the part.

### *Tar-water.*

Pour a gallon of water on two pounds of Norway tar, and ſtir them ſtrongly together with a wooden rod. When they have ſtood to ſettle two days, pour off the water for uſe.

This water was formerly celebrated in many diſeaſes, acute as well as chronic; and though its virtues were exaggerated by men of great eminence, it is ſtill acknowledged to be a valuable medicine. It excites appetite, promotes digeſtion, and increaſes the ſecretions, particularly that of urine.

### *Cinnamon-water.*

Steep one pound of cinnamon-bark, bruiſed in a gallon and a half of water, and one pint of brandy, for two days; and then diſtil off one gallon.

This is an agreeable aromatic water, highly endowed with the fragrance and cordial virtues of the ſpice.

Great care ſhould be had in the choice of the cinnamon, to avoid the too common impoſition of ſubſtituting caſſia-bark in its room. The latter yields a water much leſs agreeable than that of cinnamon, and the flavour of which is manifeſtly empyreumatic. The two drugs may be eaſily diſtinguiſhed from one another by their manner of breaking. Caſſia-bark breaks over ſmooth, while cinnamon ſplinters. The former has likewiſe a ſlimy and mucilaginous taſte, without any thing of the roughneſs of the true cinnamon.

### *Pennyroyal-water.*

Take of pennyroyal leaves, dried, a pound and a half; water, from a gallon and a half to two gallons. Draw off by diſtillation one gallon.

This water is endowed with the ſmell, taſte, and medicinal virtues of the plant. It is employed in juleps and mixtures adapted to the hyſteric diſorder.

An infuſion of the herb in boiling water may be uſed with nearly equal advantage.

### *Peppermint-water, and Spearmint-water.*

Both theſe may be prepared in the ſame manner as the preceding.

They are much uſed as ſtomachic waters, in ſickneſs at the ſtomach and vomiting; particularly where the cauſe of theſe complaints is indigeſtion, or cold viſcid phlegm. They are alſo employed in ſome colicky complaints, the gout in the ſtomach, &c. In the laſt of theſe, eſpecially, the peppermint-water is the moſt powerful.

### *Roſe-water.*

Take of roſes freſh gathered, ſix pounds; water, two gallons. Diſtil off one gallon.

This water is chiefly regarded on account of its agreeable flavour.

*Jamaica Pepper water.*

Take of Jamaica pepper, half a pound; water, a gallon and a half. Diſtil off one gallon.

This water is generally found agreeable both in flavour and taſte, and may anſwer the purpoſes of the more coſtly aromatic waters.

## SPIRITUOUS DISTILLED WATERS.

*Spirituous Cinnamon-water.*

Take of cinnamon-bark, one pound; proof ſpirit, and common water, of each one gallon. Steep the cinnamon in the liquor for two days; then diſtil off one gallon.

*Spirituous Jamaica Pepper water.*

Take of Jamaica pepper, half a pound; proof ſpirit, three gallons; water, two gallons. Diſtil off three gallons.

This is a ſufficiently agreeable cordial, and may ſupply the place of the *aromatic water.*

## WHEYS.

*Alum Whey.*

Boil two drachms of alum, powdered, in a pint of milk, till it is curdled; then ſtrain out the whey.

This whey is uſed with advantage in an immoderate flow of the *menſes*, and in a *diabetes*, or exceſſive diſcharge of urine.

It is taken in the quantity of two, three, or four ounces, according as the ſtomach will bear it, three times a day. If it ſhould occaſion vomiting, it may be diluted.

*Muſtard Whey.*

Take milk and water, of each a pint; muſtard-ſeed, bruiſed, an and a half. Boil them together till the curd is perfectly ſeparated; afterwards ſtrain the whey through a cloth.

This preparation of muſtard warms and invigorates the ſyſtem, and promotes the different ſecretions. It will often ſupply the place of wine in the low ſtate of nervous fevers; and is alſo uſeful in the chronic rheumatiſm, palſy, dropſy, &c. It may be rendered more agreeable to the palate by the addition of a little ſugar.

The uſual doſe is an ordinary tea-cupful four or five times a-day.

### *Scorbutic Whey.*

Take of the ſcorbutic juices, half a pint; milk, a quart. Boil them till the curd be ſeparated.

The ſcorbutic plants are chiefly brook-lime, garden ſcurvy-graſs, and water-creſſes.

Many other wheys may be prepared in nearly the ſame manner; ſuch as orange-whey, cream of tartar whey, vinegar-whey, &c. Theſe are cooling pleaſant drinks in fevers, and may be rendered cordial, when neceſſary, by the addition of wine.

## WINES.

Wine is not only an article, at table, and where it can be procured genuine, one of the moſt uſeful cordials, but is alſo employed as a *menſtruum* for extracting the virtues of other medicinal ſubſtances. Being itſelf a natural compound of water, inflammable ſpirit, and acid, it acts both upon vegetable and animal ſubſtances; diſſolving likewiſe ſome bodies of the mineral kind, ſuch as antimony, iron, &c. Whence it becomes impregnanted with their reſpective virtues.

### *Antimonial Wine.*

Take a glaſs of antimony, reduced to a fine powder, half an ounce; Liſbon wine, eight ounces. Digeſt, without heat, for three or four days, now and then ſhaking the bottle: afterwards filter the wine through paper.

The doſe of this wine is regulated according to the intention for which it is preſcribed. As an alterative and diaphoretic, it may be taken from ten to fifty or ſixty drops. In a large doſe it generally proves purgative, or excites vomiting.

### *Aloetic Wine.*

Take of ſocotorine aloes, one ounce; ginger, three drachms, Digeſt them for a week in a pint of mountain wine, and half a pint of brandy, frequently ſhaking the bottle; and afterwards ſtrain off the tincture.

This compoſition, taken from one to two ounces, is a uſeful purge for perſons of a phlegmatic habit; but is more commonly uſed in ſmall doſes as an alterative.

### *Ipecacuanha Wine.*

Take of ipecacuanha, in powder, one ounce; mountain wine, a pint. Infuſe for three or four days; then filter the tincture.

This is a ſafe vomit, and is well adapted for thoſe whoſe ſtomachs are too irritable to bear the ingredient in powder.

The doſe is from one ounce to an ounce and a half.

### *Chalybeate or Steel Wine.*

Take filings of iron, two ounces; cinnamon and mace, of each two drachms: Rheniſh wine, two pints. Infuſe for three or four weeks, frequently ſhaking the bottle; and afterwards paſs the wine through a filter. Inſtead of Rheniſh wine may be uſed Liſbon, ſharpened with half an ounce of cream of tartar, or a ſmall quantity of the vitriolic acid.

### *Stomachic Wine.*

Take of Peruvian bark, groſsly powdered, one ounce; orange-peel, bruiſed, half an ounce. Infuſe in a bottle of Liſbon wine for five or ſix days; and then ſtrain off the wine.

This wine is not only uſeful in a weakneſs of the ſtomach and inteſtines, but may alſo be taken as a preventive, by perſons liable to intermitting fevers, or who reſide in places where the diſeaſe is prevalent; and will likewiſe be of advantage to thoſe who recover ſlowly after fevers of any kind, by promoting digeſtion, and reſtoring the general ſtrength. A glaſsful of it may be taken two or three times a-day.

## *Familiar Explanation of the Nature of ACIDS, ABSORBENTS, ALKALINE and NEUTRAL SALTS.*

THESE ſubſtances being of great importance in the cure of diſeaſes, it ſeems proper to give the reader a general idea of their nature and medicinal effects upon the body.

### ACIDS.

Every ſubſtance is ſaid to be acid which excites the ſenſation of ſourneſs upon the organs of taſte; will change certain blue vegetable colours into red, as the juice of turnſole, ſyrup of violets, &c. and will, in common, though not univerſally, effervefce with alkalies. Acids are animal, vegetable, and mineral. The vegetable are the native, ſuch as the juice of lemons, citrons, &c. or the product of fermentation, as vinegar. The mineral are thoſe of ſulphur or vitriol, nitre, and common ſalt. The animal is obtained from ants, and ſome other inſects, in conſiderable quantities. It is alſo contained in human fat, and in the ſuet of animals that ruminate.

The medicinal effects of acids, duly diluted, and exhibited in proper doſes, are to cool, quench thirſt, correct a tendency to putrefaction, and allay inordinate motions of the blood. By theſe qualities, in hot bilious temperaments and inflammatory diſorders, they frequently reſtrain immoderate hæmorrhages, and promote the natural ſecretions. In ardent fevers they correct the inflammatory diſpoſition of the fluids, and excite a diaphoreſis, more certainly, and with greater ſafety, than any other ſpecies of medicine. In fainting, lethargic, and hyſteric paroxyſms, vinegar, in particular, if applied to the noſe and mouth, often affords great relief: and, in many inſtances, more than by volatile alkaline ſpirits, or fœtid gums.

Vegetable acids, particularly the native juices of certain plants and fruits, have ſome degree of ſaponaceous quality, by means of which they attenuate or diſſolve viſcid phlegm, and deterge the veſſels, and thus prove ſerviceable in various chronical diſorders. Great effects have been experienced from their continued uſe in inveterate ſcurvies, eſpecially when given in conjunction with medicines of the acrid or pungent kind; and it is found that the latter have much better effects when thus managed than when exhibited by themſelves.

The mineral acids inſtantly coagulate the blood; but the vegetable dilute it, even when inſpiſſated or thickened by heat; in which ſtate watery liquors alone will not properly mingle with it. Hence, in ſome fevers, where water runs off by the kidneys almoſt as pale and inſipid as when drunk, vegetable acids renders the urine of the due colour and quality. A like effect is produced by mineral acids, the ſpirit of nitre in particular, combined with vineous ſpirits.

Acids, however, are prejudicial in cold, pale, phlegmatic habits, where the veſſels are lax, the circulation languid, and the bile deficient in quantity. In theſe conſtitutions an acid is often generated too copiouſly in the ſtomach, from milk and vegetable food, which occaſions uneaſineſs in that organ, flatulencies, ſometimes pain, likewiſe, of the bowels, and vomiting or purging.

## ABSORBENTS.

Abſorbents, taken in a general ſenſe, are all ſuch medicines as have the power of drying up redundant humours, either internally or externally; but this denomination is now generally reſtricted to certain earths ſuited to take acids into their pores, and at the ſame time to deſtroy their acid quality. Theſe ſubſtances are—oyſter-ſhells, crabs' claws, coral, chalk, limeſtone, ſome marles, &c. By deſtroying acidities in the firſt paſſages, they conſequently remove ſuch diſorders as proceed from that cauſe. When united with the acid they form a neutral, ſaline compound, endowed with ſome degree of an aperient and detergent quality, though too inconſiderable to exert much power in theſe reſpects.

In children, and adults of a weak conſtitution, and whoſe food is chiefly of the vegetable aceſcent kind, various complaints of the bowels, as have been already obſerved, are occaſioned by acidities. Thoſe diſorders generally diſcover themſelves by ſour eructations, a pale colour of the face, and in children by the ſour ſmell and green colour of the fæces, which are ſometimes ſo manifeſtly acid as to raiſe a ſtrong efferveſcence with alkaline ſalts. In theſe caſes, and theſe only, the uſe of abſorbent earths is indicated: for the theory is now exploded, which aſcribed to theſe ſubſtances any primary virtue in the cure of fevers, the extinction of poiſons, or any other medicinal quality.

When there are no acidities in the ſtomach or bowels, abſorbents are apt to form concretions with the mucous matter uſually lodged in the firſt paſſages, into hard, indiſſoluble maſſes, which have ſometimes been thrown up by vomit, or found in the ſtomach upon diſſection. Hence ariſe obſtructions of the bowels, and other diſorders. Inſtances are recorded, in which the ſtomach and inteſtines have been found lined with a cruſt, as it were, of theſe earthy ſubſtances; which muſt not only have prevented the ſeparation of the gaſtric juices, but likewiſe cloſed the orifices of the lacteal veſſels, ſo as to obſtruct the paſſage of the chyle into the maſs of blood.

All the abſorbents, particularly thoſe of the animal kind, contain, beſides their alkaline earth, a portion of glutinous matter. Of this we meet with an inſtance in crabs' eyes. If theſe be macerated in the weaker acids, or the ſtronger ſufficiently diluted with water, the earthy part will be diſſolved, and the animal glue remain in the form of a ſoft tranſparent mucilage. This glutinous ſubſtance increaſes their tendency to concrete in the ſtomach; and hence thoſe which contain the leaſt of it ſhould be preferred to the others. The mineral earths are found to contain the leaſt of this kind of matter; and ſome of them are very eaſy of ſolution; for inſtance chalk; which may therefore be given with greater ſafety than the animal abſorbents.

Theſe ſubſtances, diveſted of their glutinous matter by means of fire, are reduced into acrimonious calces or limes, and thus become medicines of a different claſs.

The teeth, bones, hoofs, and horns of animals, conſiſt of the ſame principles with the animal abſorbents, above mentioned, but combined in different proportions. The quantity of gelatinous matter is ſo large, as to defend the earthy part from the action of weak acids; while the earth, in its turn, protects the gluten from being eaſily diſſolved by watery liquors. Hence thoſe bodies in their crude ſtate, though recommended as poſſeſſing ſingular virtues, are in fact found to be utterly devoid of any virtue.

## FIXED ALKALINE SALTS.

Alkaline ſalts are either fixed or volatile. We ſhall firſt conſider the former. The aſhes of moſt vegetables, ſteeped or boiled in water, give out to it a ſaline ſubſtance, ſeparable in a ſolid form by evaporating the water. This kind of ſalt never pre-exiſts in the vegetable, but is always generated during the burning. The ſalt thus obtained is called fixed alkaline ſalt. The herb kali, which grows on the ſea-coaſts, when dried and burnt, affords a lixivium, or ley, which, if evaporated yields the fixed alkaline ſalt; and hence the name *alkali* has been given to the fixed ſalt of all plants. Fixed alkaline ſalts, from whatever vegetables they may be obtained, are ſcarcely diſtinguiſhable from each other, at leaſt in their effects as medicines. On this account the ſalt of tartar is as much uſed medicinally as any other.

Salt of tartar, or ſolutions of it in water, raiſe an effervefcence on being mixed with acid liquors, and deſtroy their acidity; the alkali and acid uniting together into a compound of new qualities called *neutral*. Earthy ſubſtances, and moſt metallic bodies, previouſly diſſolved in the acid, are precipitated from it by the alkali.

Solutions of this ſalt liquefy all the animal juices, except milk. They corrode the fleſhy part into a kind of mucous matter; concrete with animal fats and vegetable oils, into ſoap; and diſſolve ſulphur into a red liquor, eſpecially if aſſiſted by a boiling heat, and mingled with quick-lime, which greatly promotes their activity.

The medicinal virtues of this ſalt are, to attenuate the juices, reſolve obſtructions, and promote the natural ſecretions. A dilute ſolution of it drunk warm in bed generally excites ſweat; but if that evacuation be not favoured, its ſenſible operation is by urine. Where acidities abound in the firſt paſſages, this ſalt abſorbs the acid, and unites with it into a mild aperient neutral ſalt. As one of its principal effects is to render the animal fluids more thin, it is obvious that where they are already colliquated, as in ſcurvies, and in all putrid diſorders in general, this medicine is improper. The common doſe of the ſalt is from two or three grains to a ſcruple; in ſome circumſtances it has been extended to a drachm, in which caſe it muſt always be largely diluted with watery liquors.

## VOLATILE ALKALINE SALTS.

As fixed alkaline ſalts are produced in the burning of vegetables, and remain behind in the aſhes, ſo volatile alkaline ſalts are produced by a like degree of heat from animal ſubſtances, and riſe in diſtillation along with the other volatile principles; the admiſſion of air, neceſſary for the production of the former, is not needful for the latter. Thoſe ſalts are obtainable alſo from ſome vegetable matters, and from vegetable and animal ſoot. They are produced in urine by putrefaction, without fire; without fire alſo they exhale from it.

Volatile alkaline ſalts, and their ſolutions, called ſpirits, agree, in many reſpects, with fixed alkalies, and their ſolutions or lyes. They efferveſce with, and neutralize acids; liquefy the animal juices, and corrode the fleſhy parts; ſo as, when applied to the ſkin, and prevented by a proper covering from exhaling, to act as cauſtics. Their principal difference from the fixed alkalies ſeems to confiſt in their volatility. They exhale or emit pungent vapours, in the coldeſt ſtate of the atmoſphere; and by their ſtimulating ſmell they prove ſerviceable in languors and faintings. Taken internally, they diſcover a greater colliquating as well as ſtimulating power; the blood drawn from a vein, after their uſe has been continued for ſome time, being obſerved to be remarkably more fluid than before. They are likewiſe more diſpoſed to operate by perſpiration, and to act on the nervous ſyſtem. They are particularly uſeful in lethargic caſes, and hyſterical and hypochondriacal diſorders; and in the languors, head-achs, inflations of the ſtomach, flatulent colics, and other ſymptoms which attend them. They are generally found more ſerviceable in aged perſons, and in phlegmatic habits, than in the oppoſite circumſtances. In ſome fevers, particularly thoſe of the low kind, accompanied with a cough, hoarſeneſs, redundance of phlegm and ſizineſs of the blood, they are of great advantage; liquefying the viſcid juices, raiſing the vital power, and exciting a ſalutary perſpiration; but in putrid fevers, ſcurvies, and wherever the maſs of blood is thin and acrimonious, they are evidently hurtful. In vernal intermittents, particularly thoſe of the ſlow kind, and where the blood is denſe or ſizy, they are experienced to be an efficacious remedy. They have often been found to carry off ſuch diſorders, without any previous evacuation, but are generally more effectual if a purge be premiſed; and where the patient is plethoric, or there are any inflammatory ſymptoms, bleeding ſhould likewiſe take place before theſe medicines are adminiſtered.

Volatile ſalts are moſt commodiouſly taken in a liquid from, largely diluted; or in that of a bolus, which ſhould be made up only as it is wanted. The doſe is from one or two grains, to ten or twelve. Ten drops of a well-made ſpirit are reckoned to contain about a grain of the ſalt. In intermittents, fifteen or twenty drops of the ſpirit are given in a tea-cupſul of cold ſpring water, and repeated five or ſix times during each intermiſſion.

## NEUTRAL SALTS.

When any acid and alkaline ſalts are mixed together, in ſuch proportion as that neither of them may predominate, they form by their coalition a new compound, called neutral. The ſalts of this denomination have a more extenſive uſe in medicine than any other kind. In general, their operation is by ſtool, urine and perſpiration. In ſome circumſtances they are likewiſe accounted antiſpaſmodics. They greatly conduce to attenuate a viſcid ſtate of the humours, and to reſolve obſtructions in the veſſels and glands.

## Table of DOSES *for different Ages.*

[*The Common Dose being taken at one Drachm.*]

| | Ages. | Parts of the Common Dose. | Proportions of a Drachm. | |
|---|---|---|---|---|
| Weeks | 7 | $\frac{1}{15}$ | 4 | grains. |
| Months | 7 | $\frac{1}{12}$ | 5 | |
| | 14 | $\frac{1}{8}$ | $7\frac{1}{2}$ | |
| | 28 | $\frac{1}{5}$ | 12 | |
| Years | $3\frac{1}{2}$ | $\frac{1}{4}$ | 15 | |
| | 5 | $\frac{1}{3}$ | 20 | |
| | 7 | $\frac{1}{2}$ | 30 | |
| | 14 | $\frac{2}{3}$ | 40 | |
| | 21 | common dose. | one drachm. | |
| | 63 | $\frac{11}{12}$ | 55 | grains. |
| | 77 | $\frac{5}{6}$ | 50 | |
| | 100 | $\frac{4}{6}$ | 40 | |

### *Denominations of Apothecaries' Weights and English Wine Measures.*

| | | |
|---|---|---|
| A pound | contains | twelve ounces. |
| An ounce | contains | eight drachms. |
| A drachm | contains | three fcruples. |
| A fcruple | contains | twenty grains. |
| A gallon | contains | eight pints. |
| A pint | contains | fixteen ounces. |
| An ounce | contains | eight drachms. |

A table-fpoonful is the meafure of half an ounce.

# A GLOSSARY,

*Or Explanation of the Technical Words or Phrases which could not always be avoided in the Progress of this Work.*

## A.

*Abdomen.* The belly.

*Absorbent vessels.* Those that convey the nourishment from the intestines, and the secreted fluids from the various cavities into the mass of blood.

*Absorbent medicines.* Kinds of earths suited to take acids into their pores, and at the same time destroy their acid quality.

*Acrimony.* Corrosive sharpness.

*Acute.* This term is applied to a disease which is violent, and tends to a speedy termination.

*Adult.* Of mature age.

*Alexipharmic.* A medicine supposed to expel poison or noxious humours through the pores of the skin.

*Alterative.* A medicine suited to clear the blood from certain impurities with which it is supposed to be tainted.

*Antiscorbutic.* Good against the scurvy.

*Anthelmintic.* Destructive to worms

*Antispasmodic.* Whatever tends to prevent or remove spasm.

*Aperient.* Opening.

*Aphthæ.* Small whitish ulcers appearing in the mouth, and generally known by the name of *thrush*.

*Astringent.* Binding.

*Aqueous.* Watery.

## B.

*Bile, or gall.* A fluid secreted by the liver into the gall-bladder, and thence discharged into the intestines, for the purpose of promoting digestion.

## C.

*Cachectic.* An unhealthy state of body.

*Calculous.* Stoney or gravelly.

*Carminative.* Good for expelling wind.
*Caries.* A rottenneſs of any bone.
*Clorotic.* Relating to the green-ſickneſs.
*Chyle.* A milky fluid, formed chiefly of the aliments, and conveyed by the abſorbents from the inteſtines into the blood, to repair the waſte of the body.
*Chronic.* An epithet applied to a diſeaſe, the progreſs of which is ſlow.
*Circulation.* The motion of the blood, which is propelled by the heart through the arteries, and returns by the veins.
*Comátoſe.* Inclined to ſleep.
*Contagion.* Infectious matter.
*Criſis.* A certain period in a diſeaſe, at which there happens a deciſive alteration either for the better or the worſe.
*Critical.* Deciſive or important.
*Cutaneous.* Of or belonging to the ſkin.

## D.

*Delirium.* A temporary diſorder of the mental faculties, uſual in fevers.
*Deobſtruent.* Adapted to remove obſtructions.
*Detergent.* Cleanſing.
*Diaphragm.* A membrane which ſeparates the cavity of the cheſt from that of the belly.
*Diaphoretic.* Promoting perſpiration.
*Diuretic.* Whatever promotes the ſecretion of urine.
*Dyſpeptic.* Belonging to bad digeſtion.

## E.

*Emetic.* What excites vomiting.
*Emmenagogue.* Whatever promotes the menſtrual diſcharge.
*Emunctories.* Paſſages by which any thing is diſcharged from the body.
*Empyema.* A collection of purulent matter in the cavity of the breaſt, the conſequence of an inflammation.
*Epidemic.* Infectious.
*Errhine.* What excites ſneezing.
*Exacerbation.* The increaſe of any diſeaſe.

## F.

*Farinaceous.* Mealy.
*Febrifuge.* Removing fever.

*Fæces.* Excrements.
*Fœtid.* Emitting an offensive smell.
*Fœtus.* The child before birth, or when born before the proper period.
*Flatulent.* Producing wind.
*Fungus.* Proud flesh.

G.

*Gangrene.* Mortification.
*Gelatinous.* Gluey, Viscid.

H.

*Hectic Fever.* A slow consuming fever, generally attending the absorption of purulent or other acrid matter into the blood.
*Hæmorrhage.* A discharge of blood.
*Hæmorrhoids.* The piles.
*Hydropic.* Dropsical.
*Hypochondriac Disease.* Low spirits, sometimes accompanied with a depraved imagination.
*Hydragogue.* What carries off water by purging.

I.

*Ichor.* Thin matter, of an acrid kind.
*Imposthume.* A collection of purulent matter.
*Inflammation.* An increased action of the blood-vessels.

L.

*Ligament.* A strong tendinous membrane binding the joints of the bones.
*Ligature.* A bandage.

M.

*Mesentery.* A double membrane, connecting the intestines with the back-bone.
*Miliary eruption.* An eruption of small pustules, resembling the seeds of millet.
*Morbid.* Diseased.
*Morbific.* Causing disease.
*Mucus.* The matter discharged from the nose, lungs, &c.
*Mucous.* Resembling the matter discharged from the nose, lungs, &c.

## N.

*Narcotic.* What excites ſleep.
*Nauſea.* An inclination to vomit.
*Nephritic.* Belonging to the kidneys.
*Nervous.* Irritable.
*Nodes.* Enlargements of the bones, ariſing from the venereal diſeaſe.

## O.

*Obtund.* To blunt.

## P.

*Paroxyſm.* A fit.
*Pectoral.* Medicines adapted to cure diſeaſes of the breaſt.
*Peritonæum.* A membrane lining the cavity of the belly, and covering the inteſtines.
*Perſpiration.* The matter diſcharged from the pores of the ſkin in the form of vapour or ſweat.
*Phlegmatic.* Relaxed and abounding with phlegm.
*Phthiſical.* Conſumptive.
*Pituitous.* Phlegmatic.
*Plethoric.* Full of blood.
*Pulmonary.* Belonging to the lungs.
*Pus.* Matter contained in a boil, the conſequence of inflammation.

## R.

*Rectum.* The ſtraight gut in which the fæces are contained.
*Regimen.* Regulation of diet.
*Reſpiration.* The act of breathing.
*Reſtringent.* Binding.
*Reticular.* Made in the form of a net.

## S.

*Saliva.* The fluid ſecreted by the glands of the mouth.
*Sanies.* A thin, and generally acrid matter, diſcharged from an ill-conditioned ſore.
*Schirrous.* A diſeaſed hardneſs of glandular parts.
*Slough.* A part ſeparated from a cavity by ſuppuration.
*Spaſm.* A cramp, or diſeaſed contraction.
*Spine.* The back bone.
*Styptic.* A medicine for ſtopping the diſcharge of blood.

## T.

*Temperament.* A peculiar habit of body, of which there are reckoned four kinds, viz. the ſanguine, the bilious, the melancholic, and the phlegmatic.

*Tonic.* What increaſes the tone, or elaſticity of the fibres.

## U.

*Ulcer.* A ſore, generally ill conditioned.

*Umbilical.* Belonging to the navel.

*Ureters.* Two ſmall canals which convey the urine from the kidneys to the bladder.

*Urethra.* The canal which conveys the urine from the bladder.

## V.

*Vertigo.* Giddineſs.

*Viſcera.* Bowels.

*Vulnerary.* Healing.

# INDEX.

## A.

## B.

*Bleeding*, operation of, 317. By leeches, ibid. By cupping, 318, 319. At the nose, 292. Is proper in the inflammatory fever, 132. In the pleurisy, 181. In what circumstances to be admitted in an inflammation of the lungs, 184. Not to be practised in the nervous fever: nor, without great caution, in the putrid fever, 136. The same caution is likewise requisite in the miliary fever, 142. When necessary in the small-pox, ibid. When serviceable in the measles, 129. Is not suitable in the remittent or bilious fever, unless there be evident signs of inflammation, 147. Can be employed in the erysipelas only in certain circumstances, 162. Method of using it in an inflammation of the brain, 164. And in that of the eyes, 166. Under what circumstances to be employed in a cough, 177. And in the hooping-cough, 107. Essential in an inflammation of the stomach, 199. The same in the inflammation of the intestines, 200. In an inflammation of the liver, 204. In an inflammation of the kidneys, 208. In that of the bladder, 208. And of the womb, 209. Advisable in a suppression of urine, 288. Beneficial in a violent fit of the asthma, 256. Of great service in the acute rheumatism, 273. And in the apoplexy, in a person of a full habit of body, 235.

*Bleeding*, at the nose, spontaneous, ought not to be suddenly checked in persons abounding with blood, 292. How to restrain it when necessary, 293, 294.

*Blisters*, when proper in the inflammatory fever, 133. Admissible in the putrid fever only in certain circumstances, 137. Particularly serviceable in the nervous fever, 140. When proper in the miliary fever, 142. A powerful remedy in an obstinate inflammation of the eyes, when applied to the temples, or behind the ears, and kept open for some time, 166. A successful application in the quinsey, 170. Of advantage in a violent hooping-cough, 108. Highly beneficial in inflammation of the stomach, 199. Successfully employed in the tooth-ach, 213. Used with great advantage in an incontinency of urine, when applied to the *os sacrum*, or the lowermost part of the back-bone, 288.

*Blood*, spitting or coughing of, 184. Causes of, 184, 185. Method of cure, 186. Vomiting of, 294. Treatment of, 295.

*Blood*-shot eye, method of cure, 310.

*Bloody*-flux. See *Dysentery*.

*Boluses*, rules for preparing, 450. Astringent bolus, ibid. Diaphoretic bolus, 451. Pectoral bolus, ibid. Purging bolus, ibid.

*Bones*, broken, treatment of the patient after the accident, 334. Tight bandages prejudicial, 335. The limb ought to be kept a little bent, ibid. The most proper external applications, ibid.

## C.

D.

E.

## F.

G.

H.

## I.

## K.



## L.

M.

## N.



## O.

## P.

## S.

## T.

## U.



## V.

W.

Y.



Z.

BOOKS *lately published, and for sale, by* JAMES ORAM,
No. 102, Water-Street, New-York.

CICERO's Select Orations translated into English, with the original Latin. By WILLIAM DUNCAN. The First American Edition, carefully revised and corrected by MALCOLM CAMPBELL, Teacher of Languages, *New-York.*

---

The New American Latin Grammar, by *E. RIGG*, Late Teacher of a Grammar School, in *New-York*—corrected by *Malcolm Campbell.*

---

Selectæ é Veteri Testamento Historiæ.
Corrected by *Malcolm Campbell.*

---

Corderii Colloquiorum Centuria Selecta.
Corrected by *Malcolm Campbell.*

---

An Introduction to the making of Latin, comprising, after an easy, compendious method, the substance of the Latin Syntax. With proper English Examples, most of them translations from the Classic Authors. By JOHN CLARKE.—Corrected by *Malcolm Campbell.*

---

An Introduction to Latin Syntax. By *J. MAIR.* To which is subjoined an Epitome of Ancient History, from the Creation to the Birth of Christ.

---

*Campbell's* Narrative of his extraordinary Adventures and Sufferings by Shipwreck and Imprisonment; comprising the occurrences of four Years, and five days, in an overland Journey to India.

The History of Modern Europe, with an account of the Decline and Fall of the Roman Empire, in 5 vols. 8vo.— By WILLIAM RUSSELL, L. L. D.—Alſo, his Ancient Europe, in 2 vols. 8vo.

---

New Practical Navigator, improved and corrected. And other Nautical Works in general uſe.

---

MACKENZIE's Voyages from Montreal through the Continent of America—one to the Frozen Ocean—the other to the Waters of the Great Pacific; with a very particular and intereſting account of the Fur Trade. A new and valuable Work.

---

Travels into the Interior of Southern Africa, performed in the Years '97 and '98. By JOHN BARROW, late Secretary to the Earl of Macartney, and Auditor-General of public Accounts at the Cape of Good Hope.—A Work of great merit.

---

An Introduction to the Practice of Midwifery. By THOMAS DENMAN.

---

The Shipwreck. By *Falconer*, an Engliſh Seaman. This intereſting and much eſteemed Poem is handſomely printed & embelliſhed with four Copperplate Engravings.

---

LEWIS's Catechism, for the Use of the Episcopal Church. Reviſed by the Rev. Biſhop *Moore*.

---

The FREEMASON's Monitor: or, Illustrations of Maſonry. By *Thomas S. Webb*. A new and greatly improved Edition.—This Work is completely arranged and digeſted, agreeably to our working order, from the Entered Apprentice to the Higher Degrees incluſive.

Family Physician.
Thomson, Alexander
New York: 1802
National Library of Medicine
Bethesda, MD 20894

CONDITION ON RECEIPT·

The full leather binding had been crudely repaired with cloth tape. The boards were reversed in the repair. The internal hinges were also repaired with cloth tape. The sewing was broken in places, and the text block was split into pieces. Most of the pages were very dirty and discolored Many were very water stained A few pages had small tears at the edges; many were torn along the spine fold The title page and front pastedown were marked with graphite pencil and colored crayon The title page was also marked with stamp ink. The red crayon was soluble in water. A book plate was adhered to the front board

TREATMENT PROVIDED

The pH was recorded before and after treatment· before 6 0, after 7 0 The volume was collated and disbound. The inks were tested for solubility The head, tail, and pages were dry cleaned where necessary; the pages were washed and then buffered (deacidified) with magnesium bicarbonate solution. The front pastedown was incorporated into the text block. Tears were mended and folds guarded where necessary with Japanese kozo paper and wheat starch paste The volume was sewn on linen tapes with linen thread The volume was case bound in full cloth and titled using a gold stamped leather label.

Northeast Document Conservation Center
June 2001

Lightning Source UK Ltd.
Milton Keynes UK
UKHW011240061118
331831UK00004B/186/P

9 780331 076400